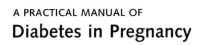

A PRACTICAL MANUAL OF
Diabetes in Pregnancy

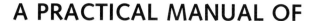

A PRACTICAL MANUAL OF
Diabetes in Pregnancy

Edited by

David R. McCance BSc, MD, FRCP, DCH
Consultant Physician/Honorary Professor of Endocrinology
Regional Centre for Endocrinology and Diabetes
Royal Victoria Hospital
Belfast, Northern Ireland

Michael Maresh MD, FRCOG
Consultant Obstetrician
St Mary's Hospital for Women
Manchester, UK

David A. Sacks MD, FACOG
Adjunct Investigator
Department of Research
Southern California Permanente Medical Group
Pasadena, California;
Clinical Professor
Department of Obstetrics and Gynecology
Keck School of Medicine
University of Southern California
Los Angeles, California, USA

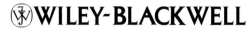

A John Wiley & Sons, Ltd., Publication

This edition first published 2010, © 2010 by Blackwell Publishing Ltd

Blackwell Publishing was acquired by John Wiley & Sons in February 2007. Blackwell's publishing program has been merged with Wiley's global Scientific, Technical and Medical business to form Wiley-Blackwell.

Registered office: John Wiley & Sons Ltd, The Atrium, Southern Gate, Chichester, West Sussex, PO19 8SQ, UK

Editorial offices: 9600 Garsington Road, Oxford, OX4 2DQ, UK

The Atrium, Southern Gate, Chichester, West Sussex, PO19 8SQ, UK

111 River Street, Hoboken, NJ 07030-5774, USA

For details of our global editorial offices, for customer services and for information about how to apply for permission to reuse the copyright material in this book please see our website at www.wiley.com/wiley-blackwell

The right of the author to be identified as the author of this work has been asserted in accordance with the Copyright, Designs and Patents Act 1988.

Wiley also publishes its books in a variety of electronic formats. Some content that appears in print may not be available in electronic books.

Designations used by companies to distinguish their products are often claimed as trademarks. All brand names and product names used in this book are trade names, service marks, trademarks or registered trademarks of their respective owners. The publisher is not associated with any product or vendor mentioned in this book. This publication is designed to provide accurate and authoritative information in regard to the subject matter covered. It is sold on the understanding that the publisher is not engaged in rendering professional services. If professional advice or other expert assistance is required, the services of a competent professional should be sought.

The contents of this work are intended to further general scientific research, understanding, and discussion only and are not intended and should not be relied upon as recommending or promoting a specific method, diagnosis, or treatment by physicians for any particular patient. The publisher and the author make no representations or warranties with respect to the accuracy or completeness of the contents of this work and specifically disclaim all warranties, including without limitation any implied warranties of fitness for a particular purpose. In view of ongoing research, equipment modifications, changes in governmental regulations, and the constant flow of information relating to the use of medicines, equipment, and devices, the reader is urged to review and evaluate the information provided in the package insert or instructions for each medicine, equipment, or device for, among other things, any changes in the instructions or indication of usage and for added warnings and precautions. Readers should consult with a specialist where appropriate. The fact that an organization or Website is referred to in this work as a citation and/or a potential source of further information does not mean that the author or the publisher endorses the information the organization or Website may provide or recommendations it may make. Further, readers should be aware that Internet Websites listed in this work may have changed or disappeared between when this work was written and when it is read. No warranty may be created or extended by any promotional statements for this work. Neither the publisher nor the author shall be liable for any damages arising herefrom.

Library of Congress Cataloging-in-Publication Data
A practical manual of diabetes in pregnancy / edited by David R. McCance, Michael Maresh, David A. Sacks.
        p. ; cm.
    Includes bibliographical references and index.
    ISBN 978-1-4051-7904-1
  1. Diabetes in pregnancy–Handbooks, manuals, etc.   I. McCance, David R.
II. Maresh, Michael.   III. Sacks, David A.
    [DNLM: 1. Pregnancy in Diabetics.   WQ 248 P895 2010]
    RG580.D5P73 2010
    618.3′646–dc22
                                                    2009029881

A catalogue record for this book is available from the British Library.

Set in 9.25 on 11.5 pt Minion by Toppan Best-set Premedia Limited
Printed and bound in Singapore by Fabulous Printers Pte Ltd

1   2010

Contents

Contributors

Nazia Arfin MSc, RGN
Diabetes Specialist Nurse
Manchester Diabetes Centre
Manchester, UK

Anita Banerjee MRCP
Specialist Registrar in Diabetes, Endocrinology and
    Obstetric Medicine
Queen Charlotte's & Chelsea Hospital
Imperial College NHS HealthCareTrust
London, UK

Marshall W. Carpenter MD
Staff Perinatologist
St. Elizabeth's Medical Center
Boston, Massachusetts, USA

Emily Y. Chew MD
Chief of Clinical Trials
Deputy Director, Division of Epidemiology and Clinical
    Applications
National Eye Institute of National Institutes of Health
Bethesda, Maryland, USA

Peter Damm MD, DMSC
Professor and Consultant in Obstetrics
Center for Pregnant Women with Diabetes
Departments of Obstetric and Endocrinology
Rigshospitalet
Faculty of Health Sciences
University of Copenhagen
Copenhagen, Denmark

Gernot Desoye PhD
Professor
Department of Obstetrics and Gynecology
Medical University of Graz
Graz, Austria

Archana Dixit MD, MRCOG
Consultant Obstetrician and Gynaecologist
West Middlesex University Hospital NHS Trust
Isleworth, Middlesex, UK

Anne Dornhorst DM, FRCP, FRCPath
Consultant Diabetologist
Queen Charlotte's & Chelsea Hospital,
Imperial College NHS HealthCareTrust
London, UK

Francine H. Einstein MD
Assistant Professor
Division of Maternal-Fetal Medicine
Department of Obstetrics & Gynecology and Women's
    Health
Diabetes Research and Training Center
Albert Einstein College of Medicine and Montefiore
    Medical Center
Bronx, New York, USA

Denice S. Feig MD, MSc, FRCPC
Associate Professor
Department of Medicine
University of Toronto;
Head, Diabetes in Pregnancy Program
Division of Endocrinology
Mount Sinai Hospital
Toronto, Ontario, Canada

Robert Fraser MD, FRCOG
Reader
Reproductive & Developmental Medicine
University of Sheffield
Sheffield, UK

Joanna Girling MRCP, FRCOG
Consultant Obstetrician and Gynaecologist
West Middlesex University Hospital NHS Trust
Isleworth, Middlesex, UK

David R. Hadden MD, FRCP
Honorary Professor of Endocrinology
Queen's University of Belfast
Honorary Consultant Physician
Regional Endocrinology and Diabetes Centre
Royal Victoria Hospital
Belfast, Northern Ireland, UK

Jane M. Hawdon MA, MBBS, MRCP, FRCPCH, PhD
Consultant Neonatologist and Honorary Senior
   Lecturer
UCL EGA Institute for Women's Health
University College London Hospitals NHS
   Foundation Trust
London, UK

Ursula Hiden Mag Dr rer nat
Junior Scientist
Department of Obstetrics and Gynecology
Medical University of Graz
Graz, Austria

Valerie A. Holmes RGN, BSc, PGCHET, PhD
Lecturer in Health Sciences
School of Nursing and Midwifery
Queen's University Belfast
Belfast, Northern Ireland, UK

Gretta Kearney RGN RM
Diabetes Specialist Midwife
St Mary's Hospital for Women
Manchester, UK

Siri L. Kjos MD, MSEd
Professor
Department of Obstetrics & Gynecology
Harbor UCLA Medical Center
Torrance, California, USA

Michael Maresh MD, FRCOG
Consultant Obstetrician
St Mary's Hospital for Women
Manchester, UK

Elisabeth R. Mathiesen MD, DMSc
Associate Professor and Consultant in Endocrinology
Center for Pregnant Women with Diabetes
Departments of Obstetrics and Endocrinology
Rigshospitalet
University of Copenhagen
Faculty of Health Sciences
Copenhagen, Denmark

David R. McCance BSc, MD, FRCP, DCH
Consultant Physician/Honorary Professor of
   Endocrinology
Regional Centre for Endocrinology and Diabetes
Royal Victoria Hospital
Belfast, Northern Ireland, UK

Ciara McLaughlin MB BCh, BAO, MRCP
Specialist Registrar
Regional Centre for Endocrinology and Diabetes
Royal Victoria Hospital
Belfast, Northern Ireland, UK

Jorge H. Mestman MD
Professor of Medicine and Obstetrics and Gynecology
Keck School of Medicine
University of Southern California
Los Angeles, California, USA

Catherine B. Meyerle MD
Staff Clinician
Clinical Trials Branch
National Eye Institute of National Institutes of Health
Bethesda, Maryland, USA

Jenny E. Myers PhD, MRCOG
Clinical Lecturer
Maternal & Fetal Health Research Centre
St Mary's Hospital
Manchester, UK

Lene Ringholm Nielsen MD PhD
Specialist Registrar
Center for Pregnant Women with Diabetes
Departments of Obstetric and Endocrinology
Rigshospitalet
Faculty of Health Sciences
University of Copenhagen
Copenhagen, Denmark

David J. Pettitt MD
Senior Scientist
Sansum Diabetes Research Institute
Santa Barbara, California, USA

Susan Quinn RGN, RM, BA
Diabetes Specialist Midwife
St Mary's Hospital for Women
Manchester, UK

Martin K. Rutter MD, FRCP
Senior Lecturer and Honorary Consultant Physician
Manchester Diabetes Centre
Manchester, UK

David A. Sacks MD
Adjunct Investigator
Department of Research
Southern California Permanente Medical Group
Pasadena, California;
Clinical Professor
Department of Obstetrics and Gynecology
Keck School of Medicine
University of Southern California
Los Angeles, California, USA

Penina Segall-Gutierrez MD, MSc
Assistant Director, Fellowship in Family Planning
    Assistant Professor of Clinical Obstetrics and
    Gynecology
Department of Obstetrics and Gynecology
Keck School of Medicine
University of Southern California
Los Angeles, California, USA

Kirsty Shaw B Nutrition and Dietetics
Diabetes Dietician
Manchester Diabetes Centre
Manchester, UK

Baha M. Sibai MD
Professor
Department of Obstetrics & Gynecology
University of Cincinnati College of Medicine
Cincinnati, Ohio, USA

David Simmons FRCP, FRACP, MD
Consultant Diabetologist
Institute of Metabolic Science
Cambridge University Hospitals NHS Foundation Trust
Addenbrookes Hospital
Cambridge, UK

Rosemary C. Temple MB, BS, MA, FRCP
Consultant Physician and Honorary Senior Lecturer
Elsie Bertram Diabetes Centre
Norfolk and Norwich University Hospital NHS Trust
Norwich, Norfolk, UK

Bob Young MMSc, MD, FRCP
Consultant Diabetologist
Diabetes Centre
Salford Royal Hospital
Salford, UK

Foreword

This is a "practical manual". The editors, and the authors of the individual chapters, envisage that you will keep *A Practical Manual of Diabetes in Pregnancy* on the front line – in the hospital, in the outpatient clinic, in the doctor's office, – rather than on your bookshelf at home, or in the university library. It is intended to be used in all parts of the world – excess glucose has the same effects during pregnancy in all women, in all countries, although specific obstetric risks may vary. The contributors represent best practice in the USA, and throughout Europe, including Denmark, Austria and the United Kingdom.

To that end most of the chapters start with four or five "practice points" – things you should think about while seeing your patient. These are followed by a relevant case history which tells a story and sets the scene for the rest of the chapter. After the review of the evidence and advice on appropriate guidelines, there is a conclusion, followed by some thoughts for the future, and a full updated reference list. The layout is divided by frequent subheadings so that a specific question should quickly find an answer. The style is professional, and evidence based, and will appeal to the busy doctor, nurse or health care worker who is actually seeing the patient and needs to be fully informed. The editors are recognised worldwide experts in this rapidly expanding field – two practicing obstetricians and an endocrinologist. All three have contributed widely to the development of knowledge in this rather specialised area.

Diabetes in pregnancy involves a team of many of us – primarily the pregnant diabetic mother herself, who will have a considerable interest in how it will affect her baby and her own future. The diabetes specialist nurse and midwife, the nutritionist or dietician, the biochemical laboratory staff, even the hospital or clinic administrator, will need special interest and training to take part in this team approach. Clinical practice in this multidisciplinary speciality varies in different countries, and even in the same country. In general the obstetrician or maternal/fetal medicine specialist will head the team and make the decisions as the pregnancy proceeds; the endocrinologist or diabetologist, often with the primary care physician or general practitioner may set the desired standards, and supervise the ongoing control of the diabetes. The neonatologist and intensive care nursery staff may be involved to a greater or lesser degree; the paediatrician, family doctor and follow up social services will all have a part to play; even the academic epidemiologist and the public health service will need to understand the rapidly developing background to the care of the diabetic woman.

A diabetic woman having a baby has always been considered to be a high risk pregnancy – it still is, but it is now clear that good team care will bring good results. This book is for the whole team.

Professor David R Hadden MD, FRCP
Honorary Professor of Endocrinology
Queen's University of Belfast
Honorary Consultant Physician
Royal Victoria Hospital, Belfast, Northern Ireland, UK.
January 2010

Preface

Although the outlook for the woman with diabetes has greatly improved since the discovery of insulin, the goal of the St. Vincent Declaration (1989), that the outcome of diabetic pregnancy should approximate that of non diabetic pregnancy, has still not been realised. This is certainly through no lack of interest or effort, but until recently progress has been hampered by limited scientific evidence and at times has been driven by differing research goals and agendas.

Against this background, the publication of a number of landmark trials in the last five years is truly remarkable, but the translation of some of these observational and randomised trial data into clinical practice has proved difficult. In addition, the changing epidemiology of diabetes in pregnancy, an expanding therapeutic armamentarium and increasing awareness of the long term implications of diabetic pregnancy for both mother and baby present new challenges for clinical care, scientific research and public health.

Practically, the management of diabetes in pregnancy remains demanding for both the patient and clinician. A multidisciplinary model of care is now accepted as the ideal but the diverse backgrounds of the stakeholders have contributed to the difficulty in achieving a uniform approach to the management of these patients. On the other hand, few would dispute that medicine is both an art and a science (grounded in knowledge, evidence and experience), and one can never legislate for every individual patient.

When an answer to a particular question is sought, the scientist will often turn to an original manuscript, or one of a number of books which are now available on the subject. Many of the latter however represent a series of research monographs rather than a comprehensive review of the key issues and their practical implications. It seemed to us therefore that there was a need for a practical manual which offered concise, contemporary guidance to the health care provider or trainee alike, while at the same time highlighting the pertinent problems, the areas of controversy and future directions for research. It was with such an aim and intention that this book has been written. Most of the chapters are prefaced with an illustrative case history, intended immediately to engage the reader, followed by a series of key questions which are then answered in the ensuing chapter. The layout of each chapter is to allow rapid appreciation of the salient facts and interminable lines of prose hopefully have been kept to a minimum. Each chapter also lists relevant original references and review articles.

The book draws on the opinion and experience of key international experts in the field, and is designed to reflect practice and perspective on both sides of the Atlantic Ocean. To that extent we hope that it will have a wide relevance and appeal.

David R. McCance
Michael Maresh
David A. Sacks
January 2010

Section 1

Epidemiology and pathophysiology

1

Epidemiologic context of diabetes in pregnancy

David Simmons

Institute of Metabolic Science, Cambridge University Hospitals NHS Foundation Trust, Addenbrookes Hospital, Cambridge, UK

PRACTICE POINTS

- The prevalence of all forms of diabetes in pregnancy, namely Type 1, Type 2, and gestational diabetes mellitus (GDM), ranges from below 2% to over 20%, although variations in definition, screening, and diagnostic criteria of GDM make comparisons difficult.
- The prevalence of Type 2 diabetes, GDM, and probably Type 1 diabetes in pregnancy is increasing and varies significantly between ethnic groups and between locations.
- The prevalence of some risk factors for GDM and Type 2 diabetes in pregnancy (e.g. obesity) is increasing.
- Adverse pregnancy outcomes are generally increased 2–7-fold in women with pre- existing diabetes and are similar for Type 1 and Type 2 diabetes.
- There is good evidence that intervention for diabetes in pregnancy can reduce adverse pregnancy outcomes: it has been estimated that for every US$1 invested in diabetes in pregnancy, there is a saving of US$3–4 on downstream health costs.
- The health, social, and economic impacts of intergenerational transmission of diabetes are unknown.

BACKGROUND

Historically, the study of diabetes in pregnancy has focused on either women with Type 1 diabetes, whose poor obstetric outcomes once led to an editorial entitled "They give birth astride the grave"[1] or GDM, an entity which remains contentious,[2,3] with variable approaches to definition, screening, and diagnosis.[4] The current epidemic of obesity and diabetes among children, adolescents, and non-pregnant adults[5] has changed the situation, leading to growing numbers with Type 2

A Practical Manual of Diabetes in Pregnancy, 1st Edition.
Edited by David R. McCance, Michael Maresh and David A. Sacks.
© 2010 Blackwell Publishing

diabetes in pregnancy and GDM (including undiagnosed Type 2 diabetes).[6–8] In parallel, our understanding of the impact of diabetes in pregnancy for future generations,[9] and our increasing ability to reduce pregnancy complications,[10] and postpone, if not prevent, diabetes after GDM,[11] have emphasized the epidemiologic and public health importance of diabetes in pregnancy.

OUTCOMES FROM DIABETES IN PREGNANCY

That there is no common unique pathognomonic complication of diabetes in pregnancy, combined with the apparent continuous relationship between glucose and fetal macrosomia, has resulted in a lack of consensus on the diagnosis of GDM. While diabetes in pregnancy is associated with increased obstetric risk compared with normal pregnancy, the overall contribution of diabetes to most obstetric and neonatal complications on a population basis is actually relatively low, with the largest impact being on shoulder dystocia (through GDM). Table 1.1 shows examples of odds ratios for each obstetric and neonatal complication by diabetes type and the proportion that diabetes in pregnancy contributes on a population basis.[12–15]

Apart from malformations, which are likely to have resulted from preconceptional or periconceptional hyperglycemia, improvements in obstetric practice have led to major reductions in adverse outcomes. Avoidance of such outcomes may dictate the need for complex obstetric decision-making, with the inevitable increase in fetal monitoring (see chapter 12) and which is strongly influenced by the preconceptional and antenatal management of hyperglycemia (see chapters 8 and 10). The importance of other metabolic factors, such as obesity[16–19] and hypertriglyceridemia,[20] in pregnancy are also now increasingly being recognized.

Table 1.1 Examples of odds ratios of diabetes for each obstetric and neonatal complication and the proportion that diabetes in pregnancy contributes on a population basis.[12–15]

	Odds ratio	Type 1 diabetes (%)	Type 2 diabetes (%)	Gestational diabetes (%)	No known diabetes (%)
Perinatal mortality	3	0.2	0.9	1.7	97.2
Malformations[1]	7	2.5		0[2]	97.5
Cesarean Section[1]	2	1.6		4.3	94.1
Birthweight ≥ 4.5 kg[1]	3	2.6		7.3	90.1
Shoulder dystocia[1]	3	<0.1[3]		23.5	76.5

[1] Type 1 and Type diabetes combined
[2] Those with malformations considered undiagnosed Type 2 diabetes, small numbers otherwise
[3] Very few on a population basis; many who will likely develop shoulder dystocia are delivered by cesarean section

The long-term implications of diabetes in pregnancy for the offspring, particularly obesity and Type 2 diabetes, are discussed in chapter 25. While there is early evidence that optimal management of diabetes during pregnancy may reduce excess adiposity in the offspring (and hopefully, ergo, subsequent diabetes),[21] this urgently requires confirmation. As yet there is no evidence that poorer neurodevelopmental outcomes, which may be associated with GDM, are amenable to change.[22] Such analyses can be confounded by the associations between socioeconomic status and both GDM and achievement.[23]

DIAGNOSIS OF GESTATIONAL DIABETES MELLITUS

While it is generally accepted that severe hyperglycemia in pregnancy is associated with adverse maternal fetal outcome, the significance of lesser degrees of hyperglycemia, along with the lack of common pathognomonic sequelae, and the apparent continuum between glucose and, for example, fetal macrosomia[24] have fuelled the lack of consensus on the optimal glycemic threshold for diagnosis of hyperglycemia in pregnancy. This is discussed in chapter 6, but essentially involves deriving a glycemic threshold above which the benefits of intervention outweigh any harm and are cost-effective.

Outside of pregnancy, the 75-g 2-hour oral glucose tolerance test (OGTT) is used. Diabetes and prediabetes are defined by their association with macrovascular and microvascular complications, the clinical appearance of the latter (retinopathy) being largely unique to diabetes. As a result, diabetes in non-pregnant adults has a globally agreed definition, as does impaired glucose tolerance (IGT) (Table 1.2). There remains disagreement between the World Health Organization (WHO) and the American Diabetes Association (ADA) definition of impaired fasting glucose (Table 1.2). As GDM is defined as carbohydrate/glucose intolerance first identified/with new onset in pregnancy, intuitively it would be thought that by definition, the criteria for diagnosis of GDM would include a fasting glucose of greater than or equal 5.6 or 6.1 mmol/L (≥101–110 mg/dL) (ADA or WHO) and/or a 2-hour glucose greater than or equal to 7.8 mmol/L (140 mg/dL), with potentially some modification should pregnancy outcomes be quantitatively worse below these cut-off points. This is discussed more fully in chapter 6.

There have been multiple attempts to define the glycemic thresholds for fetal and maternal outcomes (i.e. diagnostic criteria) for GDM (Table 1.2). These have traditionally been based upon a fasting blood glucose test, 50–100-g glucose load,[4] followed by 1–3 hours of blood glucose testing, and involving interpretation of the results either singly or in combination.

A global move to standardize the diagnostic criteria was the rationale for the Hyperglycaemia and Adverse Pregnancy Outcomes (HAPO) study, a large study among 25 000 women across continents and, importantly, involving many ethnic groups.[24] Of importance is the fact that this study showed that the impact of hyperglycemia for maternal/fetal outcome was applicable to all ethnic groups[24] and independent of maternal obesity, a recognized risk factor *per se* for large babies.[16–19] Further analysis of data from the HAPO study will address the important question of whether different glycemic thresholds are needed to predict a greater risk of glucose-sensitive adverse outcomes.

Table 1.2 Summary of international guidelines for the screening and diagnosis of gestational diabetes (primarily from Cutchie et al[4]).

Organization	Screening	Diagnosis Fasting (mmol/L [mg/dL])	1h (mmol/L [mg/dL])	2h (mmol/L [mg/dL])	3h (mmol/L [mg/dL])	Abnormal values for diagnosis
WHO (non-pregnant)	No recommendation	Diabetes ≥ 7.0 [126] IGT <7.0 [126] IFG 6.1–6.9 [110–124]	and/or	≥11.1 [200] 7.8–11.0 [140–198] <11.1 [200]		One
ADA (non-pregnant)	All ≥ 45 years If < 45 years: BMI ≥ 25 and one other risk factor Fasting glucose: OGTT if FBG ≥ 5.6 mmol/L (≥100 mg/dL)	Diabetes ≥ 7.0 [126] IGT <7.0 [126] IFG 5.6–6.9 [100–124]	and/or	≥11.1 [200] 7.8–11.0 [140–198] <11.1 [200]		One
ADA	All except low risk High risk: proceed to OGTT Moderate risk: 50 g GCT; if 1-h BGL ≥ 7.8 mmol/L (≥140 mg/dL), proceed to OGTT 75-g or 100-g OGTT	5.3 [95]	10.0 [180]	8.6 [155]	7.8 [140] (100 g only)	Two or more values
ACOG	Either screen all except low risk or universal screening. 50-g GCT; if 1-h BGL ≥7.8 mmol/L (≥140 mg/dL), proceed to OGTT. 100-g OGTT	C&C 5.3 [95] NDDG 5.8 [104]	10.0 [180] 10.6 [191]	8.6 [155] 9.2 [166]	7.8 [140] 8.0 [144]	Two or more values
CDA	Screen all with a 50-g GCT at 24–28 weeks, but in first trimester if high risk. 1-h glucose >10.3 mmol/L (>185 mg/dL), diagnostic for GDM. If 1-h glucose 7.8–10.2 mmol/L (140–184 mg/dL) proceed to 75-g OGTT	5.3 [95]	10.6 [191]	8.9 [160]		Two (if only one abnormal defined as IGT of pregnancy)
BCRCP	All except low risk. 50 g GCT. If ≥7.8 mmol/L (≥140 mg/dL), 100-g OGTT. If >10.3 mmol/L (>185 mg/dL), diagnostic for GDM	5.3 [95]	10.0 [180]	8.6 [155]	7.8 [140]	Two or more values

Table 1.2 *Continued*

Organization	Screening	Diagnosis Fasting (mmol/L [mg/dL])	1 h (mmol/L [mg/dL])	2 h (mmol/L [mg/dL])	3 h (mmol/L [mg/dL])	Abnormal values for diagnosis
DUK	No routine screening 75-g OGTT	7.0 [126]	and/or	7.8 [140]	–	One
SIGN	All. Random glucose at 28 weeks 75-g OGTT	5.5 [99]	–	9.0 [162]	–	One
CREST	All. Random glucose at 28 weeks 75-g OGTT	5.5 [99]	–	9.0 [162]	–	One
IDF	All except low risk 75-g OGTT	5.3 [95] (75 g)	–	8.6 [155]	–	
JDA	All by casual plasma glucose 75 g OGTT	5.5 [99]	10.0 [180]	8.3 [149]	–	Two or more values
ADIPS	All unless resources are limited. 50 g	5.5 [99]	–	75 g 8.0 [144](Aus) 9.0 [162] (NZ)	–	One
RANZCOG	GCT; if 1-h BGL ≥7.8 mmol/L proceed to 75-g OGTT					
WHO (if pregnant)	All except low risk 75-g OGTT	≥7.0 [126]	and/or	≥7.8 [140]	–	One
NICE (2008)	Select ethnic groups, BMI ≥30, first-degree family history, previous GDM, previous baby ≥4.5 kg	≥7.0 [126]		≥7.8 [140]		One

WHO, World Health Organization; ADA, American Diabetes Association; ACOG, American College of Obstetrics and Gynaecology; C&C, Carpenter and Coustan; NDDG, National Diabetes Diagnostic Group; CDA, Canadian Diabetes Association; BCRCP, British Columbia Reproductive Care Program; DUK, Diabetes UK; SIGN, Scottish Intercollegiate Guidelines Network; CREST, Clinical Resource Efficiency Support Team; IDF, International Diabetes Federation; JDA, Japanese Diabetic Association; ADIPS, Australasian Diabetes in Pregnancy Society; RANZCOG, Royal Australasian College of Obstetrics and Gynaecology; NICE, National Institute for Health and Clinical Excellence, OGTT, oral glucose tolerance test; GCT, glucose challenge test; IGT, impaired glucose tolerance; IFG, impaired fasting glucose; GDM, gestational diabetes mellitus; FBG, fasting blood glucose; BGL, blood glucose level; BMI, body mass index

PREVALENCE OF PREGESTATIONAL DIABETES IN PREGNANCY

The prevalence of Type 1 and Type 2 diabetes in pregnancy would be expected to reflect the rates of diabetes in the background population.[25,26] However, the standard fertility ratio (SFR) is low in Type 1 diabetes (0.80, 95% CI 0.77–0.82), and is particularly low among women with retinopathy, nephropathy, neuropathy, or cardiovascular complications (0.63, 0.54, 0.50, and 0.34, respectively).[27] While fertility rates in Type 2 diabetes have not been reported, they would also be expected to be low (particularly in view of the additional associated obesity, polycystic ovarian syndrome [PCOS], and vascular disease).

The incidence of Type 1 and the prevalence of Type 2 diabetes has been increasing over time,[28] with a reduction in the age at diagnosis of Type 2 diabetes. Both of these factors predict an increasing number of women with pregestational diabetes. However, the more rapid increase in Type 2 diabetes in pregnancy has resulted in some diabetes clinics now seeing a predominance of Type 2 over Type 1 diabetes, which has been accentuated further by ethnicity. In the US, the ratio of women with Type 1 to Type 2 diabetes has shifted from 3:1 to 1:2 between 1980 and 1995.[28] This may be partly due to changes in the population (e.g. in Birmingham, UK the ratio of Type 1 to Type 2 diabetes was 1:2 in South Asians but 11:1 in Europeans[29]). Meanwhile, there have been other important changes. Women with diabetes in pregnancy are now expected to survive. The perinatal mortality for pregnancies complicated by Type 1 diabetes has also dropped from 40% to much nearer the background rate.[23,28] In Type 2 diabetes, the evolving evidence suggests that perinatal mortality and the frequency of congenital malformations are similar to those of Type 1 diabetes,[23] including in those women diagnosed with GDM but found to have Type 2 diabetes postnatally.[6,29] While these trends are more often seen in women of non-European descent, it is likely that a similar picture will be seen in all groups eventually.

To date there are few reports of the prevalence of monogenetic forms of diabetes or secondary diabetes in pregnancy. Glucokinase mutations are present in up to 5–6% of women with GDM and up to 80% of women with persisting fasting hyperglycemia outside pregnancy, a small glucose increment during the OGTT, and a family history of diabetes.[30] Cystic fibrosis is associated with a doubling in the prevalence of diabetes outside of pregnancy, with a further increase during pregnancy (e.g. from 9.3% at baseline to 20.6% during pregnancy, and 14.4% at follow-up).[31]

PREVALENCE OF GESTATIONAL DIABETES

The prevalence of GDM globally in 1998 was examined by King et al.[32] An epidemiologic comparison between studies is difficult for the reasons shown in Fig. 1.1 and discussed more fully in chapters 5 and 6. In addition, screening too early (before 24 weeks) will result in fewer cases of GDM being detected. Some women achieve the criteria for GDM only later in pregnancy and will not be diagnosed with the conventional screening approach, which occurs between 24 and 28 weeks.

As highlighted above, there are differences in the rates of GDM when diagnosed by different criteria,[33] both within and between populations (Fig. 1.2). Notwithstanding the different diagnostic criteria, there are major differences in prevalence of GDM between ethnic groups, reflecting both the background prevalence of Type 2 diabetes and the age at onset (the "underwater volcano hypothesis" [Fig. 1.3]).[34] This hypothesis proposes that GDM is more common in people who are temporally closer to developing Type 2 diabetes.

These prevalence rates vary within the same ethnic group in different locations, with migrant populations generally having a higher prevalence than those remaining in traditional rural areas, probably relating to lifestyle change (higher energy diet, less physical activity) and greater adiposity. The prevalence has also generally increased over time (Fig. 1.4).[7,35] While this most likely reflects the epidemics of obesity and Type 2 diabetes in the non-pregnant state, an additional feature is likely to be the increasing age at which pregnancy occurs, and for some total populations, the immigration of high-risk ethnic groups (e.g. in Auckland, New Zealand, numbers of women with GDM doubled over 4 years due to a combination of these factors[36]). Such data need careful scrutiny to recognize these factors and to ensure that no change in ascertainment (e.g. screening approaches) or diagnostic criteria have occurred.

All populations apart from those of non-European descent (and even including some European populations), are now considered at such high risk that most guidelines suggest that these ethnic groups require universal screening.[4] The growth and clinical importance of undiagnosed Type 2 diabetes in pregnancy (i.e. the high end of GDM) also supports a universal screening approach in these populations, both at first antenatal assessment and at the more traditional 24–28 weeks of gestation. With the growing numbers of women with

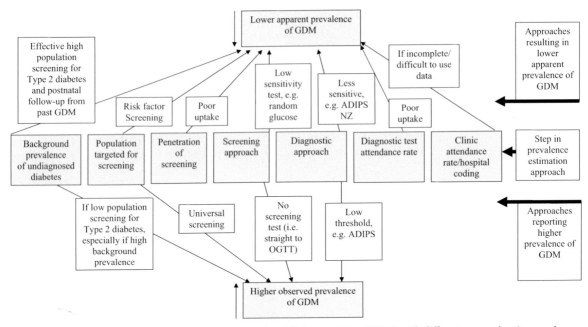

Fig. 1.1 Difficulties in comparing prevalence data in gestational diabetes mellitus (GDM) with different approaches (personal observations). ADIPS, Australian Diabetes in Pregnancy Society.

GDM, including undiagnosed Type 2 diabetes in pregnancy, the case for universal screening is becoming persuasive.[37] Prior to the most recent data, the 4th Chicago Workshop on GDM[38] recommended screening of all but those at very low risk (i.e. under 25 years, slim, no risk factors), a group of women who are becoming increasingly uncommon in modern pregnancy clinics. Surprisingly, during an obesity and diabetes epidemic, the latest recommendations from the National Institute for Health and Clinical Excellence (NICE) in the UK,[39] recommend screening using very few risk factors, even excluding older women and those with PCOS from those warranting screening. Decisions underlying these recommendations have been informed by erroneous economic analyses, including the exclusion of (1) identifying women at high risk of future diabetes who could benefit from diabetes preventative intervention, (2) the benefits in the offspring from reduced exposure to maternal hyperglycemia, and (3) future pregnancies complicated by undiagnosed diabetes, as well as an underestimate of reduced benefits when using complex screening approaches.

Risk factors for gestational diabetes mellitus

While obesity, ethnicity, maternal age, and a family history of diabetes are the major risk factors for GDM, other more traditional factors have been used in selective screening approaches[40] (Table 1.3), including parity and a previous macrosomic baby. Some studies have suggested that multifetal pregnancies (e.g. twins and triplets) may be at increased risk of GDM, although others have not confirmed this.[40] There is increasing evidence of the importance of PCOS as a risk factor for both GDM and undiagnosed Type 2 diabetes in pregnancy. It therefore has been suggested in some countries that prior to treating PCOS with, for example, metformin or clomiphene to assist conception, women should have an OGTT.[41]

Another group of women at risk of GDM are those with a previous history of GDM,[42] particularly in association with excess weight/weight gain between pregnancies and where previous GDM was diagnosed early in pregnancy and required treatment with insulin.[43]

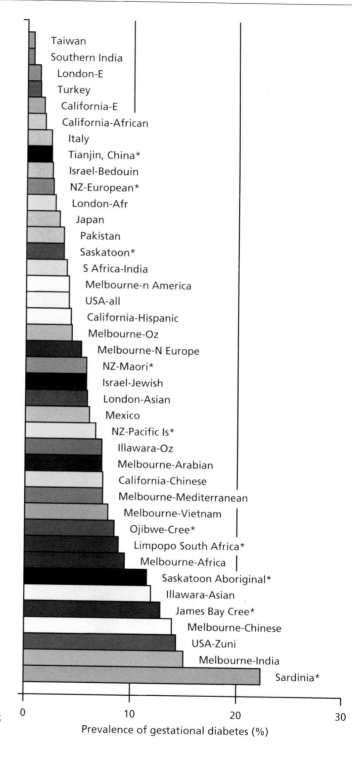

Fig. 1.2 Prevalence of gestational diabetes in different populations at different times (*since King 1998,[32] includes[63–70]).

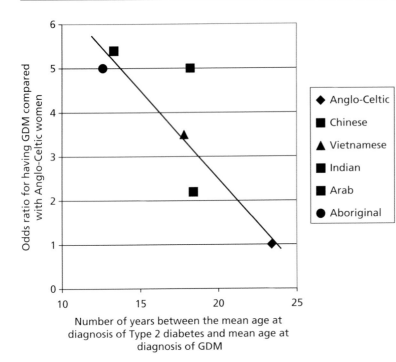

Fig. 1.3 "Underwater volcano" hypothesis: Relationship between risk of gestational diabetes mellitus (GDM) in comparison with Anglo-Celtic women and time between mean age at diagnosis of Type 2 diabetes and diagnosis of gestational diabetes mellitus.[34]

LONG-TERM IMPLICATIONS OF DIABETES IN PREGNANCY FOR THE MOTHER

The original study by O'Sullivan, from which the current US diagnostic criteria are derived, focused on the long-term risk of permanent diabetes in the mother who had hyperglycemia during pregnancy.[44] The overall literature would suggest a 5–28-year risk of developing permanent diabetes (predominantly Type 2 diabetes) of 17–63%.[45] Approximately 50% of those with autoantibodies develop Type 1 diabetes,[46] and a small number with antibodies are at least initially considered to have Type 2 diabetes.[47] The excess risk of diabetes among those with previous GDM is now seen in all populations studied, with an estimated odds ratio of 6.0 and population attributable risk of 0.10–0.31.[45] Evidence also now suggests that women with additional pregnancies may have an accelerated progression to Type 2 diabetes, as shown in one study by a relative risk of 3.34 (1.80–6.19).[48] This proposal has biologic plausibility in that an additional 9 months of insulin resistance are imposed upon a woman who already has a degree of insulin resistance. Other risk factors for progression to permanent diabetes are largely related to the level of antenatal glycemia, gestational age at diagnosis of GDM, and weight gain.[49]

The incidence of progression to frank diabetes increases markedly in the first 5 years postpartum and then plateaus after approximately 10 years.[49] Such progression to diabetes among women with past GDM can be reduced, as was shown in the Diabetes Prevention Project through both lifestyle- and medication-based interventions beyond the postpartum period.[10] Currently, systems are generally not in place to provide follow-up or intervention. Postnatal follow-up rates can be poor, even for women with Type 2 diabetes, possibly because of family demands.[50]

DIABETES IN FUTURE GENERATIONS

A small number of babies may experience long-term sequelae from congenital malformations and birth trauma (Table 1.1); however, the impact of growing in an adverse intrauterine milieu is now becoming increasingly evident.[9] Long-term studies of pregnancies complicated by Type 1 diabetes, Type 2 diabetes, and GDM, including different ethnic groups and countries, suggest that exposure to a "diabetic" intrauterine environment is associated with an increase in risk of future obesity, IGT, and diabetes (see chapter 25).[51] Among Pima Indians, diabetes is much more common in the offspring of women with maternal diabetes occurring during rather than after pregnancy[52] (see chapter 25).

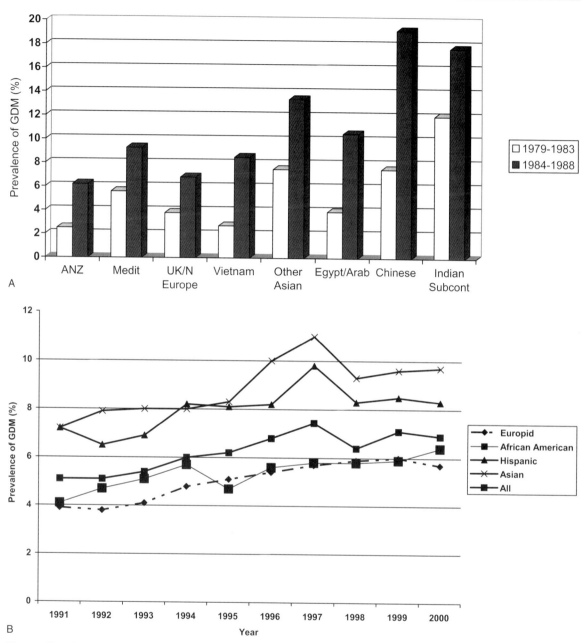

Fig. 1.4 Changing prevalence of gestational diabetes mellitus (GDM) over time in different populations. (A) Increasing prevalence of GDM in Melbourne, Australia 1979–1988.[35]

(B) Increasing prevalence of GDM among different groups in Northern California between 1991 and 2000.[7]

It is not known if intervention during or before pregnancy will ameliorate this "potential amplifier" for the current epidemic of obesity and diabetes. Obtaining long-term data will take many decades. In one small, non-randomized study, adiposity was found less often in the offspring of mothers with GDM treated with insulin than in the offspring of mothers treated with diet alone, but further evidence is needed on whether preconcepion/

antenatal interventions are of benefit.[21] However, if intrauterine exposure to diabetes is known, then the offspring can be identified as high risk, followed up, and have childhood-based interventions implemented as they become practicable.

HEALTH ECONOMIC IMPLICATIONS

A thorough health economic analysis regarding diabetes in pregnancy will require an examination of each transitional probability between clinical states and the cost and benefit from each intervention. Table 1.4 summarizes the stages in management and possible interventions. For diabetes in pregnancy, uniquely, such analyses need to include the costs of any long-term effects (beneficial or harmful) on the offspring. Preconception management of Type 1 and Type 2 diabetes, including tight glucose control, has been shown to be cost-effective, with a cost–benefit ratio of 1:3.5[53] for each US dollar invested. While there is also information on obstetric complications (e.g. brachial nerve palsy), it is unknown whether intervention reduces the future risk of obesity, Type 2 diabetes, and neurodevelopmental sequelae. Any such cost–benefit analysis is therefore likely to be incomplete. This is of particular importance in the debate over screening for GDM. Furthermore, implementation costs and uptake need to be included in any analysis, with an awareness that the more complex an approach, the less likelihood that uptake will be complete. The cost-effectiveness of whether or not and how to screen for GDM has been a longstanding issue.[54] It has been suggested that

Table 1.3 Risk factors for gestational diabetes mellitus (GDM).

Maternal demographic and physical factors
- Ethnicity (non-European)
- Increasing age
- Family history of diabetes
- Short stature
- Low birthweight
- Parity

Maternal clinical factors
- Overweight/obesity
- Diet high in red and processed meat
- Pregnancy weight gain
- Physical inactivity
- Polycystic ovarian syndrome
- α-Thalassemia trait
- High blood pressure
- Multiple pregnancy

Past obstetric history
- Macrosomia
- Stillbirth
- Past GDM

Table 1.4 Cost components in diabetes in pregnancy and potential savings from intervention.

	Interventions	Potential savings
Type 1 and Type 2 diabetes		
Preconception	Optimization of metabolic control, folate therapy, medication optimization	Malformations Fetal loss sequelae
Antenatal management	Optimization of metabolic control Optimization of obstetric management	Neonatal, maternal birth complications Offspring risk of diabetes, obesity
Retinal management	Retinal screening, laser if needed	Vitreous surgery, cesarean section
Gestational diabetes mellitus (GDM)		
Diagnosis of GDM	Screening and diagnosis program	
Antenatal management	Optimization of metabolic control Optimization of obstetric management	Neonatal, maternal birth complications Offspring risk of diabetes, obesity
Retinal management	Retinal screening if likely undiagnosed Type 2 diabetes, laser if needed	Vitreous surgery, cesarean section (rare)
Postnatal screening and intervention	Screening Primary prevention (lifestyle, drugs)	Prevention of permanent diabetes Prevention of undiagnosed Type 2 diabetes in pregnancy

approximately US$3–4 would be saved for every US$1 expended.[55,56] Improvements in outcomes in the intensive group in the Australian Carbohydrate Intolerance in Pregnancy Study (ACHOIS) suggest that benefits would be even greater if quality of life measures were included, particularly the benefits on postnatal depression.[10] This study has now shown GDM management to be cost-effective with an incremental cost per additional serious perinatal complication of US$27 503, per perinatal death prevented of US$60 506, and per discounted life year gained of US$2988.[57] One small study showed that case management (i.e. allocation of a health professional to manage closely individual cases on a day-by-day basis) of women with diabetes in pregnancy was associated with reductions in the need for hospitalization (a major cost of care), as well as improved glycemic control and increased uptake of a postnatal OGTT.[58]

Intervention to prevent progression from prediabetes to diabetes using either lifestyle measures or medication in women with previous GDM was shown to be cost-effective in the Diabetes Prevention Project.[59] With the population attributable fraction for diabetes estimated at 10–31%, such an approach could have a significant impact on the current diabetes epidemic.[45]

Postpartum screening

Kim and colleagues examined the efficacy and cost of postpartum screening strategies for diabetes among women with previous GDM and concluded that an OGTT every 3 years had the lowest cost per case of detected diabetes.[60]

THE WAY FORWARD

Epidemiologically, the way ahead differs to some extent according to the type of diabetes. Much is already known about Type 1 diabetes in pregnancy, where the diagnosis is clear and extensive research databases exist. For Type 2 diabetes, there is a growing body of literature regarding prevalence and outcomes, but this remains insufficient for many populations, and relatively little is known of the impact of undiagnosed Type 2 diabetes. Further research must focus on GDM given the current evidence which suggests that this condition has a large population health impact on future diabetes for both mother and offspring.

An epidemiologic comparison of the prevalence of diabetes in pregnancy among various populations is becoming increasingly difficult. The identification and collation of such descriptive studies is difficult. The recent UK Confidential Enquiry into Maternal and Child Health (CEMACH) study showed that it is possible (with a great deal of effort and good will) to describe a national epidemiologic snapshot of Type 1 and Type 2 diabetes in pregnancy and the related outcomes.[23] This study was able to link outcome with health service quality improvement and audit processes. A similar attempt to develop an Australasian database and benchmarking service has been piloted successfully, involving testing paper, and standalone and networked electronic methods for collecting data.[61] The ultimate goal would be to develop a global database, possibly under the auspices of the International Association of Diabetes in Pregnancy Study Groups, to allow easy description of the epidemiology of diabetes in pregnancy, to benchmark prevalence and outcomes, and to compare process (e.g. proportion of women receiving folate therapy, and proportion of women screened for GDM). This would also support the existence of such databases within nations and facilitate linkage to evaluate and support interventions from preconception counseling to postnatal OGTT follow-up in GDM.

The second major area for development remains how to best manage GDM on a population basis. A universally agreed set of diagnostic criteria derived from the HAPO study[24] will be a major step forward. Systematic screening, prevention, monitoring, and quality assurance programs are increasingly being implemented alongside the growth in evidence-based clinical practice. While long-term follow-up studies of the offspring are planned, data from these will take many years and possibly decades to emerge.

If we are, finally, to introduce a systematic approach to the screening for and diagnosis of GDM, similar to screening for syphilis, rubella immunity, and other conditions, with a high penetration, then there will be implications for health providers. The numbers of women diagnosed with GDM will increase dramatically in those places without good penetration of systematic screening currently. Those at the "lower end" of the GDM glycemia range have very different needs from those at the "higher end". Many of the former may be suitable for obstetric management in the community, rather than specialist clinics, as found in California.[62] Criteria for triaging and referral need further development. If models of care are to shift, then there is an urgent need to implement quality assurance now, so that any changes in trends from the resulting changes in practice and the increase in demands can be monitored and acted upon.

A systematic approach to the follow-up of women with previous GDM and the offspring of all women with diabetes in pregnancy also needs to be put in place. Whether this follow-up is through a centralized (e.g. cervical cancer), devolved (e.g. hypertension) or hybrid approach will depend on the individual health system. Whatever system is implemented, there needs to be linkage with approaches to preventing obesity, promoting physical activity, and preventing or delaying progression to Type 2 diabetes.

In conclusion, the epidemiology of diabetes in pregnancy is constantly changing. The growth in information management, evidence for clinical management, and consensus on how to detect, manage, and follow-up diabetes in pregnancy will clearly continue into the future.

REFERENCES

1 Drury ML. "They give birth astride of a grave". *Diabet Med* 1989;**6**:291–8.

2 Jarrett RJ. Gestational diabetes: a non entity? *Br Med J* 1993;**306**:37–8.

3 Harris MI. Gestational diabetes may represent discovery of preexisting glucose tolerance. *Diabetes Care* 1988;**11**: 401–11.

4 Cutchie W, Simmons D, Cheung NW. Comparison of international and New Zealand guidelines for the care of pregnant women with diabetes. *Diabet Med* 2006;**23**:460–8.

5 Zimmet P, Alberti KGMM, Shaw J. Global and societal implications of the diabetes epidemic. *Nature* 2001;**414**: 782–7.

6 Feig DS, Palda VA. Type 2 diabetes in pregnancy: a growing concern. *Lancet* 2002;**359**:1690–2.

7 Ferrara A. Increasing prevalence of gestational diabetes: a public health perspective. *Diabetes Care* 2007;**30** (Suppl 2): S141–S146.

8 Lawrence JM, Chen W, Contreras R, Sacks D. Trends in the prevalence of preexisting diabetes and gestational diabetes mellitus among a racially/ethnically diverse population of pregnant women 1999–2005. *Diabetes Care* 2008;**31**:899–904.

9 Freinkel N. Banting Lecture 1980. Of *pregnancy* and *progeny*. *Diabetes* 1980;**29**:1023–35.

10 Crowther CA, Hiller JE, Moss JR, McPhee AJ, Jeffries WS, Robinson JS. Effect of treatment of gestational diabetes on pregnancy outcomes. Australian Carbohydrate Intolerance Study in Pregnant Women (ACHOIS) Trial Group. *N Engl J Med* 2005;**352**:2477–88.

11 Ratner RE. Prevention of Type 2 diabetes in women with previous gestational diabetes. *Diabetes Care* 2007;**30** (Suppl 2):S242–S245.

12 Cundy T, Gamble G, Townend K, Henley PG, MacPherson P, Roberts AB. Perinatal mortality in Type 2 diabetes mellitus. *Diabet Med* 2000;**17**:33–9.

13 Lang U, Künzel W. Diabetes mellitus in pregnancy. management and outcome of diabetic pregnancies in the state of Hesse, F.R.G.; a five-year-survey. *Eur J Obstet Gynecol Reprod Biol* 1989;**33**:115–29.

14 Remsberg KE, McKeown, McFarland KF, Irwin LS. Diabetes in pregnancy and cesarean section. *Diabetes Care* 1999;**22**: 1561–7.

15 Tan YY, Yeo GS. Impaired glucose tolerance in pregnancy – is it of consequence? *Aust N Z J Obstet Gynecol* 1996; **36**:248–55.

16 Ricart W, Lopez J, Mozas J, *et al.* Spanish Group for the Study of the Impact of Carpenter and Coustan GDM Thresholds. Body mass index has a greater impact on pregnancy outcomes than gestational hyperglycaemia. *Diabetologia* 2005;**48**:1736–42.

17 Jensen DM, Ovesen P, Beck-Nielsen H, *et al.* Gestational weight gain and pregnancy outcomes in 481 obese glucose-tolerant women. *Diabetes Care* 2005;**28**:2118–22.

18 Simmons D. Relationship between maternal glycaemia and birthweight among women without diabetes from difference ethnic groups in New Zealand. *Diabet Med* 2007;**24**:240–4.

19 Catalano PM. Obesity and pregnancy – the propagation of a vicious cycle? *J Clin Endocrinol Metab* 2003;**88**:3505–6.

20 Knopp RH, Magee MS, Walden CE, Bonet B, Benedetti TJ. Prediction of infant birth weight by GDM screening tests. Importance of plasma triglyceride. *Diabetes Care* 1992;**15**: 1605–13.

21 Simmons D, Robertson S. Influence of maternal insulin treatment on the infants of women with gestational diabetes. *Diabet Med* 1997;**14**:762–5.

22 Ornoy A. Wolf A, Ratzon N, Greenbaum C, Dulitzky M. Neurodevelopmental outcome at early school age of children born to mothers with gestational diabetes. *Arch Dis Child* 1999;**81**:10F–14F.

23 Confidential Enquiry into Maternal and Child Health (CEMACH). *Pregnancy in Women with Type 1 and Type 2 Diabetes in 2002–2003, England, Wales and Northern Ireland.* London: CEMACH, 2005.

24 The HAPO Study Cooperative Research Group. Hyperglycemia and adverse pregnancy outcomes. *N Engl J Med* 2008;**358**:1999–2002.

25 World Health Organisation [homepage on the Internet]. Definition, diagnosis and classification of Diabetes Mellitus and its complications, 1999. whqlibdoc.who.int/hq/1999/WHO_NCD_NCS_99.2.pdf

26 IDF Diabetes Atlas. Brussels: International Diabetes Federation Brussels, Belgium, 2006. www.eatlas.idf.org/Prevalence

27 Jonasson JM, Brismar K, Sparen P, *et al.* Fertility in women with Type 1 diabetes: A population-based cohort study in Sweden. *Diabetes Care* 2007;**30**:2271–6.

28 Engelgau MM, Herman WH, Smith PJ, German RR, Aubert RE. The epidemiology of diabetes and pregnancy in the U.S., 1988. *Diabetes Care* 1995;**18**:1029–33.

29 Dunne FP, Brydon PA, Proffit M, Smith T, Gee H, Holder RL. Fetal and maternal outcomes in Indo-Asian compared to Caucasian women with diabetes in pregnancy. *Q J Med* 2000;**93**:813–18.

30 Ellard S, Beards F, Allen LIS, *et al.* A high prevalence of glucokinase mutations in gestational diabetic subjects selected by clinical criteria. *Diabetologia* 2000;**43**:250–3.

31 McMullen AH, Pasta D, Frederick P, *et al.* Impact of pregnancy on women with cystic fibrosis. *Chest* 2006;**129**: 706–11.

32 King H. Epidemiology of glucose intolerance and gestational diabetes in women of childbearing age. *Diabetes Care* 1998;**21**:B9–B13.

33 Agarwal, MM, Dhatt GS, Punnose J, Koster G. Gestational diabetes: dilemma caused by multiple international diagnostic criteria. *Diabet Med* 2005;**22**:1731–6.

34 Yue DK, Molyneaux LM, Ross GP, Constantino MI, Child AG, Turtle JR. Why does ethnicity affect prevalence of gestational diabetes? The underwater volcano theory. *Diabet Med* 1996;**13**:748–52.

35 Beischer NA, Oats JN, Henry OA, Sheedy MT, Walstab JE. Incidence and severity of gestational *diabetes* mellitus according to country of birth in women living in Australia. *Diabetes* 1991;**40** (Suppl 2):35–8.

36 National Women's Annual Clinical Report 2005. Auckland: National Women's Health, Auckland District Health Board.

37 Simmons D, Rowan J, Campbell N, Reid R. Screening, diagnosis and services for women with Gestational Diabetes Mellitus in New Zealand: A Technical Report from the National GDM Technical Working Party. *N Z Med J* 2008; **121**:74–86.

38 Metzger BE, Coustan DR (eds). Summary and recommendations of the Fourth International Workshop Conference on Gestational Diabetes Mellitus. *Diabetes Care* 1998;**21** (Suppl 2):B161–B167.

39 The Guideline Development Group. Guidelines: Management of diabetes from preconception to the postnatal period: summary of NICE guidance. *BMJ* 2008;**336**:714–17.

40 Ben Haroush A, Yogev Y, Hod M. Epidemiology of gestational diabetes mellitus and its association with Type 2 diabetes. *Diabet Med* 2004;**21**:103–13.

41 Simmons D, Walters BNJ, Rowan JA, McIntyre HD. Metformin therapy and diabetes in pregnancy. *Med J Aust* 2004;**180**:462–4.

42 Kim, C, Berger DK, Chamany S. Recurrence of gestational diabetes mellitus: A systematic review. *Diabetes Care* 2007;**30**:1314–19.

43 Major CA, de Veciana M, Weeks J, Morgan MA. Recurrence of gestational diabetes mellitus: who is at risk? *Am J Obstet Gynecol* 1998;**179**:1038–42.

44 O'Sullivan JB. Diabetes mellitus after GDM. *Diabetes* 1991;**40**:131–5.

45 Cheung NW, Byth K. Population health significance of gestational diabetes. *Diabetes Care* 2003;**26**:2005–9.

46 Nilsson C, Ursing D, Torn C, Aberg A, Landin-Olsson M. Presence of GAD antibodies during gestational diabetes mellitus predicts Type 1 diabetes. *Diabetes Care* 2007; **30**:1968–71.

47 Jarvela IY, Kulmala P, Juutinen J, *et al.* Gestational diabetes identifies women at risk for permanent type 1 and type 2 diabetes in fertile age. *Diabetes Care* 2006;**29**:607–12.

48 Peters RK, Kjos SL, Xiang A, Buchanan TA. Long-term diabetogenic effect of single pregnancy in women with previous gestational diabetes mellitus. *Lancet* 1996;**347**:227–30.

49 Kim C, Newton K, Knopp R. Gestational diabetes and incidence of Type 2 diabetes mellitus: a systematic review. *Diabetes Care* 2002;**26**:1862–8.

50 Simmons D, Fleming C. Prevalence and characteristics of diabetic patients with no ongoing care in South Auckland. *Diabetes Care* 2000;**23**:1791–3.

51 Clausen TD, Mathiesen ER, Hansen T, *et al.* High prevalence of Type 2 diabetes and pre-diabetes in adult offspring of women with gestational diabetes mellitus or Type 1 diabetes: The role of intrauterine hyperglycemia. *Diabetes Care* 2008;**31**:340–6.

52 Pettitt DJ, Aleck KA, Baird HR, Carraher MJ, Bennett PH, Knowler WC. Congenital susceptibility to NIDDM. Role of intrauterine environment. *Diabetes* 1988;**37**:622–8.

53 Klonoff DC, Scwartz DM. An economic analysis of interventions for diabetes. *Diabetes Care* 2000;**23**:390–404.

54 Kitzmiller JL. Cost analysis of diagnosis and treatment of gestational diabetes mellitus. *Clin Obstet Gynaecol* 2000;**43**:140–53.

55 Jovanovic-Peterson L, Bevier W, Peterson CM. The Santa-Barbara County Health Care Services program: Birth weight change concomitant with screening for and treatment of glucose intolerance of pregnancy: a potential cost effective intervention. *Am J Perinatol* 1997;**14**:221–8.

56 Langer O, Conway D, Berkus M, Xenakis EMJ. Conventional versus intensified therapy: Cost/benefit analysis. *Am J Obstet Gynecol* 1998;**178** (Suppl 1):S58.

57 Moss JR, Crowther CA, Hiller JE, Willson KJ, Robinson JS. Costs and consequences of treatment for mild gestational diabetes mellitus – evaluation from the ACHOIS randomised trial. *BMC Pregnancy Childbirth* 2007;**7**:27.

58 Simmons D, Conroy C, Scott DJ. Impact of a diabetes midwifery educator on the diabetes in pregnancy service at Middlemore Hospital. *Prac Diabet Int* 2001;**18**:119–22.

59 Herman WH, Hoerger TJ, Brandle M, *et al.* The cost-effectiveness of lifestyle modification or metformin in preventing type 2 diabetes in adults with impaired glucose tolerance. *Ann Intern Med* 2005;**142**:323–32.

60 Kim C, Herman WH, Vijan S. Efficacy and cost of postpartum screening strategies for diabetes among women with

histories of gestational diabetes mellitus. *Diabetes Care* 2007;**30**:1102–6.

61 Simmons D, Cheung NW, Lagstrom J, *et al.* for the ADIPS National Diabetes in Pregnancy Audit Project team. The ADIPS Pilot National Diabetes in Pregnancy Audit Project. *Aust NZ J Obstet Gynaecol* 2007;**47**:198–206.

62 Weiderman WC, Marcuz L. Gestational diabetes: a triage model of care for rural perinatal providers. *Am J Obstet Gynecol* 1996;**174**:1719–23.

63 Yapa M, Simmons D. Screening for gestational diabetes mellitus in a multiethnic population in New Zealand. *Diabetes Res Clin Pract* 2000;**48**:217–23.

64 Rodrigues S, Robinson E, Gray-Donald K. Prevalence of gestational diabetes mellitus among James Bay Cree women in northern Quebec. *CMAJ* 1999;**160**:1293–7.

65 Murgia C, Berria R, Minerba L, *et al.* Gestational diabetes mellitus in Sardinia. *Diabetes Care* 2006;**29**:1713.

66 Yang X, Hsu-Hage B, Zhang H, *et al.* Gestational diabetes mellitus in women of single gravidity in Tianjin city, China. *Diabetes Care* 2002;**25**:847–51.

67 Dyck R, Klomp H, Tan LK, Turnell RW, Boctor MA. A comparison of rates risk factors and outcomes of gestational diabetes between Aboriginal and non-Aboriginal women in the Saskatoon Health District. *Diabetes Care* 2002;**25**: 487–93.

68 Erem C, Cihanyurdu N, Deger O, *et al.* Screening for gestational diabetes mellitus in northeastern Turkey, Trabazon City. *Eur J Epidemiol* 2002;**18**:39–43.

69 Harris S, Caulfield LE, Sugamori ME, Whalen EA, Henning B. The epidemiology of diabetes in pregnant native Canadians. *Diabetes Care* 1997;**20**:1422–5.

70 Mamabolo RL, Alberts M, Levitt NS, Delemarre-van de Waal HA, Steyn NP. Prevalence of gestational diabetes mellitus and the effect of weight on measures of insulin secretion and insulin resistance in third-trimester pregnant rural women residing in the Central Region of Limpopo Province, South Africa. *Diabet Med* 2007;**24**: 233–9.

2 Pathophysiology of diabetes in pregnancy

Francine H. Einstein

Albert Einstein College of Medicine and Montefiore Medical Center, Department of Obstetrics & Gynecology and Women's Health, Division of Maternal Fetal Medicine, Bronx, NY, USA

PRACTICE POINTS

- Insulin resistance and compensatory hyperinsulinemia are adaptations to normal pregnancy.
- The etiology of insulin resistance in pregnancy is multifactorial and likely to include placental factors, such as human placental growth hormone and tumor necrosis factor-alpha (TNF-α), as well as body composition changes and nutrient excess.
- Glucose intolerance and gestational diabetes result when pancreatic beta cell function fails to adequately compensate for the degree of insulin resistance in pregnancy.
- Metabolic plasticity during pregnancy allows for protection of the fetus during periods of limited maternal resources.

MATERNAL METABOLIC ADAPTATION TO PREGNANCY

Pregnancy is a period of significant maternal metabolic adaptations. Teleologically, the changes in maternal anatomy and physiology are thought to occur to support the growth and development of the fetus and prepare the mother for the physiological demands of pregnancy and lactation. The composite of changes are dynamic and evolve throughout the pregnancy.

Normal metabolic homeostasis

Metabolic fuels are derived from carbohydrates, fats, and proteins in the diet. All cells require a constant supply of fuel to provide energy for the production of ATP and cellular maintenance. After a meal, dietary components (glucose, free fatty acids, and amino acids) are delivered to tissues, taken up by cells, and oxidized to produce energy. Any dietary fuel that exceeds the immediate needs of the body is stored, mainly as triglycerides in adipose tissue, or glycogen in the liver, muscle and other cells, or to a lesser extent as protein in muscle. Between meals, substrates are drawn from stores and used as needed to provide energy. The regulation of body fuels is a complex interaction of nutrients and hormones that ensure a continuous supply of energy substrates with intermittent refueling or feeding.

Insulin and glucagon are the two major hormones that regulate fuel mobilization and storage. Insulin is a polypeptide synthesized as proinsulin in β-cells of the pancreatic islets and cleaved into insulin and c-peptide. Its primary role is to orchestrate the metabolism of not only glucose, but also of lipids and amino acids, which are vital for energy homeostasis. Insulin has anabolic and anticatabolic properties. In the liver, insulin promotes glycogen and fat synthesis, while suppressing glycogenolysis, and ketogenesis. In adipose tissue, it promotes fat storage and glycerol synthesis, and suppresses lipolysis. In muscle, insulin promotes glycolysis, glycogen and protein synthesis, and suppresses proteolysis. Glucagon, synthesized in the alpha cells of the pancreas, is a major counter-regulatory hormone of insulin. It is elevated when plasma glucose levels are low and promotes glucose production through glycogenolysis and gluconeogenesis. Epinephrine and cortisol are also insulin counter-regulatory hormones due to their anti-insulin effects.

Postabsorptive state

In the postabsorptive or fasting state, glucose-dependent tissues, like the brain, renal medulla, and certain formed blood cells, continually oxidize glucose as the primary fuel for energy. Because glucose is the preferred substrate for the brain, the maintenance of an adequate plasma glucose level is a physiologic priority. Low insulin levels result in a decrease in peripheral glucose uptake in tissues, such as adipose tissue and muscle. Initially, liver glycogen

A Practical Manual of Diabetes in Pregnancy, 1st Edition.
Edited by David R. McCance, Michael Maresh and David A. Sacks.
© 2010 Blackwell Publishing

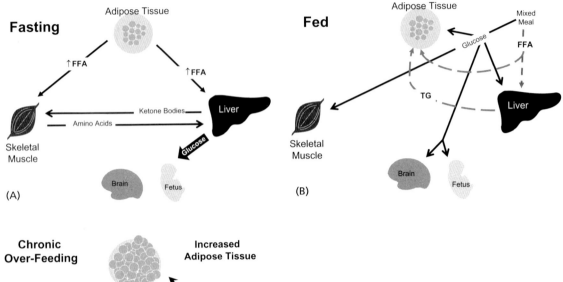

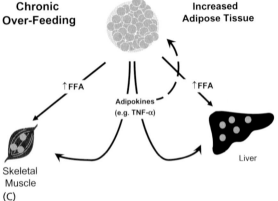

Fig. 2.1 (A) In the fasting state, glucose for dependent tissues, like the brain and the fetus, is derived from the breakdown of hepatic glycogen stores. Once this reserve is depleted, glucose is produce *de novo* from amino acids released from protein stores in muscle. Free fatty acids (FFA) are released from adipose tissue, converted to ketone bodies in the liver and used to prevent excessive glycolysis in non-glucose dependent tissues. (B) Fed state. After the ingestion of a mixed meal, carbohydrates are broken down into glucose and other monosaccharides and taken up by all tissues. Any glucose that is not needed immediately for glycolysis is converted to glycogen or triacylglyerol and stored in liver, muscle, and adipose tissue for later use. Lipids are hydrolyzed to fatty acids, resynthesized to triacylglyerol (TG), and stored in adipose tissue. (C) Chronic over-feeding. Chronic over-nutrition and obesity can lead to adipocyte dysfunction and cellular inflammation. The release of various adipokines, including tumor necrosis factor (TNF)-α, results in insulin resistance in adipose tissue, skeletal muscle and liver. Insulin resistance in adipose tissue leads to lipolysis and increased FFA release, even in the presence of relatively increased insulin levels. With continued nutrient excess the capacity of adipocyte storage capacity is exceeded and lipid "overflows" to other tissues, such as muscle and liver, worsening insulin resistance and resulting in lipotoxicity and metabolic inflexibility.

is degraded to provide glucose for glucose-dependent tissues. Approximately 70 g of glycogen is stored in the liver,[1] while the total basal consumption of glucose is 200–250 g/day,[2] well in excess of stored hepatic glycogen. When the limited stores of glycogen are depleted, the liver uses carbon from lactate, glycerol, and amino acids to synthesize glucose through gluconeogenesis. Decreased insulin levels promote gluconeogenesis, and glucagon plays an additional role in the maintenance of continuous endogenous glucose supply. Glycogenolysis and gluconeogenesis increase to match the basal need for glucose for glucose-dependent tissues during fasting (Fig. 2.1A).

Insulin levels impact on the availability of all nutrients, including amino acids and fatty acids during periods of fasting. Low insulin levels allow for the increase in proteolysis and the augmentation of the release of amino acids from skeletal muscle, the primary reservoir of protein stores. The net flux of amino acids is from the muscle to the liver, with the gluconeogenic precursors, alanine and glutamine, accounting for the largest proportion of amino acids released.[3] In adipose tissue, insulin inhibits hormone-sensitive lipase, which catalyzes the hydrolysis of stored triglycerides to free glycerol and free fatty acids. The consumption of free fatty acids in skeletal muscle is an important factor in limiting muscle glycolysis and glucose oxidation.

Post-absorptive state in pregnancy

Pregnant women have an added burden of supplying the growing fetus with energy substrates during periods of fasting. Glucose is the primary energy source for the fetus and the fetus is obligated to obtain most of the glucose it utilizes from maternal plasma due to the absence of significant gluconeogenesis.[4] A carrier-mediated transport system (GLUT1)[5] meets the high fetal demand with rapid transfer of glucose from the maternal compartment to the fetus. Maternal plasma glucose concentration and uterine/placental blood flow determine glucose supply to the fetus. Glucose transfer across the placental barrier is a relatively rapid process and has been defined as a flow-limited process.[6]

Fasting in pregnancy is more metabolically challenging for the mother due to the growing fetal demand for glucose as an energy substrate. During maternal fasting, plasma glucose levels decrease progressively with increasing gestational age.[7] With short intervals of fasting, human pregnancy is marked by increased fasting plasma insulin levels and increased basal hepatic glucose production.[8,9] A reduced insulin-induced suppression of hepatic glucose production may provide increased endogenous glucose production and therefore augments the supply of glucose for the mother and fetus between meals. Felig et al[3] studied healthy women who were scheduled to undergo termination of pregnancy in the second trimester and healthy non-pregnant controls during a prolonged 84-hour fast. The fasted pregnant women had lower concentrations of plasma glucose and insulin, and greater ketone concentrations with prolonged fasting compared to the non-pregnant women. Felig's work in the 1970s led to the concept of "accelerated starvation"

in pregnancy. The higher plasma ketones found in the fasted pregnant women were seen only in the presence of decreased insulin levels and presumably resulted from increased lipolysis.

Why are fasting glucose levels lower in pregnancy despite increased endogenous glucose production? The mechanism for this is not well understood. Decreased fasting glucose does not appear to be a result of decreased maternal protein catabolism based on urinary nitrogen excretion in pregnant compared to non-pregnant women.[10] Maternal plasma alanine levels are decreased in fasted pregnant women compared to non-pregnant women and may represent the fetal siphoning of glucogenic precursors. Although protein catabolism is increased in pregnancy, increased utilization by the placenta and fetus is likely to cause a decrease in circulating glucogenic precursors.[11] Some have suggested that the suppression of hepatic glucose production is not impaired in late pregnancy, but rather that the set point for plasma glucose levels is decreased.[12]

Postprandial state, non-pregnant

The changes in response to ingestion of a mixed macro-nutrient meal are based on homeostatic mechanisms that allow immediate usage or storage of fuel in expectation of periods of fasting (Fig. 2.1B). Incretin peptides, such as glucose-dependent insulinotropic polypeptide (GIP) and glucagon-like peptide-1 (GLP-1), are secreted from the gastrointestinal tract into the circulation in response to the ingestion of a meal, which enhances glucose-stimulated insulin secretion. Insulin release in the first phase acts predominately in the liver to decrease or shut down hepatic glucose production.[13] Glucose uptake in the splanchnic bed is largely a result of increases in glucose availability, most of which will pass through the liver.[14] Subsequently, increased insulin levels mediate peripheral glucose uptake, mainly in the muscle and adipose tissue.[15] Larger amounts of insulin are required to affect peripheral glucose uptake than are needed to suppress hepatic glucose production.[13] The repletion of muscle nitrogen depends on the net uptake of amino acids in muscle following a meal. In addition to its other functions, insulin acts to suppress proteolysis and accelerates the uptake of triglycerides, promoting fat synthesis and storage in adipose tissue and the liver. Postprandial increases in insulin levels promote the storage of all nutrients (glucose, amino acids, and fatty acids) for later use.

Postprandial state in pregnancy

In addition to the short-term (hour-to-hour) management of fuels, pregnant women have to regulate long-term energy balance that occurs with the changing metabolic demands of the mother and fetus throughout the pregnancy and during lactation. Early pregnancy is marked by storage of nutrients (anabolic state) in preparation for the later use of stored resources in the third trimester and during lactation when energy requirements increase (catabolic state). The energy balance adaptations in early to mid pregnancy probably result from large increases in estrogen, progesterone, and the lactogens (human placental lactogen and prolactin) (reviewed by Freemark[16]). The lactogens and progesterone increase appetite and induce hyperphagia, resulting in a 10–15% increase in food intake. Progesterone facilitates fat storage and the decline in pituitary growth hormone plays a permissive role in the deposition of body fat. The roles of lactogens and estrogen in lipogenesis are less clear and studies have been conflicting.[16] Human placental lactogen stimulates hyperplasia and hypertrophy of beta islet cells. The resulting enhanced insulin secretion with normal peripheral and hepatic insulin sensitivity in early pregnancy promotes the storage of energy substrates through the inhibition of lipolysis, proteolysis, and glycogenolysis.

Overall, insulin sensitivity decreases progressively during pregnancy. Early and late pregnancy changes differ significantly. Although some debate exists about insulin action in early pregnancy, Catalano *et al* found no change in peripheral and hepatic insulin sensitivities in early pregnancy using the hyperinsulinemic–euglycemic clamp technique and glucose tracer, but glucose tolerance was improved.[7,8,17] In early pregnancy, insulin secretion increases, while insulin action is variable and therefore, glucose tolerance may increase in some women.

Insulin resistance and a compensatory hyperinsulinemia are hallmarks of late pregnancy. Insulin-induced peripheral glucose uptake decreases 56% by the third trimester compared to the prepregnancy period, and insulin secretion increases 3–3.5 fold.[7] Some animal[18,19] and human studies[20,21] have shown a reduction in insulin-induced suppression of hepatic glucose production in pregnancy, in contrast to others.[12,22] Methodologic differences during insulin clamps are the likely explanation for the discrepancy, but the weight of evidence suggests that insulin's ability to suppress hepatic glucose production is impaired in late pregnancy. Obese women with normal glucose tolerance have an impaired insulin-induced decrease in hepatic glucose production compared to lean counterparts.[21] In pregnant rodents, the accumulation of visceral fat contributes to the development of hepatic insulin resistance, an effect that may be modulated through the accumulation of hepatic triglycerides.[23]

INSULIN RESISTANCE IN PREGNANCY

The etiology of insulin resistance in pregnancy is not completely understood and is likely to be multifactorial. Historically, placental hormones have been implicated for many reasons. The extent of insulin resistance in pregnancy corresponds to the growth of the placenta and many placental hormones induce insulin resistance when given to non-pregnant individuals, including human placental lactogen (hPL),[24,25] human placental growth hormone (hPGH),[26] and progesterone.[27,28] hPGH induces insulin resistance by antagonizing insulin action through regulation of p85 expression in adipose tissue.[29] hPGH has been shown to cause severe insulin resistance in transgenic mice that express high levels of the hormone, similar to levels found in late human gestation.[26] However, the transgenic mice in this study were also obese compared to wild-type animals, and the contribution of other factors, like visceral adiposity, have not been examined. Placental factors clearly have a role in the development of insulin resistance in pregnancy. Some hormones, such as hPGH, may directly affect insulin action; other factors may contribute indirectly to the insulin resistance through increased food intake and the promotion of lipogenesis.

The obesity epidemic and the increasing prevalence of the metabolic syndrome have spurred intense investigation into the adverse effects of increased adipose tissue and nutrient excess. An increase in adipose tissue, particularly an increase in visceral fat, is a key component of the metabolic syndrome[30,31] and adipose tissue is no longer considered to be solely an energy storage depot. Normal pregnancy shares many common features with the metabolic syndrome, including increased adiposity, insulin resistance, hyperinsulinemia, and hyperlipidemia. Maternal body fat increases on average more than 3 kg[32] over a relatively short time interval. Epidemiologic[33,34] and animal[23] studies suggest that visceral fat in particular increases in pregnancy, although descriptions of human body composition changes are limited due to increases in total body water and the restrictions of measurement modalities that can be used during pregnancy.[35–38]

Adipose tissue plays a role in regulating food intake, energy balance, and metabolic homeostasis through the production of fat-derived peptides. Several of these biologically active peptides affect energy homeostasis, such as leptin, which is expressed and secreted primarily by adipocytes. Leptin signals the adequacy of adipose stores to the hypothalamus, providing the afferent limb in energy homeostasis.[39,40] The human placenta produces and secretes leptin into both maternal and fetal circulation,[41] and the concentrations of leptin are elevated in pregnancy compared to the non-pregnant state, irrespective of body mass index,[42] which may seem paradoxical because food intake is increased. "Lipostatic" signals, including leptin, become secondary and do not play a role in behavioral regulation of food intake if the energy supply (i.e. glucose) to the brain is threatened. As such, hyperphagia accompanies hypoglycemia independent of adipose mass.[43] This phenomenon is termed "leptin resistance" and pregnancy is a "leptin-resistant" state. That the resistance to leptin in pregnancy is centrally mediated is supported by emerging evidence.[44,45]

Although adipocyte production of adipokines has a critical role in metabolic homeostasis, some adipokines may mediate the harmful biologic effects of increased adiposity. For example, TNF-α is associated with decreased insulin sensitivity in a number of conditions outside of pregnancy, including obesity[46] and aging.[47] In pregnancy, TNF-α plasma concentration is more predictive of insulin sensitivity than cortisol, human chorionic gonadotropin (hCG), estradiol, hPL, and prolactin.[48] Although 95% of TNF-α produced by the human placenta is released into the maternal compartment,[48] TNF-α is secreted by both the placenta and adipose tissue, and the relative contribution of each source is uncertain.

Other adipokines (resistin, interleukin [IL]-1, and [IL]-6) have also been implicated as mediators of insulin resistance.[49] Resistin, a newly discovered adipokine, decreases insulin sensitivity and increases plasma glucose levels.[50,51] Higher plasma levels of resistin are found in women late in gestation compared to non-pregnant women, and term placentas have higher resistin mRNA expression compared with first trimester chorionic villi.[52] However, the exact role of resistin and many other adipokines in pregnancy has yet to be determined.

Some adipokines improve insulin sensitivity (leptin, adiponectin. and peroxisome proliferator-activated receptor [PPAR]-γ). Little is known about the role of adiponectin during pregnancy. Although expression of adiponectin is specific to adipose tissue, plasma levels are lower in obesity.[53] Serum adiponectin levels are lower in pregnant compared to non-pregnant women. However,

no difference is found after correction for hemodilution.[54] The roles of many adipokines and fat-derived peptides in pregnancy have yet to be elucidated.

NUTRIENT EXCESS AND METABOLIC DYSFUNCTION

The expansion of adipose tissue due to chronic over-nutrition and obesity can lead to adipocyte dysfunction, cellular inflammation, and insulin resistance (Fig. 2.1C). In addition to the metabolic dysfunction caused by excess adipose tissue, the process of accumulating excess adipose tissue leads to metabolic dysregulation. Gregor and Hotamisligil[55] have proposed that a pathologic excess of nutrients and excessive lipid storage in the adipocyte leads to loss of mitochondrial function and endoplasmic reticular stress. Adipocyte dysfunction results in insulin resistance, which may be mediated through the activation of c-jun N-terminal kinase (JNK) activation, inflammation, and oxidative stress. Further, when continued nutrient excess exceeds adipocyte storage capacity, lipid then "overflows" into other tissues.[56] The oversupply of lipids into the liver, skeletal muscle and pancreatic islets results in a tissue-specific insulin resistance and impaired insulin secretion, generally termed "lipotoxicity".[56] In 1963, Randle et al[57] proposed that increased fatty acid oxidation inhibits glucose oxidation and later, McGarry et al[58] showed that hyperglycemia inhibits fatty acid oxidation. As a result of these two concepts, the concept of "metabolic inflexibility" has arisen, which proposes that in the setting of chronic over-nutrition, muscle tissue is unable to select the appropriate substrate for oxidation (glucose vs fatty acids) in response to the current nutrient supply,[59] resulting in metabolic dysregulation in skeletal muscle, the primary tissue for peripheral glucose uptake in the non-pregnant state. This theory applied to pregnancy, a state of hyperphagia and rapid increases in maternal body fat, may have important implications.

INSULIN RESISTANCE AND GLUCOSE INTOLERANCE

The terms insulin resistance and glucose intolerance are often erroneously used interchangeably and should be differentiated. *Insulin resistance* refers to the reduced ability of insulin to act on target tissues. In the most basic terms, insulin is less effective in suppressing hepatic glucose production and greater amounts of insulin are needed to induce peripheral glucose uptake in the muscle and adipose tissue. In insulin-resistant states, more insulin is required to maintain glucose homeo-stasis. *Glucose-intolerant states* generally include some degree of insulin resistance and hyperinsulinemia, but the secretion of insulin is relatively inadequate for the degree of insulin resistance and the result is a mild fasting and/or transient postprandial elevations in plasma glucose levels.

In normal pregnancy, despite a well-demonstrated insulin resistance, the large compensatory increase in insulin secretion maintains maternal plasma glucose levels within a relatively narrow margin.[20] Continuous glucose monitoring, which included more than 700 glucose measurements in a 72-hour period, demon-strated that normal weight, glucose-tolerant women at around 29 weeks of gestation had a mean fasting glucose level of 4.0 ± 0.7 mmol/L (72.1 ± 13 mg/dL) and a peak postparandial level of 5.9 ± 0.9 mmol/L (106.2 ± 16 mg/dL).[60] Thus, although pregnancy is marked by insulin resistance, normal-weight women maintain serum glucose levels within a narrow margin. Women who are unable to compensate with increased insulin secretion become glucose intolerant. Further, glucose tolerance is a continuum. The detection of ges-tational diabetes is aimed at identifying pregnancies at risk for perinatal morbidity and to some extent to identify women at risk for Type 2 diabetes later in life. The threshold for maternal glycemia at which the risks for the fetus begin is unknown and is currently being debated (see chapters 6 and 7).

The relationship between insulin sensitivity and insulin secretion is reciprocal and non-linear in nature (Fig. 2.2). In order for glucose tolerance to remain unchanged, changes in insulin sensitivity must be matched by a pro-portionate yet opposite change in circulating insulin levels. With decreasing insulin sensitivity, as is seen in pregnancy, insulin secretion must increase for glucose tolerance to remain unchanged. Failure to secrete ade-quate amounts of insulin for the degree of insulin resist-ance results in a shift of the curve to the left and impaired glucose tolerance. This process underlies the develop-ment of diabetes.

Increasing insulin resistance and a compensatory hyperinsulinemia are progressive throughout the preg-nancy. If insulin secretion cannot compensate for increased insulin resistance, glucose intolerance ensues. Many have used the analogy of the pick-up truck with a load in the bed of the truck. The engine of the truck symbolizes the pancreas and insulin secretion, and the load is insulin resistance. When the engine of the truck is normal (no defects in insulin secretion), the small load

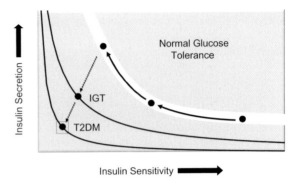

Fig. 2.2 To maintain normal glucose tolerance, insulin secretion must increase to compensate for decreasing insulin sensitivity during pregnancy (solid arrows). Failure to secrete adequate amounts of insulin for the degree of insulin resistance results in a shift of the curve to the left and impaired glucose tolerance (dotted arrows). This process underlies the development of diabetes (both gestational [IGT] and Type 2 [T2DM]). (Adapted from Kahn *et al. Nature* 2006;**444**:840–6, with permission.)

of insulin resistance from pregnancy itself is relatively inconsequential and does not affect the movement of the truck (glucose tolerance is normal). If other factors, like obesity, increased visceral fat or prolonged nutrient excess, contribute to a larger load, then the truck may be slowed, so that postprandial glucose levels are higher and may have a delayed return to baseline, allowing for increased transfer of glucose to the fetus. When the load is excessive, and the engine of the truck can no longer compensate or the engine is defective (beta cell dysfunc-tion), overt diabetes results.

METABOLIC PLASTICITY IN PREGNANCY

Maternal metabolic plasticity during pregnancy may allow for protection of the fetus during periods of limited resources. While the complex factors that determine the balance between the competing needs of the mother and fetus are incompletely understood, the study of a unique population of women in the resource-poor country of Gambia has offered some insight. In 1993, Poppitt and colleagues[61] performed a longitudinal study using whole-body calorimetry in a cohort of Gambian women who had limited resources. The women were lean, but not underweight, and had mean weight gain during pre-gnancy below the Institute of Medicine recommenda-tions, and yet the mean birthweight was normal in this small cohort. From the beginning of pregnancy, the Gambian women had a decrease in basal metabolic rate and when corrected for lean body mass, the women maintained a basal metabolic rate below their prepregnancy rate, even late in the third trimester. This study demonstrated that in an environment in which food intake cannot be increased, pregnant women have "metabolic plasticity" and adapt in order to conserve energy, presumably for the developing fetus.

In an environment with ample resources, an increase in nutrient intake results in a positive energy balance throughout the pregnancy. In sharp contrast to the women in Gambia, women in more affluent countries maintain an increased basal metabolic rate throughout pregnancy.[62] These findings suggest that the increased energy demands of pregnancy can be met through many means, such as increased intake, decreased activity, and deceased fat storage. Further, the total energy costs of pregnancy (fetus, fat deposition, and maintenance) in women from affluent and poor countries are strongly correlated with prepregnancy body fat and weight gain.[62] "Metabolic plasticity" in women who are unable to increase food intake may be protective for the fetus. Therefore, recommendations for the adequacy of caloric intake are variable and largely dependent on the resources available and the nutritional status of the mother at the start of pregnancy.

SUMMARY AND FUTURE DIRECTIONS FOR RESEARCH

The physiologic adaptations that occur in pregnancy provide adequate energy and substrates for the growing fetus and prepare the mother for the increased burden of pregnancy and lactation. Insulin resistance is progressive throughout gestation and a compensatory increase in insulin secretion maintains plasma glucose levels within a relatively narrow window. Placental factors contribute to insulin resistance directly (e.g. hPGH and TNF-α) and indirectly through the increase in appetite and weight gain. A chronic positive energy balance results in adipose tissue accretion that may be used later for increased fetal demands in late pregnancy and lactation. However, excessive amounts of adiposity before pregnancy or excessive weight gain during pregnancy may have deleterious effects on insulin action and glucose tolerance. Definitions of a healthy amount of adiposity, ideal weight gain or the necessary degree of insulin resistance required for normal fetal growth are unclear and likely to be the focus of future research.

REFERENCES

1 Hultman E. Carbohydrate metabolism normally and under trauma. *Nord Med* 1971;**85**:330–46.

2 Rothman DL, Magnusson I, Katz LD, Shulman RG, Shulman GI. Quantitation of hepatic glycogenolysis and gluconeogenesis in fasting humans with 13C NMR. *Science* 1991;**254**:573–6.

3 Felig P, Lynch V. Starvation in human pregnancy: hypoglycemia, hypoinsulinemia, and hyperketonemia. *Science* 1970;**170**:990–2.

4 Baumann MU, Deborde S, Illsley NP. Placental glucose transfer and fetal growth. *Endocrine* 2002;**19**:13–22.

5 Teasdale F, Jean-Jacques G. Morphometric evaluation of the microvillous surface enlargement factor in the human placenta from mid-gestation to term. *Placenta* 1985;**6**:375–81.

6 Illsley NP, Lin HY, Verkman AS. Lipid domain structure correlated with membrane protein function in placental microvillus vesicles. *Biochemistry* 1987;**26**:446–54.

7 Catalano PM, Tyzbir ED, Roman NM, Amini SB, Sims EA. Longitudinal changes in insulin release and insulin resistance in nonobese pregnant women. *Am J Obstet Gynecol* 1991;**165**:1667–72.

8 Catalano PM, Tyzbir ED, Wolfe RR, Roman NM, Amini SB, Sims EA. Longitudinal changes in basal hepatic glucose production and suppression during insulin infusion in normal pregnant women. *Am J Obstet Gynecol* 1992;**167**:913–9.

9 Cowett RM, Susa JB, Kahn CB, Giletti B, Oh W, Schwartz R. Glucose kinetics in nondiabetic and diabetic women during the third trimester of pregnancy. *Am J Obstet Gynecol* 1983;**146**:773–80.

10 Felig P, Lynch V. Starvation in human pregnancy: hypoglycemia, hypoinsulinemia, and hyperketonemia. *Science* 1970;**170**:990–2.

11 Felig P. Maternal and fetal fuel homeostasis in human pregnancy. *Am J Clin Nutr* 1973;**26**:998–1005.

12 Nolan CJ, Proietto J. The set point for maternal glucose homeostasis is lowered during late pregnancy in the rat: the role of the islet beta-cell and liver. *Diabetologia* 1996;**39**:785–92.

13 Rizza RA, Mandarino LJ, Gerich JE. Dose-response characteristics for effects of insulin on production and utilization of glucose in man. *Am J Physiol* 1981;**240**:E630–9.

14 Sherwin RS, Hendler R, DeFronzo R, Wahren J, Felic P. Glucose homeostasis during prolonged suppression of glucagon and insulin secretion by somatostatin. *Proc Natl Acad Sci U S A* 1977;**74**:348–52.

15 Sacca L, Cicala M, Trimarco B, Ungaro B, Vigorito C. Differential effects of insulin on splanchnic and peripheral glucose disposal after an intravenous glucose load in man. *J Clin Invest* 1982;**70**:117–26.

16 Freemark M. Regulation of maternal metabolism by pituitary and placental hormones: roles in fetal development and metabolic programming. *Horm Res* 2006;**65** (Suppl 3):41–9.

17 Catalano PM, Tyzbir ED, Wolfe RR, *et al*. Carbohydrate metabolism during pregnancy in control subjects and women with gestational diabetes. *Am J Physiol* 1993;**264**: E60–7.

18 Hauguel S, Gilbert M, Girard J. Pregnancy-induced insulin resistance in liver and skeletal muscles of the conscious rabbit. *Am J Physiol* 1987;**252**:E165–9.

19 Rossi G, Sherwin RS, Penzias AS, *et al*. Temporal changes in insulin resistance and secretion in 24-h-fasted conscious pregnant rats. *Am J Physiol* 1993;**265**:E845–51.

20 Catalano PM, Huston L, Amini SB, Kalhan SC. Longitudinal changes in glucose metabolism during pregnancy in obese women with normal glucose tolerance and gestational diabetes mellitus. *Am J Obstet Gynecol* 1999;**180**:903–16.

21 Sivan E, Chen X, Homko CJ, Reece EA, Boden G. Longitudinal study of carbohydrate metabolism in healthy obese pregnant women. *Diabetes Care* 1997;**20**:1470–5.

22 Connolly CC, Papa T, Smith MS, Lacy DB, Williams PE, Moore MC. Hepatic and muscle insulin action during late pregnancy in the dog. *Am J Physiol Regul Integr Comp Physiol* 2007;**292**:R447–52.

23 Einstein FH, Fishman S, Muzumdar RH, Yang XM, Atzmon G, Barzilai N. Accretion of visceral fat and hepatic insulin resistance in pregnant rats. *Am J Physiol Endocrinol Metab* 2008;**294**:E451–5.

24 Samaan N, Yen SC, Gonzalez D, Pearson OH. Metabolic effects of placental lactogen (HPL) in man. *J Clin Endocrinol Metab* 1968;**28**:485–91.

25 Kalkhoff RK, Richardson BL, Beck P. Relative effects of pregnancy, human placental lactogen and prednisolone on carbohydrate tolerance in normal and subclinical diabetic subjects. *Diabetes* 1969;**18**:153–63.

26 Barbour LA, Shao J, Qiao L, *et al*. Human placental growth hormone causes severe insulin resistance in transgenic mice. *Am J Obstet Gynecol* 2002;**186**:512–7.

27 Kalkhoff RK, Jacobson M, Lemper D. Progesterone, pregnancy and the augmented plasma insulin response. *J Clin Endocrinol Metab* 1970;**31**:24–8.

28 Beck P. Progestin enhancement of the plasma insulin response to glucose in Rhesus monkeys. *Diabetes* 1969;**18**: 146–52.

29 Barbour LA, Shao J, Qiao L, *et al*. Human placental growth hormone increases expression of the p85 regulatory unit of phosphatidylinositol 3-kinase and triggers severe insulin resistance in skeletal muscle. *Endocrinology* 2004;**145**: 1144–50.

30 Alberti KG, Zimmet P, Shaw J. The metabolic syndrome – a new worldwide definition. *Lancet* 2005;**366**:1059–62.

31 Zimmet P, Alberti KG, Shaw J. Global and societal implications of the diabetes epidemic. *Nature* 2001;**414**:782–7.

32 Hytten FE. Weight gain in pregnancy – 30 year of research. *S Afr Med J* 1981;**60**:15–9.

33 Blaudeau TE, Hunter GR, Sirikul B. Intra-abdominal adipose tissue deposition and parity. *Int J Obes (Lond)* 2006; **30**:1119–24.

34 Kinoshita T, Itoh M. Longitudinal variance of fat mass deposition during pregnancy evaluated by ultrasonography: the ratio of visceral fat to subcutaneous fat in the abdomen. *Gynecol Obstet Invest* 2006;**61**:115–8.

35 Hopkinson JM, Butte NF, Ellis KJ, Wong WW, Puyau MR, Smith EO. Body fat estimation in late pregnancy and early postpartum: comparison of two-, three-, and four-component models. *Am J Clin Nutr* 1997;**65**:432–8.

36 McManus RM, Cunningham I, Watson A, Harker L, Finegood DT. Beta-cell function and visceral fat in lactating women with a history of gestational diabetes. *Metabolism* 2001;**50**:715–9.

37 Sidebottom AC, Brown JE, Jacobs DR, Jr. Pregnancy-related changes in body fat. *Eur J Obstet Gynecol Reprod Biol* 2001;**94**:216–23.

38 Sohlstrom A, Forsum E. Changes in total body fat during the human reproductive cycle as assessed by magnetic resonance imaging, body water dilution, and skinfold thickness: a comparison of methods. *Am J Clin Nutr* 1997;**66**:1315–22.

39 Campfield LA, Smith FJ, Guisez Y, Devos R, Burn P. Recombinant mouse OB protein: evidence for a peripheral signal linking adiposity and central neural networks. *Science* 1995;**269**:546–9.

40 Zhang F, Basinski MB, Beals JM, *et al*. Crystal structure of the obese protein leptin-E100. *Nature* 1997;**387**:206–9.

41 Masuzaki H, Ogawa Y, Sagawa N, *et al*. Nonadipose tissue production of leptin: leptin as a novel placenta-derived hormone in humans. *Nat Med* 1997;**3**:1029–33.

42 Finn PD, Cunningham MJ, Pau KY, Spies HG, Clifton DK, Steiner RA. The stimulatory effect of leptin on the neuroendocrine reproductive axis of the monkey. *Endocrinology* 1998;**139**:4652–62.

43 Peters A, Schweiger U, Pellerin L, *et al*. The selfish brain: competition for energy resources. *Neurosci Biobehav Rev* 2004;**28**:143–80.

44 Ladyman SR, Grattan DR. Suppression of leptin receptor messenger ribonucleic acid and leptin responsiveness in the ventromedial nucleus of the hypothalamus during pregnancy in the rat. *Endocrinology* 2005;**146**:3868–74.

45 Ladyman SR, Grattan DR. Region-specific reduction in leptin-induced phosphorylation of signal transducer and activator of transcription-3 (STAT3) in the rat hypothalamus is associated with leptin resistance during pregnancy. *Endocrinology* 2004;**145**:3704–11.

46 Hotamisligil GS, Peraldi P, Budavari A, Ellis R, White MF, Spiegelman BM. IRS-1-mediated inhibition of insulin receptor tyrosine kinase activity in TNF-alpha- and obesity-induced insulin resistance. *Science* 1996;**271**:665–8.

47 Kirwan JP, Krishnan RK, Weaver JA, Del Aguila LF, Evans WJ. Human aging is associated with altered TNF-alpha production during hyperglycemia and hyperinsulinemia. *Am J Physiol Endocrinol Metab* 2001;**281**:E1137–43.

48 Kirwan JP, Hauguel-De Mouzon S, Lepercq J, *et al*. TNF-alpha is a predictor of insulin resistance in human pregnancy. *Diabetes* 2002;**51**:2207–13.

49 Hotamisligil GS, Murray DL, Choy LN, Spiegelman BM. Tumor necrosis factor alpha inhibits signaling from the insulin receptor. *Proc Natl Acad Sci U S A* 1994;**91**:4854–8.

50 Flier JS. Diabetes. The missing link with obesity? *Nature* 2001;**409**:292–3.

51 Steppan CM, Bailey ST, Bhat S, *et al*. The hormone resistin links obesity to diabetes. *Nature* 2001;**409**:307–12.

52 Yura S, Sagawa N, Itoh H, *et al*. Resistin is expressed in the human placenta. *J Clin Endocrinol Metab* 2003;**88**:1394–7.

53 Arita Y, Kihara S, Ouchi N, *et al*. Paradoxical decrease of an adipose-specific protein, adiponectin, in obesity. *Biochem Biophys Res Commun* 1999;**257**:79–83.

54 Naruse K, Yamasaki M, Umekage H, Sado T, Sakamoto Y, Morikawa H. Peripheral blood concentrations of adiponectin, an adipocyte-specific plasma protein, in normal pregnancy and preeclampsia. *J Reprod Immunol* 2005;**65**:65–75.

55 Gregor MG, Hotamisligil GS. Adipocyte stress: The endoplasmic reticulum and metabolic disease. *J Lipid Res* 2007;**48**:1905–14.

56 Muoio DM, Newgard CB. Obesity-related derangements in metabolic regulation. *Annu Rev Biochem* 2006;**75**:367–401.

57 Randle PJ, Garland PB, Hales CN, Newsholme EA. The glucose fatty-acid cycle. Its role in insulin sensitivity and the metabolic disturbances of diabetes mellitus. *Lancet* 1963;**1**:785–9.

58 McGarry JD, Mannaerts GP, Foster DW. A possible role for malonyl-CoA in the regulation of hepatic fatty acid oxidation and ketogenesis. *J Clin Invest* 1977;**60**:265–70.

59 Kelley DE, Mandarino LJ. Fuel selection in human skeletal muscle in insulin resistance: a reexamination. *Diabetes* 2000;**49**:677–83.

60 Yogev Y, Ben-Haroush A, Chen R, Rosenn B, Hod M, Langer O. Diurnal glycemic profile in obese and normal weight nondiabetic pregnant women. *Am J Obstet Gynecol* 2004;**191**:949–53.

61 Poppitt SD, Prentice AM, Jequier E, Schutz Y, Whitehead RG. Evidence of energy sparing in Gambian women during pregnancy: a longitudinal study using whole-body calorimetry. *Am J Clin Nutr* 1993;**57**:353–64.

62 Prentice AM, Goldberg GR. Energy adaptations in human pregnancy: limits and long-term consequences. *Am J Clin Nutr* 2000;**71** (5 Suppl):1226S–32S.

3

The placenta in diabetes in pregnancy

Ursula Hiden & Gernot Desoye

Department of Obstetrics and Gynecology, Medical University of Graz, Austria

PRACTICE POINTS

- The distinct placental changes associated with diabetes mellitus depend on the gestational period during which the diabetic insult occurs and thus, on the type of diabetes.
- Early placental development may be altered by insulin and tumor necrosis factor-α (TNF-α)-induced changes in matrix metalloproteinases that degrade extracellular matrix.
- The placenta is often heavier in women with diabetes, with an increase in maternal, i.e. syncytiotrophoblast, and fetal, i.e. endothelial, surface area.
- Trophoblast proliferation is regulated by maternal insulin; hypervascularization is the collective result of fetal hypoxia.
- Glucose from the maternal to fetal circulation is unaltered in gestational diabetes mellitus (GDM). The higher flux results from the steeper maternal-to-fetal concentration gradient. Amino acid transport may be altered.
- Fetal insulin and insulin-like growth factors directly influence fetal growth, but additionally promote transplacental amino acid transport that will also sustain fetal growth.
- Leptin shares parts of its signaling pathways with insulin. It is highly expressed by the placenta and secreted into the maternal and fetal circulation. It may contribute to developmental changes in diabetes.

NORMAL DEVELOPMENT

The placenta is a complex organ that is essential for fetal growth and development. It fulfils a wide spectrum of functions, among which the transport of maternal fuels to the fetus and the synthesis of various hormones and growth factors are the foremost examples. Its development and function are tightly regulated by a range of hormones, cytokines, growth factors, and substrates present in the maternal and fetal circulation. Placenta-

derived factors affect the maternal adaptation to pregnancy as well as fetal growth and development.

After blastocyst implantation into the decidual surface, the placenta continuously develops by the differentiation and proliferation of trophoblast cells, eventually leading to placental villi of varying degrees of maturation,[1] most of which float freely in the intervillous space, i.e. the area between the placental villi (Fig. 3.1). Highly proliferative villous cytotrophoblasts fuse to form the syncytiotrophoblast that represents the outermost interface of the placenta that is in contact with the maternal circulation. The microvillous membrane of this syncytium is in contact with the maternal blood and is richly endowed with receptors,[2] enzymes[3] and transporters.[4] Maternal blood emanating from remodeled and opened spiral arteries bathes the villi.

Some villi physically anchor the placenta to the uterus, thus establishing a connection between the fetus and the maternal decidua (Fig. 3.1). These anchoring villi are formed by proliferation, differentiation, and invasion by cytotrophoblasts of the maternal lining of the decidual cavity. Extravillous cytotrophoblasts also invade the decidual spiral arteries and remodel them into low resistance arteries. The resulting increase of maternal blood flow into the intervillous space ensures adequate maternal nutrient supply to the fetus.[1] Trophoblast invasion is tightly regulated in time and space by invasion-promoting and -inhibiting factors originating from the maternal decidua or the placenta. The decidua derives from the maternal endometrium after decidualization and before implantation of the embryo. This process produces a dense extracellular matrix and a cytokine milieu that reduces trophoblast invasion.[5] Levels of these factors are altered in various pregnancy-associated pathologies and diabetes mellitus (Table 3.1).

During villous development vasculogenesis and angiogenesis result in the formation of placental vessels,

A Practical Manual of Diabetes in Pregnancy, 1st Edition.
Edited by David R. McCance, Michael Maresh and David A. Sacks.
© 2010 Blackwell Publishing

Table 3.1 Alterations in maternal levels of trophoblast invasion inhibiting and promoting factors in gestational diabetes mellitus (GDM) and Type 1 diabetes mellitus (T1DM). Tumor necrosis factor-α (TNF-α) inhibits trophoblast invasion, whereas vascular endothelial growth factor (VEGF), leptin, insulin-like growth factors 1 and 2 (IGF1, IGF2) promote trophoblast invasion.

	Invasion inhibiting	Invasion promoting				Other
	TNF-α*	VEGF	Leptin	IGF1	IGF2	Insulin
T1DM	↑[28]			↓[29] NC[58]	↑[58] NC[29]	↑[37]
GDM	↑[59]	↑[30]	↑[60]	↑[61] NC[58]	↑[58] NC[29,61]	↑[37] insulin treated ↑[62]

* Decidua-derived factors
NC, no change

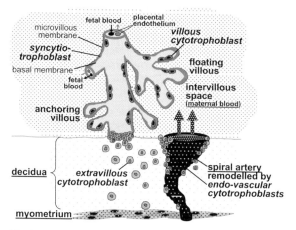

Fig. 3.1 Organization of placental villi after week 20 of gestation. The syncytiotrophoblast represents the outermost surface of the placenta and is in contact with the maternal blood via its microvillous membrane that is richly endowed with receptors, enzymes, and transport molecules. The syncytium regenerates and expands by proliferation and fusion of cytotrophoblasts lying underneath. Some cytotrophoblasts at the tips of floating villi invade the decidua, thereby anchoring the villi. A proportion of these extravillous cytotrophoblasts invade the uterine spiral arteries, leading to their remodeling into low resistance vessels. To differentiate between maternal and placental cells and tissues, maternal structures are dotted and their labelling is underlined.

a process that again is controlled by various growth factors, cytokines, and oxygen (Table 3.2), and thus can be dysregulated in diabetes.

THE PLACENTA IN DIABETES

Because of the presence of receptors and enzymes on both placental surfaces, i.e. the microvillous syncytiotro-phoblast membrane as well as the basal membrane of the syncytiotrophoblast and the placental endothelial cells, the diabetic environment may have profound effects on placental development and function. We recently proposed that these specific effects will critically depend on the time period in gestation when the insult of the diabetic environment acts upon the placenta.[6]

As glucose can stimulate and repress gene expression,[7] maternal and fetal hyperglycemia are likely to have an impact on the production of various placental proteins, but a detailed analysis is pending. Moreover, maternal and fetal hyperinsulinemia also affect placental metabolism, growth, and development.[3,8,9] However, the changes in the diabetic environment extend beyond glucose and insulin (Tables 3.1 and 3.2). Those in the mother can induce modifications in the placenta, including altered synthesis of cytokines and growth factors, which in turn may act locally in an autocrine or paracrine manner. Altered cytokines and growth factors, along with metabolites, can be secreted into both the maternal and fetal circulation, and thus affect both mother and fetus (Fig. 3.2).

Despite the improvement in maternal glycemic control over the last few decades[10] structural and functional changes of the diabetic placenta at term may occur independent of the type of diabetes.[11] Similar to fetal weight, placental weight tends to be heavier in diabetes, but the weight gain is more pronounced in the placenta than in the fetus, as is reflected in a higher placental-to-fetal weight ratio than in normal gestation.[12,13] It has remained an unresolved question whether placental overweight is the cause or consequence of fetal overgrowth in diabetes.

Intuitively, possible changes in placental transport in diabetes may be implicated. Despite altered expression of placental glucose transporters, perfusion experiments

Table 3.2 Alterations in fetal levels of pro- or anti-angiogenic factors in pregnancy with gestational diabetes mellitus (GDM) and Type 1 diabetes mellitus (T1DM). Both types of diabetes are characterized by enhanced vascularization.

| | Antiangiogenic | Proangiogenic | | | | | | | Other |
	TNF-α	VEGF	FGF2	PlGF	Leptin	IGF1	IGF2	Hypoxia	Insulin
GDM	↓[59]		↑[30]	NC[63]	↑[64]		↑[58]	↑[65]	↑[66]
T1DM		↓[67]	↑[68]	NC[63]	↑[64]	↑[29,44]	↑[44,58]	↑[69]	↑[37]

TNF-α, tumor necrosis factor-α; VEGF, vascular endothelial growth factor; FGF2, fibroblast-specific growth factor 2, PlGF, placental growth factor; IGF1, IGF2, insulin-like growth factor 1 and 2; NC, no change

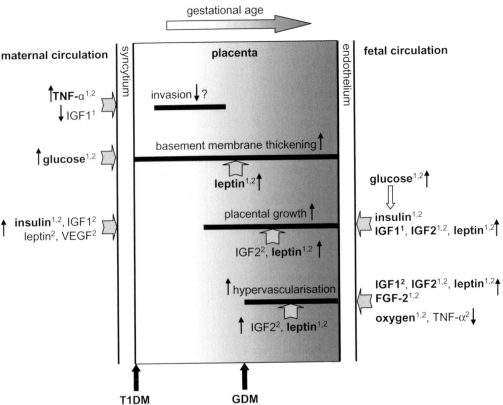

Fig. 3.2 Hypothetical model for diabetes-induced alterations in human placenta. Elevated maternal tumor necrosis factor-α (TNF-α) and reduced insulin-like growth factor 1 (IGF1) levels in Type 1 diabetes mellitus (T1DM) may inhibit placental invasion, paralleling a higher incidence of early pregnancy loss in diabetes. Maternal hyperglycemia induces thickening of the placental basement membrane, hence reducing oxygen transport. Increased levels of placental leptin may even further contribute to the excessive extracellular matrix synthesis. Various factors elevated in the placenta (IGF2, leptin), maternal (insulin, vascular endothelial growth factor [VEGF]) or fetal (insulin, IGF1, IGF2, leptin) circulations in diabetes promote proliferation and placental growth. Placental hypervascularization may be supported by elevated levels of placental IGF2 and leptin, increased fetal IGF1, IGF2, leptin, fibroblast-specific growth factor 2 (FGF2), and reduced fetal TNF-α, as well as by fetal hypoxia. These derangements in the feto-placental compartment are characteristic of gestational diabetes mellitus (GDM), overt diabetes, or both. [1]Changed in T1DM; [2]changed in GDM. Factors in bold denote similar dysregulation in T1DM and GDM.

have demonstrated an unchanged if not reduced transplacental glucose transport in GDM[14] even on a total placenta weight basis. Studies that also integrate potential structural changes argue strongly for the steeper maternal-to-fetal glucose concentration gradient as the major, if not only, reason for increased glucose fluxes across the placenta in diabetes. This conclusion is also supported by the unchanged concentration differences for glucose in umbilical arteries and veins in GDM.[15]

Syncytiotrophoblast amino acid transport systems may be altered in diabetes.[4,16] However, even for transport systems that are unaltered, when expressed per unit protein or tissue weight, an increase in total placental weight will result in increased nutrient transport. It is unclear if this will stimulate fetal growth or just serve to cover the increased fetal nutrient requirements when the overgrowth of the fetus overgrowth is driven by other factors.

In all types of diabetes, gross placental structure may be altered. In particular, the surface and exchange areas are enlarged[17] as a result of hyperproliferation and hypervascularization. The underlying mechanisms for the villous surface increase are not clear. Maternal hyperinsulinemia early in gestation is a candidate,[8] but other maternal growth factors may also contribute.

The greater placental capillary surfaces may result from feto-placental counter-regulatory mechanisms to fetal hypoxia which can be inferred from the elevated fetal erythropoietin levels, polycythemia, and increased nucleated red cells often observed in fetuses of women with diabetes.[18] Materno-placental oxygen supply may be reduced in diabetes because of:

- Decreased maternal arterial oxygen saturation and increased proportion of glycosylated hemoglobin, which has a higher affinity for oxygen than non-glycosylated hemoglobin[19]
- Thickening of the trophoblast basement membrane[20] although this is not uniformly found[21]
- Under certain instances, reduced utero-placental blood flow[22] as a result of increased flow impedance in the uterine and umbilical arteries.[23,24]

In addition to impaired oxygen supply, fetal oxygen demand is increased because aerobic metabolism is stimulated by fetal hyperinsulinemia. The resulting low fetal oxygen levels ultimately upregulate the transcriptional synthesis of proangiogenic factors in the feto-placental compartment. Established examples include fibroblast growth factor 2 (FGF2), vascular endothelial growth factor (VEGF), and leptin.[25–27] Higher levels of these factors promote placental endothelial cell prolifera-

tion, a key process in angiogenesis. The increase in placental vascular exchange area against a background of fetal hypoxia appears paradoxical in a situation of maternal nutritional oversupply and may underline the overriding importance of adequate oxygen delivery to the fetus.

Little is known about the placental changes in the first trimester, when the developing placenta is exposed to the maternal diabetic environment, i.e. hyperglycemia, hyperinsulinemia resulting from the relatively excessive insulin doses needed to maintain strict metabolic control, increased expression of TNF-α,[28] reduced insulin-like growth factor 1 (IGF1),[29] and elevated FGF2.[30] It seems reasonable to assume that the diabetic milieu will have an influence on placental development and function during this critical period when placental structures are formed, and the placenta is likely to be most sensitive to environmental derangements. Placental growth and development sometimes appear to be retarded in the first gestational weeks, probably because of a reduction of trophoblast proliferation resulting from hyperglycemia.[31,32] A higher incidence of spontaneous abortions[33] and pregnancy pathologies, such as pre-eclampsia and intrauterine growth restriction (IUGR), suggest impaired trophoblast invasion, which would result in inadequate placental anchoring and opening of the maternal spiral arteries.[34] This is further supported by the reduced uteroplacental blood flow, as observed occasionally[22] although not uniformly.[35,36]

Placental expression and activity of the matrix metalloproteinases MMP14 and MMP15, major proteases involved in tissue remodeling processes associated with invasion, angiogenesis, and proliferation, are elevated in Type 1 diabetes[3] induced by elevated maternal insulin and TNF-α.[28,37] MMP14 and MMP15 accept a remarkably wide spectrum of substrates, including components of the extracellular matrix.[38] In addition, mature and immature cytokines may become activated or inactivated, thus further contributing to the alterations in diabetes. In particular, the active form of placental MMP14, which is generated by cleavage by the protease furin, is elevated in diabetes. Furin contains a HIF1-α promoter binding site. This makes it tempting to hypothesize that hypoxic conditions in the villous placental structure in diabetes may be implicated as a cause of increased MMP14 activity. These results demonstrate the sensitivity of early placental development to changes in growth factor and cytokine levels. However, reduced trophoblast invasion in maternal diabetes still remains speculative.

Role of the insulin/insulin-like growth factor system and leptin

Maternal and fetal hyperleptinemia are well-established in diabetes and obesity. Both insulin and leptin fulfil pleiotropic roles beyond the regulation of metabolism, including stimulating growth factor activity and potency, which in turn stimulates expression of various target genes.[9,39] Resistance to insulin and leptin occurs often coincidentally in human obesity, because of the considerable overlap between their signaling pathways.[40] The extensive cross-talk between their signaling cascades may represent a major contributing factor to the diabetes-induced placental changes, especially in the first trimester of pregnancy.

Insulin, insulin-like growth factor 1 and 2

The insulin/insulin-like growth factor system is thought to have a central role in the control of fetal and placental growth and development.[41] The insulin receptor and the highly related IGF1 receptor essentially signal through two main intracellular pathways:[42] the extracellular signal-regulated kinase (ERK)1/2 pathway stimulating proliferation and the phosphoinositide 3-kinase (PI3K)/protein kinase B (AKT) pathway mainly modulating metabolic function.

The feto-placental expression of insulin, IGF1, IGF2, and their receptors is developmentally regulated in a tissue-specific manner and can be affected by nutritional and endocrine conditions.[41] Placental expression of insulin receptors undergoes a developmental shift from the trophoblasts in the first trimester to the placental endothelial cells in the third trimester.[9,43] The placental IGF1 receptor (IGF1R) is mainly expressed on the basal membrane of the syncytiotrophoblast. Hence, it is predominantly accessible for fetal IGF1 and IGF2.[2] The specific roles of these growth factors for the human placenta have not been investigated in great detail. Targeted disruption of the fetal *IGF1*, *IGF2* or *IGF1R* gene in mice resulted in retardation of fetal growth, whereas IGF2 overexpression enhanced fetal growth. IGF1 stimulates fetal growth dependent on the nutrient supply, whilst placental IGF2 is a key regulator of placental growth and nutrient transfer, thereby allowing enhancement of fetal growth.[41]

The effects of IGF1 and IGF2 can be attenuated or amplified by soluble IGF-binding proteins (IGFBPs) that influence their bioavailability. In humans, the most prevalent IGFBPs in fetal plasma and tissue are the IGFBPs 1–4. Fetal cord blood data suggest that these binding proteins may be dysregulated in diabetes in pregnancies.[44] A decrease in IGFBPs would result in higher bioavailability of IGFs and thus, indirectly might contribute to fetal overgrowth in diabetes.

The endocrine interaction between mother, fetus, and placenta is exemplified by the effect of maternal and fetal insulin on the placenta. Maternal insulin affects placental development[3] via receptors expressed on the microvillous membrane of the syncytiotrophoblast. In turn, the placenta affects the mother by secretion of hormones, cytokines, and metabolic waste products. For instance, maternal insulin upregulates leptin production in trophoblast cells[45] and, after secretion into the maternal circulation, leptin enhances maternal insulin resistance. Both leptin and insulin suppress secretion of placental growth hormone (PGH) in trophoblast cells.[46] PGH can cause maternal insulin resistance.[47] Thus, a reduction of PGH secretion by insulin and leptin may represent a materno-placental forward feedback mechanism, ultimately alleviating maternal insulin resistance.

Fetal insulin affects gene expression in endothelial cells from placental arteries and veins,[9] which will directly or indirectly affect placental and fetal development. The change of insulin receptor expression from the trophoblast in the first trimester to the endothelium at term thus enables maternal insulin to regulate placental function at the beginning of gestation, whereas as gestation advances, the fetus takes over control of placental insulin effects[9] (Fig. 3.3).

IGF1 and IGF2 stimulate trophoblast invasion[48] by upregulation of the metalloproteinases MMP2 and MMP9 that degrade gelatine and collagen, components of the extracellular matrix. Lower maternal IGF1 levels in Type 1 diabetes mellitus may thus contribute to impaired trophoblast invasion. Insulin and IGFs stimulate nutrient transport through the syncytiotrophoblast, in particular the transport of a broad range of neutral amino acids by upregulation of amino acid transporter system A.[49–51] Hence, in GDM, transplacental amino acid transport and thereby fetal growth may be promoted by the diabetes-associated increase in maternal concentrations of growth factors (Table 3.1).

Changes can also be seen in the fetal circulation (Table 3.2). However, the consequence of these changes for the fetus, apart from the well-known insulin-stimulated fat accretion, remains unclear.

Leptin

Leptin is a central hormone in metabolic control indirectly promoting insulin resistance.[52] In humans, leptin levels correlate highly with adiposity. However, the hormone has various functions beyond metabolic

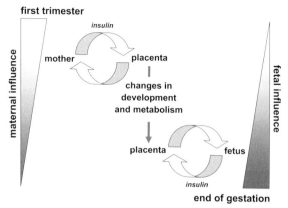

first trimester

maternal influence

insulin

mother → placenta

changes in
development
and metabolism

placenta → fetus

insulin

fetal influence

end of gestation

Fig. 3.3 Spatio-temporal change of insulin receptor expression in the placenta allows a shift in control of insulin regulation from the mother to the fetus. Insulin receptor expression shifts from the trophoblast in the first trimester to the endothelial cells in the third trimester. In the first trimester, maternal insulin influences the placenta by interaction with trophoblast insulin receptors. These may in turn affect the mother by secretion of cytokines, hormones, or metabolic waste products. Later in gestation, the fetus takes over control of insulin-dependent placental processes by fetal insulin interacting with placental endothelial cells. The effects on placental development and metabolism induced at the beginning of pregnancy by maternal insulin along with the effects of fetal insulin on the placenta later in gestation may have repercussions on fetal development and metabolism. (Reproduced from Desoye and Hauguel-de Mouzon,[6] with permission of The American Diabetes Association.)

control, such as stimulation of angiogenesis, and regulation of hematopoiesis and the inflammatory response.[53] The main source of leptin is adipose tissue, but it is also expressed in various organs of the feto-placental unit. During gestation maternal leptin concentrations rise by 30% and the placenta becomes the primary leptin source.

The predominant expression site of the leptin receptor in the placenta is the syncytiotrophoblast. Leptin induces human chorionic gonadotropin (hCG) production, enhances mitogenesis, stimulates amino acid uptake, and increases the synthesis of extracellular matrix proteins and metalloproteinases,[53] implicating a role for the hormone in the regulation of placental growth. Moreover, it might be further hypothesized that hyperleptinemia contributes to other placental changes in diabetes, e.g. basement membrane thickening, owing to its ability to alter collagen synthesis.[54] In addition, the proangiogenic effect of leptin suggests a contributing role to the diabetes-associated placental hypervascularization (see Fig. 3.2).

SUMMARY

Placental structure and function can be changed as a result of maternal diabetes. The specific nature and extent of these changes depend on the gestational period of the diabetic insult and by inference, on the type of diabetes. Some alterations[55,56] continue to occur despite improvements in maternal glycemic control over the last decades, thus indicating that hyperglycemia is not the only causal factor. However, various changes in villous morphology may improve if diabetes is well controlled.[11,57] Maternal and fetal concentrations of several growth factors, cytokines, and hormones are also altered in diabetes and may affect fetal and placental growth and development. Current research in this area is trying to identify the specific biologic effects and the detailed mechanisms underlying them.

REFERENCES

1 Aplin JD. Implantation, trophoblast differentiation and haemochorial placentation: mechanistic evidence in vivo and in vitro. *J Cell Sci* 1991;**99**:681–92.

2 Hayati AR, Cheah FC, Tan AE, Tan GC. Insulin-like growth factor-1 receptor expression in the placentae of diabetic and normal pregnancies. *Early Hum Dev* 2007;**83**:41–6.

3 Hiden U, Glitzner E, Ivanisevic M, *et al.* MT1-MMP expression in first-trimester placental tissue is upregulated in type 1 diabetes as a result of elevated insulin and tumor necrosis factor-alpha levels. *Diabetes* 2008;**57**:150–7.

4 Jansson T, Ekstrand Y, Bjorn C, Wennergren M, Powell TL. Alterations in the activity of placental amino acid transporters in pregnancies complicated by diabetes. *Diabetes* 2002;**51**:2214–9.

5 Kliman HJ. Uteroplacental blood flow. The story of decidualization, menstruation, and trophoblast invasion. *Am J Pathol* 2000;**157**:1759–68.

6 Desoye G, Hauguel-de Mouzon S. The human placenta in gestational diabetes mellitus. The insulin and cytokine network. *Diabetes Care* 2007;**30** (Suppl 2):S120–6.

7 Foufelle F, Girard J, Ferre P. Regulation of lipogenic enzyme expression by glucose in liver and adipose tissue: a review of the potential cellular and molecular mechanisms. *Adv Enzyme Regul* 1996;**36**:199–226.

8 Mandl M, Haas J, Bischof P, Nohammer G, Desoye G. Serum-dependent effects of IGF-I and insulin on proliferation and invasion of human first trimester trophoblast cell models. *Histochem Cell Biol* 2002;**117**:391–9.

9 Hiden U, Maier A, Bilban M, *et al.* Insulin control of placental gene expression shifts from mother to foetus over the course of pregnancy. *Diabetologia* 2006;**49**:123–31.

10 Younes B, Baez-Giangreco A, al-Nuaim L, al-Hakeem A, Abu Talib Z. Basement membrane thickening in the placentae from diabetic women. *Pathol Int* 1996;**46**:100–4.

11 Calderon IM, Damasceno DC, Amorin RL, Costa RA, Brasil MA, Rudge MV. Morphometric study of placental villi and vessels in women with mild hyperglycemia or gestational or overt diabetes. *Diabetes Res Clin Pract* 2007;**78**:65–71.

12 Taricco E, Radaelli T, Nobile de Santis MS, Cetin I. Foetal and placental weights in relation to maternal characteristics in gestational diabetes. *Placenta* 2003;**24**:343–7.

13 Lao TT, Lee CP, Wong WM. Placental weight to birthweight ratio is increased in mild gestational glucose intolerance. *Placenta* 1997;**18**:227–30.

14 Osmond DT, King RG, Brennecke SP, Gude NM. Placental glucose transport and utilisation is altered at term in insulin-treated, gestational-diabetic patients. *Diabetologia* 2001;**44**:1133–9.

15 Radaelli T, Taricco E, Rossi G, *et al.* Effect of gestational diabetes on fetal oxygen and glucose levels *in vivo*. *BJDG* 2009;DOI 10.1111/j.1471-0528.2009.02341.

16 Kuruvilla AG, D'Souza SW, Glazier JD, Mahendran D, Maresh MJ, Sibley CP. Altered activity of the system A amino acid transporter in microvillous membrane vesicles from placentas of macrosomic babies born to diabetic women. *J Clin Invest* 1994;**94**:689–95.

17 Mayhew TM, Sorensen FB, Klebe JG, Jackson MR. Growth and maturation of villi in placentae from well-controlled diabetic women. *Placenta* 1994;**15**:57–65.

18 Mimouni F, Miodovnik M, Siddiqi TA, Butler JB, Holroyde J, Tsang RC. Neonatal polycythemia in infants of insulin-dependent diabetic mothers. *Obstet Gynecol* 1986;**68**:370–2.

19 Madsen H, Ditzel J. Red cell 2,3-diphosphoglycerate and hemoglobin-oxygen affinity during diabetic pregnancy. *Acta Obstet Gynecol Scand* 1984;**63**:403–6.

20 al-Okail MS, al-Attas OS. Histological changes in placental syncytiotrophoblasts of poorly controlled gestational diabetic patients. *Endocr J* 1994;**41**:355–60.

21 Jirkovska M. Comparison of the thickness of the capillary basement membrane of the human placenta under normal conditions and in type 1 diabetes. *Funct Dev Morphol* 1991;**1**:9–16.

22 Nylund L, Lunell NO, Lewander R, Persson B, Sarby B. Uteroplacental blood flow in diabetic pregnancy: measurements with indium 113m and a computer-linked gamma camera. *Am J Obstet Gynecol* 1982;**144**:298–302.

23 Bracero LA, Jovanovic L, Rochelson B, Bauman W, Farmakides G. Significance of umbilical and uterine artery velocimetry in the well-controlled pregnant diabetic. *J Reprod Med* 1989;**34**:273–6.

24 Bracero LA, Schulman H. Doppler studies of the uteroplacental circulation in pregnancies complicated by diabetes. *Ultrasound Obstet Gynecol* 1991;**1**:391–4.

25 Black SM, Devol JM, Wedgwood S. Regulation of fibroblast growth factor-2 expression in pulmonary arterial smooth muscle cells involves increased reactive oxygen species generation. *Am J Physiol Cell Physiol* 2008;**294**:C345–54.

26 Grosfeld A, Andre J, Hauguel-De Mouzon S, Berra E, Pouyssegur J, Guerre-Millo M. Hypoxia-inducible factor 1 transactivates the human leptin gene promoter. *J Biol Chem* 2002;**277**:42953–7.

27 Josko J, Mazurek M. Transcription factors having impact on vascular endothelial growth factor (VEGF) gene expression in angiogenesis. *Med Sci Monit* 2004;**10**:RA89–98.

28 Abdel Aziz MT, Fouad HH, Mohsen GA, Mansour M, Abdel Ghaffar S. TNF-alpha and homocysteine levels in type 1 diabetes mellitus. *East Mediterr Health J* 2001;**7**:679–88.

29 Bhaumick B, Danilkewich AD, Bala RM. Insulin-like growth factors (IGF) I and II in diabetic pregnancy: suppression of normal pregnancy-induced rise of IGF-I. *Diabetologia* 1986;**29**:792–7.

30 Lygnos MC, Pappa KI, Papadaki HA, *et al.* Changes in maternal plasma levels of VEGF, bFGF, TGF-beta1, ET-1 and sKL during uncomplicated pregnancy, hypertensive pregnancy and gestational diabetes. *In Vivo* 2006;**20**:157–63.

31 Brown ZA, Mills JL, Metzger BE, *et al.* Early sonographic evaluation for fetal growth delay and congenital malformations in pregnancies complicated by insulin-requiring diabetes. National Institute of Child Health and Human Development Diabetes in Early Pregnancy Study. *Diabetes Care* 1992;**15**:613–9.

32 Weiss U, Cervar M, Puerstner P, *et al.* Hyperglycaemia in vitro alters the proliferation and mitochondrial activity of the choriocarcinoma cell lines BeWo, JAR and JEG-3 as models for human first-trimester trophoblast. *Diabetologia* 2001;**44**:209–19.

33 Galindo A, Burguillo AG, Azriel S, Fuente Pde L. Outcome of fetuses in women with pregestational diabetes mellitus. *J Perinat Med* 2006;**34**:323–31.

34 Desoye G, Shafrir E. The human placenta in diabetic pregnancy. *Diabetes Rev* 1996;**4**:70–89.

35 Salvesen DR, Higueras MT, Mansur CA, Freeman J, Brudenell JM, Nicolaides KH. Placental and fetal Doppler velocimetry in pregnancies complicated by maternal diabetes mellitus. *Am J Obstet Gynecol* 1993;**168**:645–52.

36 Johnstone FD, Steel JM, Haddad NG, Hoskins PR, Greer IA, Chambers S. Doppler umbilical artery flow velocity waveforms in diabetic pregnancy. *Br J Obstet Gynaecol* 1992;**99**:135–40.

37 Desoye G, Hofmann HH, Weiss PA. Insulin binding to trophoblast plasma membranes and placental glycogen content in well-controlled gestational diabetic women treated with diet or insulin, in well-controlled overt diabetic patients and in healthy control subjects. *Diabetologia* 1992;**35**:45–55.

38 d'Ortho MP, Will H, Atkinson S, *et al.* Membrane-type matrix metalloproteinases 1 and 2 exhibit broad-spectrum proteolytic capacities comparable to many matrix metalloproteinases. *Eur J Biochem* 1997;**250**:751–7.

39 Taleb S, Van Haaften R, Henegar C, *et al.* Microarray profiling of human white adipose tissue after exogenous leptin injection. *Eur J Clin Invest* 2006;**36**:153–63.

40 Myers MG, Jr. Leptin receptor signaling and the regulation of mammalian physiology. *Recent Prog Horm Res* 2004;**59**: 287–304.

41 Gicquel C, Le Bouc Y. Hormonal regulation of fetal growth. *Horm Res* 2006;**65** (Suppl 3):28–33.

42 Pirola L, Johnston AM, Van Obberghen E. Modulation of insulin action. *Diabetologia* 2004;**47**:170–84.

43 Desoye G, Hartmann M, Jones CJ, *et al.* Location of insulin receptors in the placenta and its progenitor tissues. *Microsc Res Tech* 1997;**38**:63–75.

44 Yan-Jun L, Tsushima T, Minei S, *et al.* Insulin-like growth factors (IGFs) and IGF-binding proteins (IGFBP-1, -2 and -3) in diabetic pregnancy: relationship to macrosomia. *Endocr J* 1996;**43**:221–31.

45 Coya R, Gualillo O, Pineda J, *et al.* Effect of cyclic 3',5'-adenosine monophosphate, glucocorticoids, and insulin on leptin messenger RNA levels and leptin secretion in cultured human trophoblast. *Biol Reprod* 2001;**65**:814–9.

46 Zeck W, Widberg C, Maylin E, *et al.* Regulation of placental growth hormone secretion in a human trophoblast model – the effects of hormones and adipokines. *Pediatr Res* 2008;**63**:353–7.

47 Barbour LA, Shao J, Qiao L, *et al.* Human placental growth hormone causes severe insulin resistance in transgenic mice. *Am J Obstet Gynecol* 2002;**186**:512–7.

48 Chakraborty C, Gleeson LM, McKinnon T, Lala PK. Regulation of human trophoblast migration and invasiveness. *Can J Physiol Pharmacol* 2002;**80**:116–24.

49 Constancia M, Hemberger M, Hughes J, *et al.* Placental-specific IGF-II is a major modulator of placental and fetal growth. *Nature* 2002;**417**:945–8.

50 Karl PI. Insulin-like growth factor-1 stimulates amino acid uptake by the cultured human placental trophoblast. *J Cell Physiol* 1995;**165**:83–8.

51 Karl PI, Alpy KL, Fisher SE. Amino acid transport by the cultured human placental trophoblast: effect of insulin on AIB transport. *Am J Physiol* 1992;**262**:C834–9.

52 Webber J. Energy balance in obesity. *Proc Nutr Soc* 2003;**62**:539–43.

53 Hauguel-de Mouzon S, Lepercq J, Catalano P. The known and unknown of leptin in pregnancy. *Am J Obstet Gynecol* 2006;**194**:1537–45.

54 Madani S, De Girolamo S, Munoz DM, Li RK, Sweeney G. Direct effects of leptin on size and extracellular matrix components of human pediatric ventricular myocytes. *Cardiovasc Res* 2006;**69**:716–25.

55 Evers IM, de Valk HW, Mol BW, ter Braak EW, Visser GH. Macrosomia despite good glycaemic control in Type I diabetic pregnancy; results of a nationwide study in The Netherlands. *Diabetologia* 2002;**45**:1484–9.

56 Pietryga M, Brazert J, Wender-Ozegowska E, Dubiel M, Gudmundsson S. Placental Doppler velocimetry in gestational diabetes mellitus. *J Perinat Med* 2006;**34**:108–10.

57 Mayhew TM, Jairam IC. Stereological comparison of 3D spatial relationships involving villi and intervillous pores in human placentas from control and diabetic pregnancies. *J Anat* 2000;**197**:263–74.

58 Gelato MC, Rutherford C, San-Roman G, Shmoys S, Monheit A. The serum insulin-like growth factor-II/mannose-6-phosphate receptor in normal and diabetic pregnancy. *Metabolism* 1993;**42**:1031–8.

59 Ategbo JM, Grissa O, Yessoufou A, *et al.* Modulation of adipokines and cytokines in gestational diabetes and macrosomia. *J Clin Endocrinol Metab* 2006;**91**:4137–43.

60 Vitoratos N, Salamalekis E, Kassanos D, *et al.* Maternal plasma leptin levels and their relationship to insulin and glucose in gestational-onset diabetes. *Gynecol Obstet Invest* 2001;**51**:17–21.

61 Hughes SC, Johnson MR, Heinrich G, Holly JM. Could abnormalities in insulin-like growth factors and their binding proteins during pregnancy result in gestational diabetes? *J Endocrinol* 1995;**147**:517–24.

62 Homko C, Sivan E, Chen X, Reece EA, Boden G. Insulin secretion during and after pregnancy in patients with gestational diabetes mellitus. *J Clin Endocrinol Metab* 2001;**86**:568–73.

63 Loukovaara M, Leinonen P, Teramo K, Andersson S. Concentration of cord serum placenta growth factor in normal and diabetic pregnancies. *BJOG* 2005;**112**:75–9.

64 Lea RG, Howe D, Hannah LT, Bonneau O, Hunter L, Hoggard N. Placental leptin in normal, diabetic and fetal growth-retarded pregnancies. *Mol Hum Reprod* 2000;**6**: 763–9.

65 Salvesen DR, Brudenell JM, Snijders RJ, Ireland RM, Nicolaides KH. Fetal plasma erythropoietin in pregnancies complicated by maternal diabetes mellitus. *Am J Obstet Gynecol* 1993;**168**(1 Pt 1):88–94.

66 Westgate JA, Lindsay RS, Beattie J, *et al.* Hyperinsulinemia in cord blood in mothers with type 2 diabetes and gestational diabetes mellitus in New Zealand. *Diabetes Care* 2006;**29**:1345–50.

67 Lassus P, Teramo K, Nupponen I, Markkanen H, Cederqvist K, Andersson S. Vascular endothelial growth factor and angiogenin levels during fetal development and in maternal diabetes. *Biol Neonate* 2003;**84**:287–92.

68 Hill DJ, Tevaarwerk GJ, Caddell C, Arany E, Kilkenny D, Gregory M. Fibroblast growth factor 2 is elevated in term maternal and cord serum and amniotic fluid in pregnancies complicated by diabetes: relationship to fetal and placental size. *J Clin Endocrinol Metab* 1995;**80**: 2626–32.

69 Teramo K, Kari MA, Eronen M, Markkanen H, Hiilesmaa V. High amniotic fluid erythropoietin levels are associated with an increased frequency of fetal and neonatal morbidity in type 1 diabetic pregnancies. *Diabetologia* 2004;**47**:1695–703.

Section 2

Impaired glucose tolerance and gestational diabetes

4 Historical context of hyperglycemia in pregnancy

David R. Hadden

Regional Endocrinology and Diabetes Centre, Royal Victoria Hospital, Belfast, Northern Ireland, UK

PRACTICE POINTS

- Historical concepts reveal the roots of today's practice.
- Diabetes as a clinical disorder has a very long history.
- It is less than 200 years since the first recorded case of pregnancy in a mother with diabetes. The prognosis then was very poor.
- One hundred years later the first case where insulin was used had a successful outcome.
- Gestational diabetes is still a concept under investigation – its roots go back to the first recorded case.

A chapter on historical concepts needs a date to set the scene. Diabetes has a very ancient bibliography, going back to the Egyptian Ebers papyrus in 1500 BC, with subsequent references in Greek by Hippocrates and Aristotle, updated by the Arabian physician Avicenna, as well as independent observations in early Hindu, Chinese, and Japanese manuscripts. Written records of human pregnancy are older still. So it is perhaps strange that the first reference to diabetes in pregnancy is as recent as 1824. The story of that patient with gestational diabetes, and her problems in delivering a stillborn 12 lb baby, was well recorded by Dr Heinrich Bennewitz in Berlin.[1] The only possible treatment was venesection, rest, and some indefinite food supplements.

In 1882 Dr J. Matthews Duncan (Fig. 4.1), then at St Bartholomew's Hospital London, emphasized the very poor outlook for both mother and fetus[2]. He summarized reports of 22 pregnancies in 15 diabetic mothers – half of the mothers and half of their babies were dead at or soon after delivery. In the USA by 1909 things were marginally more optimistic. Dr J. Whitridge Williams, Professor of Obstetrics at the recently built Johns Hopkins Hospital

in Baltimore, was concerned to emphasize that the prognosis was "not always so alarming as is frequently stated". He had made a study of the several types of glycosuria found in pregnancy, and carried out what may have been the first prospective screening program for what has become known as gestational diabetes. Although this was largely dependent on simple urine tests for reducing substances, he actually found a few cases of true glucosuria in a sample of 167 cases found to have "sugar" in their urine during their pregnancy.[3]

Dr Eliot Joslin practiced in Boston both before and after the discovery of insulin, and his textbook in its continuing editions is a demonstration of the enormous advance which insulin treatment offered. By 1915 he had treated only seven cases of diabetes and pregnancy, and only three of these mothers were still alive.[4] The subsequent legacies of several well-remembered clinicians to the historical development of present day care of the diabetic woman in pregnancy have been well summarized by their colleagues.[5-7]

One hundred years after the publication of the report by Bennewitz, another seminal publication recorded one of the first diabetic pregnancies successfully managed with insulin, which had just been discovered in 1923 by Banting and Best,[8] and was rapidly made available for clinical use. Dr George Graham (Fig. 4.2), also of St Bartholomew's Hospital (Fig. 4.3), presented his report to the Royal Society of Medicine in London in 1924, and it is worth reproducing in full as a focus for discussion on many aspects of clinical care which are still relevant over 80 years later.[9] The first case reported from the USA at the same time was on the use of insulin in diabetic coma complicating pregnancy.[10]

"The outlook of a patient with true diabetes mellitus complicating pregnancy has always been considered as being very unfavourable. Whitridge Williams reports the results of sixty-six cases; 27 per cent of the women either died at the time of labour or within two weeks of it, and 23 per cent in the next two years.

A Practical Manual of Diabetes in Pregnancy, 1st Edition.
Edited by David R. McCance, Michael Maresh and David A. Sacks.
© 2010 Blackwell Publishing

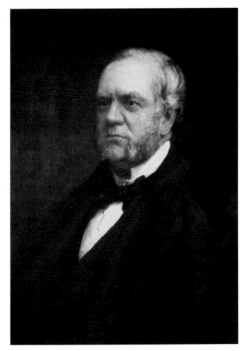

Fig. 4.1 Dr James Matthews Duncan: 1826–1890. MD Aberdeen; Physician for Diseases of Women, Royal Infirmary of Edinburgh; subsequently Professor of Midwifery, St Bartholomew's Hospital, London. (Reproduced with permission of the Royal College of Physicians of Edinburgh.)

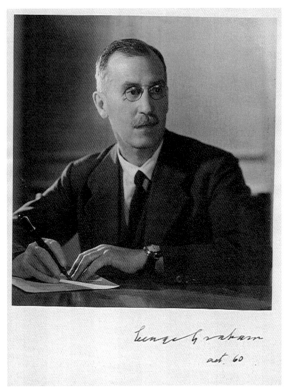

Fig. 4.2 Dr George Graham: 1882–1971. Consulting Physician, St Bartholomew's Hospital, London. He was one of the early physician biochemists, and the first to describe renal glycosuria. He was the last important UK link with the preinsulin era, remembered for his "ladder diet" of gradually increasing carbohydrate intake. (Reproduced with permission of St Bartholomew's Hospital Archives.)

Of the children, 12 per cent were born dead as the result of abortion, and of those which came to term, 33 per cent were born dead.

It is impossible to say how many of the women really had true diabetes mellitus in a severe form, as the data are lacking, but it is fairly certain that the outlook of the diabetic patient who becomes pregnant is a bad one. The introduction of insulin in the treatment of diabetes has altered the prospects of the diabetic patient, and it is important to consider how much the outlook of the pregnant woman has been altered. I have had the opportunity of watching one woman who had been treated with insulin before conception and has given birth to a healthy child.

The patient, aged 34, had already had one child. She was quite well until she had a sudden onset of thirst, and became very irritable, in October 1922. The sugar was discovered by Dr Philps about fourteen days after the onset of the symptoms. She was dieted by removal of the carbohydrates of the diet, but not very drastically, and she also did not adhere closely to the prescribed diet. I first saw her with Dr Philps in June 1923, as she had become very thin and weak. She then looked ill, and had obviously lost a great deal of weight. She was very constipated, and the abdomen was moving rather deeply with respiration, as

though she was approaching coma. The knee-jerks were active, and there was no other sign of disease. The urine contained a great deal of sugar ,and gave a brisk reaction for aceto-acetic acid. The blood sugar was not estimated then, as the diagnosis was not in doubt."

This patient must have been one of the very first to have been treated with insulin in London, in June 1923. Although aged 34, the presence of aceto-acetic acid in the urine (identified by the old ferric perchloride test, which was less sensitive but easier than the nitroprusside test for acetone), and extreme weight loss in spite of poor dietary adherence indicate what we now term Type 1 diabetes. Dr Graham continued to use the severe dietary restriction which was all that was possible before insulin – his 1350 calorie diet, giving 5% energy as carbohydrate and 78% as fat, would not please present day dietitians, but

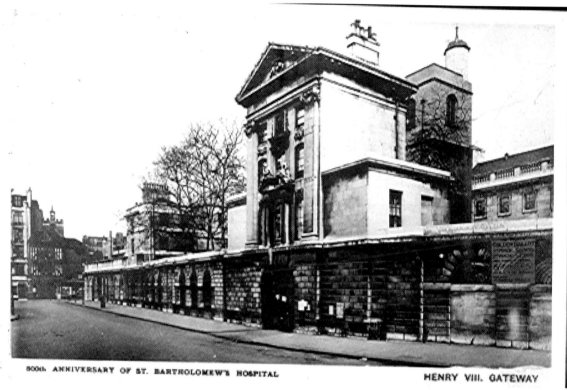

800th ANNIVERSARY OF ST. BARTHOLOMEW'S HOSPITAL

HENRY VIII. GATEWAY

Fig. 4.3 St Bartholomew's Hospital, London. The King Henry VIII gateway. (Reproduced with permission of St Bartholomew's Hospital Archives.)

it certainly worked in the short term. After 2 months he allowed a very cautious increase to 1500 calories. The small dose of insulin by present day standards (10 U short-acting insulin once a day) clearly improved her general health and strength, but the energy restriction may have been of more benefit in achieving his aim of "resting" the islets of Langerhans – there has been some renewal of interest in this concept recently.

"She was treated drastically with two starvation days, and five units of insulin on the first day. The urine was sugar-free after the second day, and the diet was gradually increased up to: protein 57 grm, fat 118 grm, sugar 16 grm, caloric value 1,360; calories per kilo 30. The blood sugar one week later was 0.11 per cent [6.1 mmol/L; 110 mg/dL], and insulin administration, 10 units, was begun on the tenth day in order to give the islets of Langerhans as little work to do as possible. She improved greatly in health and strength during the next eight weeks while she was in bed, and gained 1 lb in weight in spite of the low caloric value of the diet. The blood sugar remained between 0.1 per cent [5.5 mmol/l; 100 mg/dL] and 0.12 per cent [6.6 mmol/L, 120 mg/dL], and the diet was increased to protein 70 grm, fat 126 grm, sugar 21 grm, calories 1500 on August 29."

Although she was "in bed" for the first 8 weeks of insulin treatment – probably at home rather than in hospital – this did not interfere with conception, which must have occurred very soon after starting the new drug. There would not have been any package insert or National Institute for Health and Clinical Excellence (NICE) guideline regarding the unknown effects of this new therapy on pregnancy, but doctor, patient, and husband must all have been pleased with the outcome.

"Sometime about the third week after the insulin treatment was begun the patient became pregnant in spite of precautions. On August 29, 1923, she had missed two menstrual periods, but she seemed very well, and the blood sugar was normal. I regret now that I did not test out her sugar tolerance with a dose of 50 grm of dextrose for the sake of comparison with her present condition and with that of other patients. Until December 10, 1923, she kept very well, and was then six months pregnant, and was 9 lb heavier than in August. There did not seem any indication to interfere, especially as the parents wished for another child. Unfortunately she was developing a severe coryza that afternoon, and the blood sugar was 0.19 per cent [10.6 mmol/L; 190 mg/dL]. She was told to stay in bed, and to increase the dose

of insulin so long as she was ill, but for various domestic reasons she did not do so. The illness, which was perhaps influenza, made her quite ill, and by January 4, 1924, she had lost a good deal of weight and felt very weak. The blood sugar was 0.24 per cent [13.3 mmol/L; 240 mg/dL] although she had had 15 units of insulin six hours before the blood was collected."

As so often happens, the pregnancy may have been unplanned from Dr Graham's point of view, but the patient and her husband were clearly happy in spite of the medical opinion. When he saw her at 6 months of gestation she was developing some form of infection – this was not long after the severe pandemic of influenza throughout Europe, and he advised bed rest. But it was Christmas time, and she kept going somehow, but lost weight and became "quite ill". Infection was the main cause of uncontrolled ketoacidosis in those early days of insulin therapy – we would increase the insulin dose more today, even if we still do not have effective antiviral chemotherapy.

"*The question of terminating the pregnancy was considered in consultation with Dr. P. R. Bolus and Dr F. G. K. Philps, but it was decided not to do anything at that time as it was thought too dangerous while the diabetes was so severe. She was therefore kept in bed on a much reduced diet, and the insulin was increased to 15 units in the morning and 5 at night. On this regime she ceased to pass sugar in the urine, but the fasting blood sugar was 0.2 per cent [11.1 mmol/L; 200 mg/dL) on January 12. On January 26 the blood sugar had fallen to 0.14 per cent [7.7 mmol/L; 140 mg/dL], and the dose of insulin was reduced to 10 units in the morning and 5 at night. The diet was kept constant at protein 57 grm, fat 117 grm, sugar 16 grm, caloric value 1,360. This is the same diet she was having in July 1923, and at that time she was only having 10 units of insulin in the day and the blood sugar was normal. The insulin requirements of the patient had therefore increased by 5 units, but whether this was the result of the pregnancy or only of the influenza from which she was suffering cannot be stated with any certainty. As she was feeling better but still weak the diet was increased to protein 74 grm, fat 138 grm, sugar 23 grm, caloric value 1,600.*"

Termination of the pregnancy at 7 months was a drastic option, and his two colleagues must have been as optimistic about the pregnancy as they were afraid of the diabetes and the dreaded ketoacidosis. Cesarean section, or even premature delivery, was not possible, especially in an uncontrolled diabetic patient. Most of the maternal deaths in diabetes in pregnancy were due to the diabetes rather than obstetric problems. The small increase in the insulin dose was probably sufficient in view of the severely restricted food intake. Perhaps the nutritional deficiency helped to prevent fetal macrosomia in the last weeks of pregnancy.

"*Labour began on March 3, 1924, and was conducted by Dr Bolus. Scopolamine and morphia were given, and the labour terminated very easily. The child was quite healthy, and the patient was not unduly disturbed. During the first 10 days of the puerperium the diet was increased by 40 oz of milk, and 15 extra units of insulin were given to look after the extra sugar – protein 114 grm, fat 174 grm, sugar 65 grm, caloric value 2,250. The extra sugar was given with the object of having more sugar in the body in a form in which it could be used, so that the patient might be able to deal with any minor septic complications which might arise. Fortunately there were no complications at all.*"

Fortune favours the brave, and all went well. He made no further comment on the baby, who was presumably of normal size and appearance. With the small doses of insulin there was little risk of hypoglycemia, which does not seem to have become a problem in diabetes in pregnancy for many years, until the desire for totally normal blood glucose as well as normal food intake necessitated more insulin. Various forms of long-acting insulins have probably exacerbated the tendency to hypoglycemia, both in early gestation and postpartum.

"*The increase in the sugar caused her to excrete sugar again, as the insulin was not quite sufficient, but it was thought better to allow her to excrete sugar for a few days than to run any risk of overdosage, as the insulin requirements might have been much less as the result of the termination of the pregnancy. On the tenth day the milk was reduced to 4 oz and the insulin to 18 units in the morning and 8 units at night. She made a good recovery and has felt very well and much stronger. On March 26, 1924, the blood sugar was 0.2 per cent [11.1 mmol/L; 200 mg/dL], although she was not passing any sugar, and as it was still at this figure on April 5, the milk was stopped altogether and the insulin increased by another 2 units to 28 units.*"

The concept of allowing rather higher blood glucose immediately post delivery would still find favor today. It is not clear if the baby was breastfed, but this was probable in those days, at least initially. We would all like to know what happened in the future – this baby could now be 94 years old.

"*On reviewing the case it is clear that the sugar tolerance has diminished considerably during the past ten months, but whether this is due to the pregnancy or to the influenza it is impossible to say. The prognosis in any case of true diabetes mellitus is affected in various ways, and one of the most serious is the incidence of infections of any kind. If, therefore, a diabetic woman becomes pregnant, it seems probable that she will be liable to many more dangers than before, even if the strain of the pregnancy does not cause any ill effects. The special danger is that of sepsis during parturition, as the patient's resistance to this will probably be very small. Although the present case shows that a pregnancy can be carried through successfully on a diet of low caloric value with the help of insulin, it seems to me that the patient runs a grave risk of the diabetes being made considerably worse."*

Doctors are always inclined to dwell on the risks – his fear of long-term exacerbation of diabetes by pregnancy has not been confirmed. The reduction of the risk of infection may have been just as important as the use of insulin.

HISTORICAL ASPECTS OF DIABETES IN PREGNANCY

The most comprehensive assessment of the historical publications on diabetes and pregnancy is by Mestman, an endocrinologist and obstetric physician who has worked in Southern California since 1960.[11] Following the paper by Matthews Duncan in 1882,[2] Mestman indicates the major change which followed was the introduction of insulin, allowing a woman with diabetes to carry a full-term pregnancy and deliver a healthy infant. He documents the dramatic reduction in maternal mortality, and the more modest improvement in perinatal mortality and morbidity. It was not until the recognition of the need for a team approach, from obstetrician, diabetologist, and pediatrician, that the fetal outcome improved.[12] The gradual introduction of obstetric (or maternal/fetal medicine) tests to assess placental function,[13] fetal well-being,[14] and fetal lung maturity[15] resulted in the reduction of three of the causes of fetal loss – sudden intrauterine death, neonatal death, and birth trauma due to macrosomia. Not all of these tests have stood the test of time, but the academic interest which they generated was largely responsible for the recognition of diabetes in pregnancy as a high-risk process, requiring special supervision not available except in centers of excellence. This left congenital fetal abnormalities as the residual problem, even in these centers. Basic animal and human research then showed that poor glycemic control at the time of conception and soon after was a major cause of both congenital abnormalities and spontaneous abortion.[16] However, the provision of this degree of detailed care for all diabetic mothers at a community level has been more difficult to achieve, and a number of national surveys have shown deficiencies in many aspects of this healthcare provision.[17]

Definition of gestational diabetes

Another reason for differing results has been the actual definition of "gestational diabetes mellitus" that has been adopted. The early reports concentrated on a specific pregnancy-induced problem, which was assumed not to have been present before, and shown not to be present after the pregnancy. The most controversial topic in the early days was the significance of the finding of sugars of various types in the urine, and the role of this finding in the diagnosis of asymptomatic diabetes. J. W. Williams in Baltimore, USA came to a number of conclusions in a review of the literature up to 1909.[3] His own studies showed that between 1 and 3 g/L of sugar in the urine was most likely physiologic, but more than this suggested diabetes, particularly early in pregnancy or if symptoms were present. In 1926 Lambie in Edinburgh reviewed the problems associated with glycosuria and acetonuria in pregnancy, and discussed the details of a 50-g oral glucose tolerance test with calculations of what he termed the ketogenic–antiketogenic balance.[18] Perhaps the earliest report of glucose "intolerance" in pregnancy, quoted by Lambie, was in the thesis in Paris by Brocard in 1898, who found glycosuria 2 hours after ingesting 50 g of glucose in 50% of pregnant compared to 11% of non-pregnant women. Ten years after the discovery of insulin, a complete literature review was published by Eric Skipper of 136 pregnancies in 118 diabetic women, and of a further 37 under his own care at the London Hospital.[19] Among other important observations, he drew attention to the high fetal mortality (39%) in women where the apparent onset of the diabetes was during the pregnancy, almost as high as that with onset before pregnancy (46%). Priscilla White in 1949 (Fig. 4.4) summarized her long experience at the Joslin Clinic in Boston in a classic paper which established what became known as the "White Classification".[20] White class A indicated women with "a glucose tolerance test which deviates but slightly from the normal" either before or during the pregnancy, who were treated with diet alone, and was never synonymous with gestational diabetes, which was uncommon in the established diabetic population of the Joslin Clinic. Subsequently, J. W. Hare revised the classification to separate gestational diabetes from the alphabetic list,[5] but the overall classification has now outlived its usefulness.

Screening for hyperglycemia in pregnancy

Gradually antenatal screening for unrecognized hyperglycemia in pregnancy became established, although without an unequivocal evidence base, and the screening processes used were different in different countries.[21,22] In historical terms, different screening and diagnostic

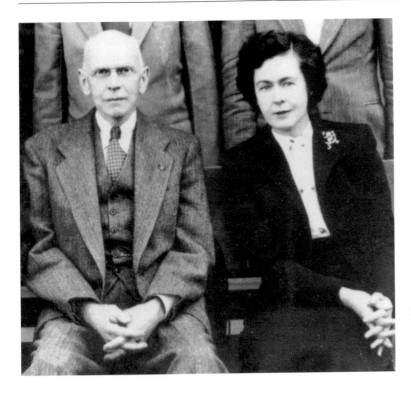

Fig. 4.4 Dr Priscilla White, with Dr Eliot Joslin, at the Joslin Clinic, Boston. (Reproduced with permission from the Joslin Archives, Joslin Diabetes Center, Boston, USA.)

procedures, even within the same country, as well as the increasing incidence of diabetes in the background populations and the rapidly altering demographic trends in human reproduction, have resulted in considerable variation in the reported prevalence. In Scandinavia the outcome of pregnancy in indigenous women has for many years been better than in other parts of Europe, and these differences are also seen in the diabetic populations. The increasing prevalence of obesity and the immigration of women from ethnically different populations have altered these findings, and recent studies are more similar to the North American experience.

Following major studies in Boston[23] and Philadelphia,[24] it became necessary for the obstetrician to identify these mildly hyperglycemic mothers during the antenatal period without knowledge of their prepregnancy glycemic status, and follow-up after delivery was only rarely attempted. A number of International Colloquia on Carbohydrate Metabolism in Pregnancy (four held in Aberdeen, Scotland between 1973 and 1988) failed to reach a transatlantic or worldwide consensus on what dose of glucose to use, how to give it, or when to measure blood glucose subsequently to test for hyperglycemia during pregnancy,[25] and it was not until the first of five Work-

shop-Conferences on Gestational Diabetes, which have been held in Chicago, USA, that the definition "carbohydrate intolerance of variable severity recognized for the first time in pregnancy" was adopted by most centers.[26] This allowed a definite subgroup of women to be identified at 28 weeks of gestation, and many outcome studies on such selected populations have been published.

The use of the term "intolerance" has concentrated both clinicians and researchers on the need for a glucose tolerance test. This perceived need to test intolerance persists in the 50-g, 1-hour screening test, which became established in the USA following the O'Sullivan papers.[27] However, there has always been a concept that fasting (or basal) hyperglycemia might be a better indicator of the disorder of diabetes mellitus than a post-glucose measurement, but in pregnancy this is confounded by the very definite fall in fasting glucose values which occurs early in the gestation and continues until late in the third trimester. So, a definition that used the fasting value might identify a different population from that using a post-glucose value – especially if the fasting value was compared to a non-pregnant baseline. This was the problem produced by the World Health Organization (WHO) definition of gestational diabetes (which was

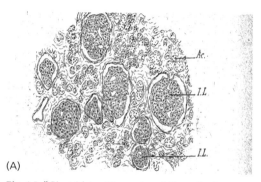

(A)

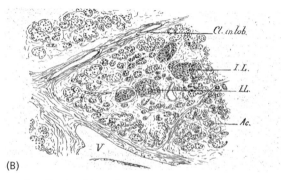

(B)

Fig. 4.5 "Giant islets of Langerhans". From the first report of the fetal islet response to maternal hyperglycaemia. (A) Pancreas of the newborn, delivered form a glycosuric

mother. IL, giant islets of Langerhans; Ac, pancreatic acini. (B) Pancreas of a normal newborn. Cl inlob, interlobular septum. (Reproduced from Dubreuil and Anderodias[32].)

pronounced by a committee which did not include an obstetrician, and assumed that non-pregnant values for hyperglycemia, both fasting and post glucose, would be those deleterious to both mother and fetus).[28]

With continuing confusion as to whether fasting or post-glucose results, or both, or any two of three which might or might not include a fasting value, the stage was set for much difficulty in reaching an international consensus or comparing results. This was best shown by the large Brazilian screening study, where concordance was poor between pregnancies identified by the WHO criteria and the adjusted Carpenter and Coustan modified O'Sullivan criteria.[29,30] The publication of the Hyperglycemia and Adverse Pregnancy Outcome (HAPO) study and the subsequent consensus conference in 2008 will allow worldwide agreement and recognition of the actual level of risk for the major outcome problems related to milder degrees of hyperglycemia.[31] Hopefully, confusion and disagreement will be relegated to the history books, and appropriate preventive measures and treatment where necessary will follow.

Stillborn infant of a glycosuric mother

There has been an interest in the histologic appearance of the islets of Langerhans in the pancreas of the infant of a diabetic mother from an early time in this field. In 1920 Dubreuil and Anderodias described strikingly large islets in a stillborn child of a glycosuric mother (Fig. 4.5), which was later confirmed by other investigators.[32] By 1938 Brandstrup and Okels in Copenhagen were able to assume that this represented fetal hyperproduction of insulin; they postulated that this might assist the mother, but could be fatal to the child by production of hypogly-

cemia.[33] The more precise definition of what is now known as the Pedersen hypothesis[34] has its roots in these earlier observations. Retrospective chart studies of birthweights of infants born to mothers who subsequently became diabetic followed these pathologic investigations, and the concept of a prediabetic period was established.[35,36] Although not all workers agreed with this concept,[37] the high prediabetic perinatal mortality rate remained an obstetric challenge,[38] which led to the concept of hyperglycemia in pregnancy or gestational diabetes as we understand it today.

CONCLUSIONS

Nearly 200 years after the first recorded pregnancy in a diabetic mother, and over 80 years since the first successful pregnancy where insulin was used, it is still interesting to revisit some of the original papers describing the failures and more recently the successes of the pioneers in this field. Whether the authors considered the pregnancy was complicating the diabetes or *vice versa* depended on whether they were diabetologists or obstetricians; eventually it became clear that both needed to work together. These authors were working with much less understanding of what was going on from a physiologic point of view, and without the therapeutic guidelines and evidence base we are now accustomed to, but the data which they recorded remain the basis of our practice today.

REFERENCES

1 Bennewitz HG. *De Diabete Mellito, Gravidatatis Symptomate.* MD Thesis, University of Berlin, 1824.

2 Duncan JM. On puerperal diabetes. *Trans Obstet Soc London* 1882;**24**:256–85.

3 Williams JW. The clinical significance of glycosuria in pregnant women. *Am J Med Sci* 1909;**137**:1–26.

4 Joslin EP. Pregnancy and diabetes mellitus. *Boston Med Surg J* 1915;**173**:841–9.

5 Hare JW. The Priscilla White legacy. In: Hod M, Jovanovic L, Di Renzo GC, de Lieva A, Langer O (eds). *Textbook of Diabetes and Pregnancy*. London: Martin Dunitz, 2003: 13–22.

6 Molsted-Pedersen L. The Pedersen legacy. In: Hod M, Jovanovic L, Di Renzo GC, de Lieva A, Langer O (eds). *Textbook of Diabetes and Pregnancy*. London: Martin Dunitz, 2003:23–9.

7 Metzger BE. The Freinkel legacy. In: Hod M, Jovanovic L, Di Renzo GC, de Lieva A, Langer O (eds). *Textbook of Diabetes and Pregnancy*. London: Martin Dunitz, 2003: 30–8.

8 Banting FG, Best CH. The internal secretion of the pancreas. *J Lab Clin Med* 1922;**7**:256–71.

9 Graham G. A case of diabetes mellitus complicated by pregnancy, treated with insulin. *Proc R Soc Med* 1923–4; **17**:102–4.

10 Reveno WS. Insulin in diabetic coma complicating pregnancy. *JAMA* 1923;**81**:2101–2.

11 Mestman JH. Historical notes on diabetes and pregnancy. *Endocrinologist* 2002;**12**:224–242.

12 Harley JMG, Montgomery DAD. Management of pregnancy complicated by diabetes. *Br Med J* 1965;**i**:14–16.

13 Rivlin MR, Mestman JH, Hall TD, *et al.* Value of estriol estimations in the management of diabetic pregnancy. *Am J Obstet Gynecol* 1970;**106**:875–84.

14 Manning F, Platt L, Sipos L. Antepartum fetal evaluation: Development of a fetal biophysical profile. *Am J Obstet Gynecol* 1980;**136**:878.

15 Bhagwanani SG, Fahmy D, Turnbull AC. Prediction of neonatal respiratory distress by estimation of amniotic fluid lecithin. *Lancet* 1972;**i**:159–62.

16 Eriksson UJ. Congenital malformations in diabetic animal models: a review. *Diabetes Res* 1984;**1**:57–66.

17 Confidential Enquiry into Maternal and Child Health. Pregnancy in women with Type 1 and Type 2 diabetes in 2002–2003; England, Wales and Northern Ireland. London: CEMACH, 2005:38.

18 Lambie CG. Diabetes and pregnancy – Part 1; Glycosuria and acetonuria in pregnancy and the puerperium. *J Obstet Gynecol Br Emp* 1926;**33**:564–81.

19 Skipper E. Diabetes mellitus and pregnancy. A clinical and analytical study, with special observations upon thirty-three cases. *QJM* 1933;**2**:353–80.

20 White P. Pregnancy complicating diabetes. *Am J Med* 1949;**5**:609–16.

21 Hadden DR. Screening for abnormalities of carbohydrate metabolism in pregnancy 1966–1977: the Belfast experience. *Diabetes Care* 1980;**3**:440–6.

22 Roberts RN, Moohan JM, Foo RLK, Harley JMG, Traub AI, Hadden DR. Fetal outcome in mothers with impaired glucose tolerance in pregnancy. *Diabetic Med* 1993;**10**: 438–43.

23 Wilkerson HLC, Remein QR. Studies of abnormal carbohydrate metabolism during pregnancy. *Diabetes* 1957;**6**: 324–9.

24 Carrington ER, Shuman CR, Reardon HS. Evaluation of the prediabetic state during pregnancy. *Obstet Gynecol* 1957;**9**:664–9.

25 Hadden DR. Glucose tolerance tests in pregnancy. In: Sutherland HW, Stowers JM (eds). *Carbohydrate Metabolism in Pregnancy and the Newborn*. Edinburgh: Churchill Livingstone, 1975:19–41.

26 Hadden DR. Geographic, ethnic and racial variations in the incidence of gestational diabetes. *Diabetes* 1985;**34** (Suppl 2):8–12.

27 O'Sullivan JB. Gestational diabetes. Unsuspected, asymptomatic diabetes in pregnancy. *N Engl J Med* 1961;**264**: 1082–5.

28 World Health Organization Expert Committee on Diabetes Mellitus. *Technical Report Series (Definition, Diagnosis and Classification) 646*. Geneva: WHO, 1980:9–14.

29 Carpenter MW, Coustan DR. Criteria for screening tests for gestational diabetes. *Am J Obstet Gynecol* 1982;**144**: 763–73.

30 Schmidt MI, Duncan BB, Reichelt AJ, *et al.* Gestational diabetes diagnosed with a 75g OGTT and adverse pregnancy outcomes. *Diabetes Care* 2001;**24**:1151–5.

31 HAPO Study Cooperative Research Group. Hyperglycemia and adverse pregnancy outcomes. *N Engl J Med* 2008;**358**: 1991–2002.

32 Dubreuil G, Anderodias. Ilôts de Langerhans géants chez un nouveau-né, issue de mère glycosurique. *Comptes Rend Soc Biol (Paris)* 1920;**83**:1490–3.

33 Brandstrup E, Okkels H. Pregnancy complicated with diabetes. *Acta Obstet Gynecol Scand* 1938;**18**:136–63.

34 Pedersen J. *Diabetes and Pregnancy. Blood Sugar of Newborn Infants*. MD Thesis. Copenhagen: Danish Science Press, 1952.

35 Miller HC. The effect of the prediabetic state on the survival of the fetus and the birthweight of the newborn infant. *N Engl J Med* 1945;**233**:376–8.

36 Hadden DR. Prediabetes and the big baby. *Diabetic Med* 2008;**25**:1–10.

37 Pirart J. The so-called prediabetic syndrome of pregnancy. *Acta Endocrinol* 1955;**10**:192–208.

38 Hoet JP. Carbohydrate metabolism during pregnancy. *Diabetes* 1954;**3**:1–12.

5 Screening for hyperglycemia in pregnancy

David A. Sacks

Department of Obstetrics and Gynecology, Kaiser Foundation Hospital, Bellflower, CA, USA

PRACTICE POINTS

- Screening tests identify women at risk for a disease, and are used to select those at higher disease risk for definitive testing for gestational diabetes mellitus (GDM).
- Currently, there is no international consensus regarding criteria for either screening or definitive testing for GDM.
- The lower the threshold glucose concentration to indicate an oral glucose tolerance test (OGTT), the greater the number of women who will need to undergo the definitive test.
- Glucose challenge tests are poorly reproducible and vary with the time of day and the time since the last meal prior to the test.
- The use of random glucose and fasting glucose as screening tests has not been shown to be superior to testing with the 50-g glucose load. The poor reproducibility of the 50-g, 1-hour glucose screening test (GST) may result in those at risk for GDM not being treated for GDM.
- Development of a simple screening and/or diagnostic test for GDM must be evaluated in the light of the HAPO study results.

- What are the current screening recommendations for GDM?
- Should this woman be treated empirically for GDM or glucose intolerance?
- Should she start home blood glucose monitoring?
- Should this woman have an OGTT now, or later in gestation? If the latter, should another 1-hour screening test be done to determine the necessity for a full OGTT?
- When in gestation should the second test(s) be given?
- Should a different screening tool be used?
- If a second screening test is selected, should the same 50-g dose be used?
- Will it make any difference at what time of day the test is performed, or whether the woman has fasted for some hours prior to taking the screening test?

CASE HISTORY

A 37-year-old woman, G3P2, presents for her first pre-natal visit at 9 weeks of gestation. She gives a history of having had insulin-requiring diabetes discovered during her last pregnancy. The latter ended in the vaginal delivery of a 4200-g neonate following induction of labor at 38 weeks. Her father and one of her two sisters are being treated for diabetes with diet and oral hypoglycemic agents. Her current body mass index (BMI) is $41 \, \text{kg/m}^2$. At this visit, she is given a 50-g, 1-hour GST, with a result of 6.7 mmol/L (121 mg/dL).

A Practical Manual of Diabetes in Pregnancy, 1st Edition.
Edited by David R. McCance, Michael Maresh and David A. Sacks.
© 2010 Blackwell Publishing

BACKGROUND

The questions posed in the case history have been addressed in several studies. Not all studies have reached the same conclusions about the same issue. Some have questioned the need for any screening for GDM. Their argument rests on the paucity of data demonstrating that the treatment of GDM causes a positive change in maternal, perinatal, or neonatal outcomes.[1] However, two randomized controlled trials have demonstrated a reduction in large for gestational age neonates and in birth trauma with treatment for GDM.[2,3]

Conventionally, a screening test is employed to determine whether a definitive diagnostic test (OGTT, in the context of GDM) is indicated. Over the years much controversy and confusion has existed over how and when to screen for GDM. A variety of screening tests and testing protocols have been recommended (Table 5.1A).[4-10] This

Table 5.1 (A) Details of protocols for screening for gestational diabetes. (B) Factors specified by different groups to define high risk.

A

Source	Selective screening	Whom to screen	When to test	Which screening test	Threshold indicating an OGTT	Glucose load (g)	Definition of GDM
						? Diagnostic test	
ADA[4]	Yes	All pregnant women Definitive test only if meet all of criteria for high risk	As soon as feasible if strong family hx of DM, obese, prior GDM, glycosuria. If no GDM, retest @ 24–28 weeks	One step: no screen		75	FPG 5.3 mmol/L (95 mg/dL) 1-h PG 10.0 mmol/L (180 mg/dL) 2-h PG 8.6 mmol/L (155 mg/dL) >2 results must be equaled or exceeded
			All others: 24–28 weeks	Two step: 50 g, 1 h	7.8 mmol/L (140 mg/dL) detects 80% of GDM 7.2 mmol/L (130 mg/dL) selects 90% of GDM	100	FPG 5.3 mmol/L (95 mg/dL) 1-h PG 10.0 mmol/L (180 mg/dL) 2-h PG 8.6 mmol/L (155 mg/dL) 3-h PG 7.8 mmol/L (140 mg/dL) (≥2 results must be equaled or exceeded)
ADIPS[5]	Yes	All patients If resources are limited, or GDM incidence low, test only those with risk factors	High suspicion of GDM: any time All others: screen @ 26–28 weeks	No screening test recommended		75	FPG >5.5 mmol/L (100 mg/dL) 2 h PG >8.0 mmol/L (144 mg/dL) (Aus) 2 h PG >9.0 mmol/L (162 mg/dL) (NZ)
CDA[6]	Yes	All but low risk (age <25, Caucasian, no personal or family hx of diabetes, no hx of large babies)	24–28 weeks	50 g, 1 h or 75 g, 1 h 50 g, 1 h	7.8 mmol/L (140 mg/dL) 8.0 mmol/L (144 mg/dL) 7.8 mmol/L (140 mg/dL)	75	FPG 5.3 mmol/L (95 mg/dL) 1-h PG 10.6 mmol/L (190 mg/dL) 2-h PG 8.9 mmol/L (160 mg/dL) (≥2 results must be equaled or exceeded) If 50 g, 1-h screening test result is ≥10.3 mmol/L (185 mg/dL), patient is assumed to have GDM
DPSGI[7]	Yes	All pregnant women	24–28 weeks	75 g, 1 h	Same as ADA	75	2-h PG 7.8 mmol/L (140 mg/dL)
NICE[8]	Yes	Prior GDM Women with risk factors and those with prior GDM not found to have GDM on earlier testing	16–18 weeks 24–28 weeks	Screen with risk factors	SMBG or OGTT	75	FPG ≥7.0 mmol/L (126 mg/dL) or 2-h PG ≥7.8 mmol/L (140 mg/dL)

Source	hx	Glycosuria	Testing recommendation		Glucose load (g)	Diagnostic criteria
SIGN[9]	Yes	Check for glycosuria every visit. If ≥2+, get RBS. RBS for all others	Every visit 28 weeks	Screen urine glucose	GTT if RBS: >5.5 mmol/L (100 mg/dL) ≥2h post-meal or >7.0 mmol/L (126 mg/dL) <2h post-meal	75	FPG >5.5 mmol/L (100 mg/dL) Or 2-h PG >9.0 mmol/L (162 mg/dL)
WHO[10]	Unclear	"... may be appropriate" to test high-risk women during 1st trimester	"Formal systematic testing for GDM is usually done between 24 and 28 weeks"	No screening test recommended		75	FPG <7.0 mmol/L (126 mg/dL) and 2-h PG ≥7.8 mmol/L (140 mg/dL) and 2-h PG <11.1 mmol/L (200 mg/dL) or FPG ≥7.0 mmol/L (126 mg/dl) or 2-h PG ≥11.1 mmol/L (200 mg/dL)

B

Source	Increased maternal age	Ethnicity	Glycosuria	Prior GDM	Overweight/obese	Family history of DM	Prior large baby	Prior adverse pregnancy outcome
ADA[4]	✓	✓		✓	✓	✓		
ADIPS[5]	✓	✓		✓	✓	✓		✓
CDA[6]	✓	✓		✓		✓		✓
DPSGI[7]							✓	
NICE[8]		✓		✓	✓	✓	✓	
SIGN[9]			✓	✓				
WHO[10]	✓	✓		✓			✓	

hx, history; FPG, fasting plasma glucose; PG, post-glucose; DM, diabetes mellitus; GDM, gestational diabetes; GTT, glucose tolerance test; OGTT, oral glucose tolerance test; ?, change to random plasma glucose (RPG) throughout; RBS, Random blood sugar; SMBG, self-monitored blood glucose; ADA, American Diabetes Association; WHO, World Health Organization; CDA, Canadian Diabetes Association; NICE, National Institute for Health and Clinical Excellence; SIGN, Scottish Intercollegiate Guidelines Network; ADIPS, Australasian Diabetes in Pregnancy Society; DSPGI, Diabetes in Pregnancy Study Group of India.

chapter will review the current issues surrounding screening for GDM. It will address concerns regarding the method, timing, and frequency of testing for hyperglycemia in pregnancy, threshold values used to indicate an OGTT, and whether a screening test need be utilized at all in deciding whether or not to perform an OGTT during pregnancy.

DEFINITIONS

The terms "screening" and "diagnosis" are often used interchangeably. In the context of detecting glucose intolerance in pregnancy, a screening test is one that identifies women at greater or lower risk for diabetes, depending upon whether the test results fall above or below a threshold glucose concentration, respectively. It does not, however, identify those who do or do not have the disease. Most testing algorithms require that women exceeding a selected threshold concentration on the screening test proceed to a definitive test (OGTT). Thus, a screening test for diabetes identifies a subgroup of the population which is at greater risk for the disease. Within this subgroup, a relatively small minority will be found to have diabetes. Conversely, within the subgroup defined as being at lesser risk, there will be another minority who, if tested, would also be found to have diabetes. In contrast to a screening test, an OGTT (the diagnostic test) will usually provide a definitive answer as to the presence or absence of diabetes.

SCREENING

Universal *versus* selective screening

There is no consensus among international bodies as to whether screening for GDM is justified, and if so, whether universal or selective screening is most appropriate (Table 1A).[4–10] The argument for selective screening is primarily one of cost savings. However, to be both cost-effective and clinically useful, a screening test must be both sensitive and specific. As will be discussed, few data exist for determining both of these important characteristics for any screening test for GDM. The ideal would be to develop a definitive test which requires little preparation and takes little time to perform, without requiring the prior interposition of a screening test, and which could be applied to the entire obstetric population. This universal approach to testing for GDM has been recommended by some.

Screening by clinical characteristics

In all likelihood, because of the time and expense of screening, criteria based on patients' demographics and medical histories have been proposed to select those patients who should receive definitive testing for GDM. This screening method is attractive, because it utilizes readily ascertainable information. Included among the risk factors used to select women for definitive testing are increased maternal age, membership of an ethnic group known or suspected to have a greater prevalence of GDM and/or of non-gestational diabetes, random glycosuria, GDM in a prior pregnancy, overweight and obesity, a family history of diabetes, and a prior large baby (Table 5.1B). Unfortunately, each of these factors is not uniformly, and is sometimes vaguely, defined. Furthermore, to determine the proportion of women with one or more of these risk factors who have GDM (positive predictive value), glucose tolerance testing has to be performed on only those women who have one or more risk factors. To determine the proportion of all women with GDM who have one or more risk factors (sensitivity), and those who have GDM but no risk factors (false negative rate), definitive (glucose tolerance) testing would have to be done on all pregnant women. Few studies with this design have been reported. Perhaps as a consequence of the lack of pertinent data, the selection of risk factors currently recommended to determine candidacy for glucose tolerance testing is not uniform (Table 5.1B).[4–10]

Screening tests using glucose loads

Screening for hyperglycemia during pregnancy using a 50-g oral glucose load followed by a blood sample for glucose concentration 1 hour later is likely the most commonly used method to determine whether or not a patient merits an OGTT. While it offers the advantages of simplicity and ease of interpretation, the test has significant drawbacks, which have become evident over the years.

History

To determine the proportion of the patient sample which will be correctly or incorrectly identified as being at risk for a given disease, both the screening and the definitive test must be administered to all subjects. In 1973, O'Sullivan *et al* published a study in which both a 50–g, 1-hour GST and a 100-g OGTT were administered to 752 unselected women, most of whom were in the second and third trimester. The authors determined that a

Table 5.2 Methodology and results of a study of the 50-g, 1-hour glucose screening test for gestational diabetes mellitus (GDM).[11]

N = 752 unselected pregnant women, all but 20 in second or third trimesters
Medium tested: venous whole blood
Glucose assay method: Somogyi–Nelson

Glucose screening test (GST)
• Load: 50 g of glucose administered in the afternoon
• Threshold defining a positive screen: 7.2 mmol/L (130 mg/dL) 1 h after ingestion of glucose load

Glucose tolerance test (GTT)
• Load: 100 g of glucose administered after 3 days of 250 g of carbohydrate for 3 days followed by an overnight fast
• Threshold defining GDM: at least two of the following values equaled or exceeded: fasting 5.0 mmol/L (90 mg/dL); 1-h 9.2 mmol/L (165 mg/dL), 2-h 8.0 mmol/L (145 mg/dl); 3-h 6.9 mmol/L (125 mg/dL)

Results

		GDM	
		Present	Absent
GST	[+]	15 (TP)	94 (FP)
	[−]	4 (FN)	639 (TN)

Sensitivity = TP/TP + FN = 15/19 = 79%
Specificity = TN/TN + FP = 639/639 + 94 = 87%
PPV = TP/TP + FP = 15/15 + 94 = 14%
NPV = TN/TN + FN = 639/639 + 4 = 99%

TP, true positives; FP, false positives, TN, true negatives; FN, false negatives; PPV = Positive predictive value, NPV, negative predictive value

threshold value of 7.2 mmol/L (130 mg/dL) detected 79% of women who subsequently had a positive OGTT, while 87% of those without GDM would not have been (unnecessarily) tested with the OGTT[11] (Table 5.2). Although multiple studies have since appeared employing a variety of screening tests for GDM, few have administered both screening and definitive tests to all subjects. This is an important omission, as it leaves unanswered the question of what proportion of the patient sample that has GDM will be detected or missed by testing only those above the threshold value selected for a particular screening test.

Screening test thresholds

It is unclear from the O'Sullivan data why a threshold of 7.2 mmol/L (130 mg/dL) was chosen for the 50-g, 1-hour screening test. Selection of a lower screening threshold results in detection of a greater proportion of women within the population who have GDM (i.e. increased sensitivity of the screening test), but at the cost of selecting for definitive testing more women without GDM (i.e. reduced specificity) (Fig. 5.1). In the O'Sullivan study, the selection of the 7.2 mmol/L (130 mg/dL) threshold

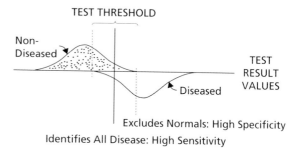

Fig. 5.1 Hypothetical distribution of results of a diagnostic test (curves) and a screening test for the disease (horizontal line). The lower end of the distribution of values is on the left, and the upper end on the right. The influence of raising or lowering the screening test threshold may be envisioned by moving the vertical line to the right or left. (Reproduced from Carpenter and Coustan,[13] with permission from Elsevier.)

provided a reasonable sensitivity of 79% and a specificity of 87%, but it should be noted that there were only 19 subjects who had GDM among the 752 studied. It is likely that a few more diabetic women on either side of the 7.2 mmol/L (130 mg/dL) threshold would have substantially altered the performance of the screening test (Table 5.2).

One of the difficulties in applying the O'Sullivan data is that over the years changes have occurred in glucose assay methods and the medium assayed. First, the less specific (Somogyi–Nelson) method, which assays for all reducing substances, has been replaced by enzyme-based assays specific for glucose (e.g. glucose oxidase, hexokinase, glucose dehydrogenase). Second, the glucose assay is now performed on plasma rather than on whole blood. The concentration of glucose in plasma is greater than that in red blood cells. Thus, based on current methodology (enzyme assay of plasma) alone, to maintain equivalence with the results obtained by O'Sullivan the GST threshold would have to be numerically lowered if only the difference in assay methods is considered, but raised if only the difference in concentration of glucose in plasma compared with that in whole blood is considered. The Carpenter–Coustan diagnostic threshold values defining GDM[12] were empirically derived by adding 14% to the O'Sullivan criteria[11] to adjust for the differences between whole blood and plasma, and subtracting 0.28 mmol/L (5 mg/dL) to adjust for the differences in assay methods. A subsequent study developed a conversion equation by comparing results using the same patients' blood specimens of glucose concentrations in whole blood assayed with the Somogyi–Nelson method with those obtained by assaying their plasma with glucose oxidase. The empirically-derived Carpenter–Coustan criteria were all found to be within the 95% confidence intervals of the glucose thresholds derived with this formula.[13]

The effect of raising or lowering the 50-g, 1-hour GST threshold on sensitivity and specificity was evaluated in a study of 704 unselected pregnant women between 24 and 28 weeks of gestation. All subjects were given a 50-g GST in the fasting state followed by a 100-g, 3-hour OGTT within 1 week of the screening test. Using receiver–operator characteristic curves, the authors found that the optimal balance of sensitivity and specificity (respectively 91% and 73%) using Carpenter–Coustan diagnostic criteria[13] was achieved at a screening test threshold of 7.8 mmol/L (141 mg/dL).[14]

The incidence of GDM among women who have had an OGTT following a 1-hour screening test result greater than or equal to 11.1 mmol/L (200 mg/dL) is reported to vary from 10% to 47%.[15–19] Thus, it seems prudent to perform an OGTT following an elevated GST result of any magnitude.

Timing of the test

Standard screening procedures make no adjustments for gestational age at testing. Some stipulate the time of day that the test is to be administered or the time of testing relative to the last meal.[5] Others state that the test should be given without regard to either.[4,6] The potential influence of gestational age was examined in a study using cross-sectional data in which women were tested serially at 20, 28, and 34 weeks. Among those whose previous test result was less than 7.8 mmol/L (140 mg/dL), the mean increment in post-challenge plasma glucose was 0.06 mmol/L/week (1.1 mg/dL/week).[20] A similar increment was noted in a further study in which all women who tested negative for GDM in the first trimester had a repeat screening test in the third trimester. In the latter study, of those patients whose first trimester result was less than or equal to 6.1 mmol/L (110 mg/dL) (56% of the 124 subjects in the study), only 10% equaled or exceeded the 7.5 mmol/L (135 mg/dL) threshold upon repeat testing in the third trimester, and none of the latter was found to have GDM on testing with the OGTT. The authors concluded that it is probably unnecessary to perform further testing for GDM if the first trimester screening test is less than or equal to 6.1 mmol/L (110 mg/dL).[21]

Two studies examined the influence of timing of the last meal prior to the GST, and demonstrated that the longer the fast prior to the glucose load, the higher the maternal glucose concentration 1 hour after loading.[22,23] One study noted a J-shaped relationship between duration of the fast prior to the test and the test result (Fig. 5.2). In the other report, screening test results of women with GDM were significantly lower if the women had been fed 1 hour prior to testing compared with those tested directly following an overnight fast. In the latter report no significant differences in post-glucose load test results were found between non-diabetic women who had or had not been fed prior to glucose loading.[23] Thus, while time of the last meal prior to administration of the 50-g glucose load does affect the GST result, the finding of improved glucose disposal following successive glucose loads (Staub–Traugott effect[24,25]) in pregnant women remains unexplained.

The time of day that the glucose load is administered may also affect the test results. Data comparing tests results when the glucose load was given in the morning with those when the GST was administered in the afternoon to demographically similar groups[26] and to the same subjects[27] demonstrated significantly elevated

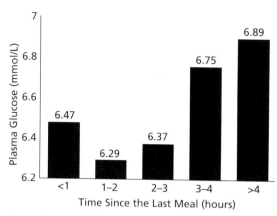

Fig. 5.2 Relationship between 50-g post-load mean maternal plasma glucose and time elapsed in hours since last meal. (Reproduced from Sermer et al,[22] with permission from Elsevier.)

post-glucose challenge maternal glucose concentrations when tested in the afternoon.

Reproducibility of screening and diagnostic tests

Two studies examined the differences in 50-g, 1-hour GST results when the same pregnant women were tested on two successive days. The first was performed under varying dietary conditions prior to testing. Regardless of whether patients were tested early (12–24 weeks) or late (24–28 weeks) in gestation, statistically significant day-to-day differences in test results were found among those tested in the fasting state on both days (first day's test results were greater than the second day's), or tested in random order, fasting one day and fed the other (test results were greater following fasting). The differences in test results were statistically significant except among those tested after having been fed on both days. Among those tested early in pregnancy, the chance of both a first and second test result exceeding a threshold of 7.2 mmol/L (130 mg/dL), 7.5 mmol/L (135 mg/dL), and 7.8 mmol/L (140 mg/dL) was 61%, 47%, and 43%, respectively. However, among those tested late in pregnancy, the likelihood of similar findings was greater than 83%.[28] In the second study, women at a mean gestational age of 27 weeks were instructed to return at the same time of day after having eaten the same foods and engaged in the same or similar activities at the same time on two successive days of testing. Among the 30 women known to have GDM but as yet untreated, three had screening test results below the 7.5 mmol/L (135 mg/dL) threshold on both days, and 10 others exceeded the threshold on only

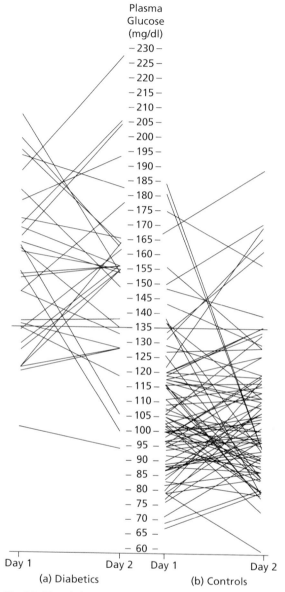

Fig. 5.3 Plot of glucose screening test results on day 1 and day 2 for GDM and control groups. A line connects values on successive days from the same individual. A threshold of 7.5 mmol/L (135 mg/dL) was used to indicate an oral glucose tolerance test. (Reproduced from Sacks et al,[29] with permission from Elsevier.)

one of the two days of testing (five on day 1 and five on day 2; Fig. 5.3). Thus, on any given testing day, potentially 27% (eight of 30) of women with GDM may have gone untested and undetected.[29] Similar data have been reported for glucose tolerance testing among women whose 1-hour GST results were greater than or equal to 7.5 mmol/L (135 mg/dL). When the same women were given OGTTs 1–2 weeks apart, 22%[30] and 24%[31] were found in two studies, respectively, to have GDM on only one of the two tests. The poor reproducibility of the definitive (glucose tolerance) test, the need for which is determined by a poorly reproducible (1-hour post-glucose) screening test, suggests that a substantial proportion of women with GDM may go undetected using the two-step approach. Alternatives include lowering the GST threshold used to indicate definitive testing, or eliminating screening altogether in favor of a single OGTT for all at-risk women.

Other means of delivery of glucose or carbohydrate loads

Because of the unpalatable side effects of the 50-g glucose-containing cola drink (e.g. nausea, headaches), other means of delivery of the glucose load have been explored. One study tested the same patients in the same sequence (cola test followed by 18 Brach jelly bean test) within 2 weeks. All subjects were given a 100-g, 3-hour OGTT. At a threshold of 7.8 mmol/L (140 mg/dL) for cola and jelly beans the respective sensitivities were 46% and 31%, and respective positive predictive values for GDM 18% and 40%.[32] In another study, subjects were given the 50-g cola and 28 Brach jelly beans in random sequence. All subjects were given an OGTT. The mean maternal glucose concentrations after cola and jelly beans were 6.5 mmol/L (116.5 mg/dL) and 6.5 mmol/L (116.9 mg/dL), respectively. However, of the five subjects found to have GDM, only one had both screening test results equal to or greater than the 7.8 mmol/L (140 mg/dL) threshold.[33] Preference for jelly beans over cola was expressed by subjects in both studies.[32,33]

The standard solution used for the 50-g glucose challenge test contains 50-g of glucose diluted in 150 ml of a flavored, carbonated liquid. To test the hypothesis that greater retention of the hyperosmolar cola in the stomach might fail to challenge the islets to produce insulin compared with the more dilute glucose-containing solution, the same patients were screened, in random order, with a 50-g, 150 ml glucola and a solution of the 50-g cola diluted with an additional 300 ml of water. The two screening tests were followed by a 100-g OGTT. In both non-diabetic and diabetic subjects, the 30-minute maternal glucose concentrations were significantly greater following ingestion of the dilute solutions. The 1-hour glucose result was significantly elevated for the diabetic women only. In both diabetic and non-diabetic women

the insulin concentrations were significantly greater following the dilute glucose solution.[34]

Assessing maternal glycemia after a standard meal seems a more physiologic approach to screening than testing after a glucose load. One group compared the glucose concentrations of the same subjects 1 hour after a 600 calorie meal with those 1 hour after a 50-g glucose load. The investigators reported detection of over 90% of GDM at a threshold of 5.6 mmol/L (100 mg/dL) for the former and 7.8 mmol/L (140 mg/dL) for the latter. Respective specificities were 74% and 88%. It must be noted, however, that GTTs in this study were performed only if the maternal glucose value equaled or exceeded 7.2 mmol/L (130 mg/dL) on the 50-g GST.[35]

The use of a glucose polymer *in lieu* of a glucose-containing challenge solution has been investigated. While reasonable concordance was found between glucose and polymer challenge test results, no comparison of GDM detection or false-positive rate was reported.[36]

Random blood glucose as a screening test

Using random blood glucose as a screening test has the advantages of simplicity, and patient tolerance and compliance with testing. In different studies the threshold selected was the 99th,[37] 97.5th,[38] or 90th[39] centile derived from the population under study. These thresholds were then applied to a second patient sample,[37,38] a portion of the first,[39] or the entire cohort[40] to determine which subjects needed an OGTT. Another study performed the OGTT only when preselected thresholds for both the random glucose and fasting glucose were equaled or exceeded.[41] While this approach allows determination of the proportion of those exceeding the threshold who have GDM (positive predictive value), it does not allow determination of the proportion of women who have GDM and who exceed the random glucose threshold (sensitivity) or the proportion of patients whose random glucose concentrations exceed the threshold but do not have GDM (false-positive rate). Two other studies have performed both random glucose and glucose tolerance testing on all pregnant women. Both studies employed multiple random blood glucose results for their calculations; in the first, a mean of five values taken on a single day during the third trimester,[42] and in the second, the highest of random samples taken throughout pregnancy.[43] Because the sensitivities and specificities of only two random blood glucose thresholds were reported in the first study,[42] it was not possible to select the optimal threshold to indicate an OGTT from these data. In the second study, the highest sensitivity (75%) was obtained at a random blood glucose of 6.5 mmol/L (117 mg/dL). The corresponding specificity was 78%. From these reports it seems reasonable to infer that an inadequate amount of data is currently available to support the use of random glucose testing as a screening test for GDM.

Fasting glucose as a screening test

Obtaining a fasting blood sample is simpler, less unpleasant, and less expensive than obtaining a timed sample after a glucose load. The results of studies using this screening tool have been inconsistent, most likely related to differences in study design, maternal and gestational age at testing, maternal glycemic thresholds used to define GDM, and the prevalence of glucose intolerance in the populations tested.

Several studies which looked at the potential use of the fasting plasma glucose (FPG) as a screening test for GDM have been reported.[44–50] At the FPG value that gave a sensitivity similar to the 79% reported by O'Sullivan[13] (range 76–87%), specificities ranged from 43% to 76%.[43–49] In all but one of these reports,[46] the fasting plasma glucose component of the GTT was used as the FPG screening test. By performing the analyses in this fashion, the underlying assumption is that there is little day-to-day variability in FPG results within the same individual. That this is not likely to be the case was suggested in a study in which the fasting plasma glucose assayed on two successive days in eight normal women at 37 weeks of gestation was significantly different.[51] As with the 50-g, 1-hour GST, poor day-to-day reproducibility of the FPG screening test may result in underdiagnosis of GDM.[28,29]

The ideal for a screening test would be one in which the test result varies little throughout gestation. The data on changes in FPG throughout gestation are not in agreement, with some showing a difference in FPG results[52] and others reporting similar FPG results with advancing gestation.[53,54] All studies were performed using normal pregnant women.

Comparisons have been made for the performance of the FPG test and the 50-g, 1-hour GST as predictors of GDM. No statistically significant difference was found in the areas under the receiver–operator characteristic curves of both screening tests.[50,55]

In summary, at FPG values that provide adequate sensitivity, some have found a high false-positive rate. There is a paucity of data regarding the reproducibility of the FPG test. In the few published comparative studies, the FPG test appears to perform as well as the 50-g, 1-hour GST.

Glycated hemoglobin and glycated albumin as screening tests

When plasma glucose is consistently elevated over time, glycation of hemoglobin takes place. The process is one of irreversible non-enzymatic attachment of a glucose molecule to the N-terminal valine on the beta chain of the hemoglobin molecule. The resulting hemoglobin A1c (HbA1c) remains in circulation for the life of the red blood cell, and thus is reflective of the patient's average blood glucose over the previous 2–3 months. The results are expressed as the percentage of total hemoglobin that has been glycated. HbA1c has been evaluated as a possible screening test for GDM. Test results in normal pregnant women vary with ethnicity and with gestational age.[56] The distribution of values of HbA1c was found to be no different between women who did and those who did not have GDM.[57] In a comparison between HbA1c and the 50-g, 1-hour glucose screen, the latter was able to discriminate between women at greater risk of maternal and perinatal morbidity, whereas the former was not.[58] Thus, HbA1c does not appear to be a useful predictor of either GDM or its attendant morbidities.

Fructosamine is a glycated albumin formed by the non-enzymatic reaction between fructose and an ammonia or an amine. It is also formed when the carbonyl group of a glucose molecule reacts with an amino group of a protein. Because the half-life of albumin is 2–3 weeks, fructosamine concentration is a reflection of glucose concentrations for that short time period. Fructosamine has been examined as a potential screening test for GDM. As with HbA1c, fructosamine concentrations vary with gestational age[59] and prevailing albumin levels.[59] Findings of fructosamine concentrations which did[60] and did not[61] differ between women who had GDM and those who did not have been reported. The area under the receiver–operator curves for the 50-g, 1-hour screening test was reported to be greater than that under the curve for fructosamine, suggesting that at most thresholds the former test was more sensitive and specific than the latter.[62] Thus, not unlike glycosylated hemoglobin, most of the published evidence suggests that glycated albumin is not a useful screening tool for GDM.

CONCLUSIONS

Although screening tests for GDM may decrease the need for definitive OGTT, they do have significant drawbacks. Depending on the threshold value selected to indicate an OGTT, a proportion of those who have GDM will not be identified, and a large proportion of those who do not have the disease will undergo definitive testing. A post-glucose test is poorly reproducible. Thus, a woman who is screened with a 50-g, 1-hour glucose challenge and who has GDM may not be detected unless screened on several occasions prior to undergoing an OGTT. A single, easy to administer, and tolerable definitive diagnostic test seems preferable to the two-step procedure. Upon universal acceptance of the criteria for defining GDM developed from data generated by the HAPO study,[63] exploration may be undertaken to attempt to develop a simple, sensitive, and specific screening test for GDM.

REFERENCES

1 Hillier TA, Vesco KK, Pedula KL, Beil TL, Whitlock EP, Pettitt DJ. Screening for gestational diabetes mellitus: a systematic review for the U.S. Preventive Services Task Force. *Ann Intern Med* 2008;**148**:766–75.

2 Crowther CA, Hiller JE, Moss JR, McPhee AJ, Jeffries WS, Robinson JS. Effect of treatment of gestational diabetes mellitus on pregnancy outcomes. *N Engl J Med* 2005;**352**: 2477–86.

3 Landon MB, Spong CY, Thom E, *et al.* A multicenter, randomized trial of treatment for mild gestational diabetes. *N Engl J Med* 2009;**361**:1339–48.

4 American Diabetes Association. Diagnosis and classification of diabetes mellitus. *Diabetes Care* 2008;**31** (Suppl 1):S55–S60.

5 Hoffman L, Nolan C, Wilson JD, Oats JJN, Simmons D. Australasian Diabetes in Pregnancy Society. Gestational diabetes-management guidelines. *Med J Aust* 1998;**169**: 93–7.

6 Meltzer S, Leiter L, Daneman D, *et al.* 1998 clinical practice guidelines for the management of diabetes in Canada. *Can Med Assoc J* 1998;**8** (Suppl):S1–29.

7 Sheshia V, Das AK, Balaji V, Joshi SR, Parikh MN, Gupta S. Gestational diabetes – Guidelines. *J Assoc Phys India* 2006; **54**:622–8.

8 National Institute for Health and Clinical Excellence. *Diabetes in pregnancy. NICE clinical guideline 63. National Collaborating Center for Women's and Children's Health,* 2008. www.nice.org.uk

9 Scottish Intercollegiate Guidelines Network. *Management of Diabetes,* 55, 2001. www.sign.org.uk

10 Alberti KJMM, Zimmet PZ. Definition, diagnosis and classification of diabetes mellitus and its complications. Part 1: Diagnosis and classification of diabetes mellitus. Provisional report of a WHO consultation. *Diabet Med* 1998;**15**: 539–353.

11 O'Sullivan JB, Mahan CM, Charles D, Dandrow RV. Screening criteria for high-risk gestational diabetic patients. *Am J Obstet Gynecol* 1973;**116**:895–900.

12 Sacks DA, Abu-Fadil S, Greenspoon JS, Fotheringham N. Do the current standards for glucose tolerance testing in pregnancy represent a valid conversion of O'Sullivan's original criteria? *Am J Obstet Gynecol* 1989;**161**:638–41.

13 Carpenter MW, Coustan DR. Criteria for screening tests for gestational diabetes. *Am J Obstet Gynecol* 1982;**144**: 768–73.

14 Bonomo M, Gandini ML, Mastropasqua A, *et al.* Which cutoff level should be used in screening for glucose intolerance in pregnancy? *Am J Obstet Gynecol* 1998;**179**:179–85.

15 Landy HJ, Gómez-Marín O, O'Sullivan MJ. Diagnosing gestational diabetes mellitus: Use of a glucose screen without administering the glucose tolerance test. *Obstet Gynecol* 1996;**87**:395–400.

16 Bobrowski RA, Bottoms SF, Micallef J-A, Dombrowski MP. Is the 50-gram glucose screening test ever diagnostic? *J Matern Fetal Med* 1996;**5**:317–20.

17 Atilano LC, Lee-Parritz A, Lieberman E, Cohen AP, Barbieri RL. Alternative methods of diagnosing gestational diabetes mellitus. *Am J Obstet Gynecol* 1999;**181**:1158–61.

18 Sacks DA, Abu-Fadil S, Karten GJ, Forsythe AB, Hackett JR. Screening for gestational diabetes with the one-hour 50-g glucose test. *Obstet Gynecol* 1987;**70**:89–93.

19 Shivers SA, Lucas MJ. Gestational diabetes. Is a 50-g screening result ≥200 mg/dl diagnostic? *J Reprod Med* 1999;**44**:685–88.

20 Watson WJ. Serial changes in the 50-g oral glucose test in pregnancy: implications for screening. *Obstet Gynecol* 1989;**74**:40–3.

21 Nahum GG, Huffaker BJ. Correlation between first- and early third-trimester glucose screening test results. *Obstet Gynecol* 1990;**76**:709–13.

22 Sermer M, Naylor D, Gare DJ, *et al.* Impact of time since last meal on the gestational glucose challenge test. *Am J Obstet Gynecol* 1994;**171**:607–16.

23 Coustan DR, Widness JA, Carpenter MW, Rotondo L, Pratt DC, Oh W. Should the fifty-gram, one-hour plasma glucose screening test for gestational diabetes be administered in the fasting or fed state? *Am J Obstet Gynecol* 1986;**154**:1031–5.

24 Staub H. Examination of sugar metabolisms in humans. *Z Klin Med* 1921;**91**:44.

25 Traugott K. In reference to the reactions of blood sugar levels in repeated and varied types of enteral sugar increases and their significance in liver function. *Klin Wochenschr* 1922;**1**:892–4.

26 McElduff A, Hitchman R. Screening for gestational diabetes: the time of day is important. *Med J Aust* 2002;**176**:136.

27 Aparicio NJ, Joao MA, Cortelezzi M, *et al.* Pregnant women with impaired tolerance to an oral glucose load in the after-

noon: evidence suggesting that they behave metabolically as patients with gestational diabetes. *Am J Obstet Gynecol* 1998;**178**:1059–66.

28 Espinoza de los Monteros A, Parra A, Cariño N, Ramirez A. The reproducibility of the 50-g, 1-hour glucose screen for diabetes in pregnancy. *Obstet Gynecol* 1993;**82**: 515–8.

29 Sacks DA, Abu-Fadil S, Greenspoon JS, Fotheringham N. How reliable is the fifty-gram, one-hour glucose screening test? *Am J Obstet Gynecol* 1989;**161**:642–5.

30 Harlass FE, Brady K, Read JA. Reproducibility of the oral glucose tolerance test in pregnancy. *Am J Obstet Gynecol* 1991;**164**:564–8.

31 Catalano PM, Avallone DA, Drago NM, Amini SB. Reproducibility of the oral glucose tolerance test in pregnant women. *Am J Obstet Gynecol* 1993;**169**:874–81.

32 Boyd KL, Ross EK, Sherman SJ. Jelly beans as an alternative to a cola beverage containing fifty grams of glucose. *Am J Obstet Gynecol* 1995;**173**:1889–92.

33 Lamar ME, Kuehl TJ, Cooney AT, Gayle LJ, Holleman S, Allen SR. Jelly beans as an alternative to a fifty-gram glucose beverage for gestational diabetes screening. *Am J Obstet Gynecol* 1999;**181**:1154–7.

34 Schwartz JG, Phillips WT, Blumhardt MR, Langer O. Use of a more physiologic oral glucose solution during screening for gestational diabetes mellitus. *Am J Obstet Gynecol* 1994; **171**:685–91.

35 Coustan DR, Widness JA, Carpenter MW, Rotondo L, Pratt DC. The "breakfast tolerance test": Screening for gestational diabetes with a standardized mixed nutrient meal. *Am J Obstet Gynecol* 1987;**157**:1113–7.

36 Reece EA, Holford T, Tuck S, Bargar M, O'Connor T, Hobbins JC. Screening for gestational diabetes: One-hour carbohydrate tolerance test performed by a virtually tasteless polymer of glucose. *Am J Obstet Gynecol* 1987;**156**: 132–4.

37 Lind T, McDougall AN. Antenatal screening for diabetes mellitus by random blood glucose sampling. *Br J Obstet Gynaecol* 1981;**88**:346–51.

38 Hatem M, Dennis KJ. A random plasma glucose method for screening for abnormal glucose intolerance in pregnancy. *Br J Obstet Gynaecol* 1987;**94**:213–16.

39 Nasrat AA, Johnstone FD, Hasan SA. Is random glucose an efficient screening test for abnormal glucose tolerance in pregnancy? *Br J Obstet Gynaecol* 1988;**95**:855–60.

40 Stangenberg M, Persson B, Norlander E. Random capillary blood glucose and conventional selection criteria for glucose tolerance testing during pregnancy. *Diabetes Res* 1985;**2**: 29–31.

41 Nielsen K, Vinther S, Birch K, Lange A. Random blood glucose sampling as an early antenatal screening test for diabetes mellitus. *Diabetes Res* 1988;**8**:31–3.

42 Jowett NI, Samanta AK, Burden AC. Screening for diabetes in pregnancy: Is a random blood glucose enough? *Diabet Med* 1987;**4**:160–3.

43 Östlund I, Hanson U. Repeated random blood glucose measurements as universal screening test for gestational diabetes mellitus. *Acta Obstet Gynecol Scand* 2004;**83**: 46–51.

44 Fadl H, Östlund I, Nilsson K, Hanson U. Fasting capillary glucose as a screening test for gestational diabetes. *Br J Obstet Gynaecol* 2006;**113**:1067–71.

45 Agarwal MM, Dhatt GS, Punnose J, Zayed R. Gestational diabetes. Fasting and postprandial glucose as first prenatal screening tests in a high-risk population. *J Reprod Med* 2007;**52**:299–305.

46 Sacks DA, Chen W, Wolde-Tzadik G, Buchanan TA. Fasting plasma glucose test at the first prenatal visit as a screen for gestational diabetes. *Obstet Gynecol* 2003;**101**:1197–203.

47 Perucchini D, Fischer U, Spinas GA, Huch R, Huch A, Lehmann R. Using fasting plasma glucose concentrations to screen for gestational diabetes mellitus: prospective population based study. *Br Med J* 1999;**319**:812–5.

48 Reichelt AJ, Spichler ER, Branchtein L, Franco LJ, Schmidt MI. Fasting plasma glucose is a useful test for the detection of gestational diabetes. *Diabetes Care* 1998;**21**:1246–9.

49 Agarwal MM, Hughes PF, Ezimokahi M. Screening for gestational diabetes in a high-risk population using fasting plasma glucose. *Int J Gynecol Obstet* 2000;**68**:147–8.

50 Rey E, Hudon L, Michon N, Boucher P, Ethier J, Saint-Louis P. Fasting plasma glucose challenge test: screening for gestational diabetes and cost effectiveness. *Clin Biochem* 2004;**37**:780–4.

51 Campbell DM, Bewsher PD, Davidson JM, Sutherland HW. Day-to-day variations in fasting plasma glucose and fasting plasma insulin levels in late normal pregnancy. *J Obstet Gynaecol Br Com* 1974;**81**:615–21.

52 Agardh C-D. Åberg A, Nordén N. Glucose levels and insulin secretion during a 75 g glucose challenge test in normal pregnancy. *J Intern Med* 1996;**240**:303–9.

53 Lind T, Billewicz WZ, Brown G. A serial study of changes occurring in the oral glucose tolerance test in pregnancy. *J Obstet Gynaecol Br Com* 1973;**80**:1033–9.

54 Kühl C. Glucose metabolism during and after pregnancy in normal and gestational diabetic women. *Acta Endocrinol* 1975;**79**:709–19.

55 Tam W-H, Rogers MS, Yip S-K, Lao TK, Leung TY. Which screening test is the best for gestational impaired glucose tolerance and gestational diabetes mellitus? *Diabetes Care* 2000;**23**:1432.

56 Loke DFM. Glycosylated haemoglobins in women with low risk for diabetes in pregnancy. *Singapore Med J* 1998;**36**: 501–4.

57 Agarwal M, Dhatt GS, Punnose J, Koster G. Gestational diabetes: a reappraisal of HBA1c as a screening test. *Acta Obstet Gynecol Scand* 2005;**84**:1159–63.

58 Cousins L, Dattel B, Hollingsworth D. Hulbert D, Zettner A. Screening for carbohydrate intolerance in pregnancy: a comparison of two tests and reassessment of a common approach. *Am J Obstet Gynecol* 1985;**153**:381–5.

59 Bor MV, Bor P, Cevik C. Serum fructosamine and fructos-amine-albumen ratio as screening tests for gestational diabetes mellitus. *Gynecol Obstet* 1999;**262**:105–11.

60 Huter O, Heinz D, Brezinka C, Soelder E, Koelle D, Patsch JR. Low sensitivity of serum fructosamine as a screening parameter for gestational diabetes mellitus. *Gynecol Obstet Invest* 1992;**34**:20–3.

61 Cefalu WT, Prather KL, Chester DL, Wheeler CJ, Biswas M, Pernoll MI. Total serum glycated proteins in detection and monitoring of gestational diabetes. *Diabetes Care* 1990;**13**: 872–5.

62 Roberts AB, Baker JR, Metcalf P, Mullard C. Fructosamine compared with a glucose load as a screening test for gestational diabetes. *Obstet Gynecol* 1990;**76**:773–5.

63 HAPO Study Cooperative Research Group, Metzger BE, Lowe LP, Dyer AR, *et al.* Hyperglyceimia and adverse pregnancy outcome. *N Engl J Med* 2008;**358**:1991–2002.

6

Diagnosis of hyperglycemia in pregnancy

Marshall W. Carpenter

St Elizabeth's Medical Center, Boston, MA, USA

PRACTICE POINTS

- Controversy surrounds the significance of the effects of minor degrees of maternal hyperglycemia on perinatal health and fetal imprinting that may lead to characteristics of the metabolic syndrome, including obesity and hyperglycemia, prior to puberty.
- Disparate diagnostic criteria for maternal glucose intolerance presently employed reflect the absence of blinded studies sufficiently large enough to identify the likely continuum of glycemic risk for fetal outcome.
- In the US, the O'Sullivan and Mahan criteria have traditionally been used, involving a 100-g, 3-hour oral glucose tolerance test (OGTT); while elsewhere a 75-g, 2-hour OGTT is frequently employed, interpreted by World Health Organization (WHO) criteria.
- A consensus has proposed that the same numerical fasting, 1- and 2-hour post-glucose thresholds be used for both the 75-g and 100-g OGTT.
- The Hyperglycemia and Adverse Perinatal Outcome (HAPO) study of gravidas without overt diabetes employed a 75-g OGTT with detailed measures of maternal and perinatal outcomes. This international study will likely provide the foundation for universal diagnostic criteria.

CASE HISTORY

Ms Smith was a 28-year-old G2P1 patient whose first pregnancy was uncomplicated. She had undergone a 100-g glucose tolerance test (GTT) at 29 weeks of gestation because her 50-g, 1-hour glucose screening test (GST) (routine practice in the US) value was 8.6 mmol/L (155 mg/dL). A subsequent 100-g, 3-hour test was normal by the 1979 National Diabetes Data Group US

A Practical Manual of Diabetes in Pregnancy, 1st Edition.
Edited by David R. McCance, Michael Maresh and David A. Sacks.
© 2010 Blackwell Publishing

standards[1] employed at that time. She underwent a normal labor and delivered a 4.1 kg (9 lb 2 oz) infant without complication. Five years later she again became pregnant. She was noted to weigh 2.3 kg (5 lb) more than her weight when she registered for care in her first pregnancy. Because of the usual practice of universal screening in the US and mindful of the birthweight of her first child, she again underwent a GTT at 27 weeks of gestation, which demonstrated glucose values similar to those in her first pregnancy. However, because the newer criteria suggested by the American Diabetes Association (ADA) were now being used, she was diagnosed with gestational diabetes. She required no medical treatment other than changes in diet and activity, and her pregnancy was uncomplicated. Her obstetrician observed normal fundal growth, but because of her previous diagnosis, ordered sonographic fetal biometry at 38 weeks. This showed an estimated fetal weight of 4432 g (9 lb 12 oz). After counseling with her obstetrician, Ms Smith underwent a primary cesarean section productive of a 3920 g (8 lb 10 oz) infant.

Ms Smith was disappointed that she had chosen a cesarean delivery and inquired why she had been counseled to undergo the surgery. Her obstetrician stated that his practice was to examine fetal weight in all women with gestational diabetes because of concerns about birth trauma. He further explained that estimates of fetal weight are inaccurate, often by as much as 15%.

- Does universal screening for maternal glucose intolerance carry any risk for maternal health?
- Is there scientific evidence supporting a lowering of the diagnostic threshold for gestational diabetes from that recommended in 1979?
- What is the relative risk of fetal macrosmia associated with maternal glucose intolerance?

Table 6.1 Consensus criteria for gestational diabetes.

Criteria	1964 O'Sullivan and Mahan[4]*		1979 NDDG[1]	1999 WHO[2]	2000 ADA[5]	2001 ADA[6]
Medium and time	Whole blood 100-g 3-h (mmol/L (mg/dL))[†]	Plasma 100-g 3-h (mmol/L (mg/dL))[†]	Plasma 100-g 3-h (mmol/L (mg/dL))[†]	Plasma 75-g 2-h (mmol/L (mg/dL))[‡]	Plasma 100-g 3-h (mmol/L (mg/dL))[†]	Plasma 75-g 2-h (mmol/L (mg/dL))[†]
Fasting	≥5.0 (90)	≥5.8 (105)	≥5.8 (105)	<7.0 (126)	≥5.3 (95)	≥5.3 (95)
1 h	≥9.2 (165)	≥10.6 (190)	≥10.6 (190)		≥10.0 (180)	≥10.0 (180)
2 h	≥8.1 (145)	≥9.2 (165)	≥9.2 (165)	>7.8 (140), ≤11.1 (200)	≥8.6 (155)	≥8.6 (155)
3 h	≥6.9 (125)	≥8.1 (145)	≥8.1 (145)		≥7.8 (140)	

ADA, American Diabetic Association; WHO, World Health Organization; NDDG, National Diabetes Data Group
* O'Sullivan and Mahan rounded mean plus 2 SD values to nearest 0.28 mmol/L (5 mg/dL) value
† Two elevated values required for diagnosis
‡ One elevated value required for diagnosis

RATIONALE FOR DIAGNOSING MATERNAL HYPERGLYCEMIA

Gestational hyperglycemia as defined by criteria for "impaired glucose tolerance" accepted by the WHO[2] or as "gestational diabetes" by the ADA[3] has been associated with stillbirth, fetal overgrowth, and injury at birth. The ADA defines gestational diabetes as "any degree of glucose intolerance with onset or first recognition during pregnancy", but provides diagnostic thresholds for fasting and post-glucose loading values[3] (Table 6.1). Gravidas with even mild hyperglycemia are at increased risk of offspring with respiratory insufficiency, hypoglycemia polycythemia, and hyperbilirubinemia. The association of measures of maternal hyperglycemia with adverse perinatal outcomes, especially stillbirth, have been recognized for decades and continue to be identified in recent reports. In 1972, Karlsson and Kjellmer[7] reported a four-fold increase in stillbirths in mothers with mean glucose values of 5.6–8.3 mmol/L (100–150 mg/dL) compared to those with lower mean values. O'Sullivan et al[4] chose statistical diagnostic criteria of maternal hyperglycemia (two or more of four values at ≥ 2 SD above the mean) from a 100-g 3-hour oral GTT. They were able to identify a subgroup of gravidas, older than 24 years of age, with a four-fold risk for stillbirth.[8] Though O'Sullivan et al's study sought diagnostic criteria predictive of later maternal Type 2 diabetes, their criteria, modified as to present assay techniques, have been adopted in the US to define gestational diabetes mellitus (GDM).[3]

More recent studies suggest that, despite improvements in obstetric care, gestational diabetes is still associated with increased stillbirth risk. Aberg et al studied the rate of stillbirth in prior pregnancies among Swedish women newly diagnosed with gestational diabetes in their subsequent pregnancy. They found a stillbirth rate of 14.9 per 1000 in the prior pregnancies (births from 1987 to 1992), a significantly increased risk (RR 1.6, 95% CI 1.1–2.2) compared to population rates.[9] Obesity is well recognized to predispose to glucose intolerance. Examination of the association of maternal obesity with stillbirth has demonstrated an increased risk of stillbirth from an RR of 1.2 (95% CI 0.6–2.2) to 3.1 (95% CI 1.6–5.9) among gravidas with a body mass index (BMI) of 25–29 and 30 or greater compared to those with BMIs of 18.5–24.9.[10] Cohorts from as late as the mid-1990s demonstrate continued increased risk of stillbirth, even among those diagnosed with GDM. Conde-Agudelo et al documented a 1.9-fold (95% CI 1.5–2.1) risk of stillbirth among gravidas with gestational diabetes compared to non-diabetic controls.[11] Consequently, it may reasonably be inferred that subclinical maternal hyperglycemia during pregnancy predisposes to late fetal death, thereby emphasizing the importance of close glycemic monitoring in diabetic pregnancy.

Glycemic monitoring and liberal use of insulin to achieve maternal euglycemia has been associated with a fall in perinatal mortality rate. Beischer et al[12] retrospectively examined a group of gravidas receiving GDM treatment (1981–1995) whose 75-g, 1-hour OGGT glucose values lay between 9 and 10 mmol/L (163–180 mg/dL) and 2-hour values between 7 and 7.8 mmol/L (127–140 mg/dL), and historical controls (1971–1980) within the same OGTT stratum who were not identified as having gestational diabetes and received only routine prenatal care. Those identified as having GDM had a perinatal mortality rate of less than one-third of the earlier control cohort (7 of 1000 *vs* 26 of 1000).

Observational studies have demonstrated an association between GDM and macrosomia at birth[13,14] and randomized trials have demonstrated that treatment of even modest maternal hyperglycemia reduces fetal macrosomia.[15,16] These data suggested that identification and treatment of women with mild degrees of glucose intolerance may reduce perinatal mortality and improve rates of perinatal morbidity.

Fetal overgrowth in the context of maternal gestational diabetes (ADA criteria) also appears to be a marker of later evidence of fetal imprinting that leads to later metabolic disorders. Offspring of mothers with GDM who demonstrate fetal overgrowth have been found to be at increased risk of obesity at 1 year of age.[17] Further, offspring of glucose intolerant mothers (ADA criteria) with a birthweight above the 90th centile demonstrate a 3.6-fold risk of developing the metabolic syndrome (two or more of the following: obesity, hypertension [systolic or diastolic], glucose intolerance, and dyslipidemia) as early as 11 years of age compared to those with a normal birthweight.[18]

Because of the attribution of fetal risk to modest maternal hyperglycemia, oral glucose testing of gravidas for glucose intolerance became widespread. In the US, such screening has taken the form of a modification of the O'Sullivan protocol, in which all patients were tested in the afternoon following a 50-g oral glucose load.[4] Current US practice allows for testing at 24–28 weeks of gestation. The glucose load may be administered at any time of day, without regard to the time elapsed since the last meal. Plasma glucose is measured 1 hour after ingestion. A 100-g, 3-hour OGTT is recommended for those with a screening test value over 7.8 mmol/L (140 mg/dL). The original O'Sullivan thresholds have been modified, based on present day use of glucose oxidase methods in venous plasma (Table 6.1).

The practice of screening for subclinical glucose intolerance has been controversial. Sermer *et al*[19] blinded patients and caregivers to glucose testing results of gravidas meeting the later, lower-threshold criteria for gestational diabetes,[20] but not the earlier, higher-threshold criteria.[1] These subjects received usual prenatal care but were not identified as having gestational diabetes. Those subjects meeting the higher-threshold criteria underwent glucose surveillance and treatment. Compared with euglycemic controls, those (untreated) subjects meeting only the lower-threshold criteria had elevated rates of fetal macrosomia (28.7% *vs* 13.7%) and cesarean delivery (29.6% *vs* 20.2%). By contrast, gravidas meeting the higher (National Diabetes Data Group [NDDG]) threshold glucose criteria and who had been treated to achieve more normal glucose values, had a reduced rate of fetal macrosomia, comparable with euglycemic controls. However, despite normal fetal weight, those labeled with gestational diabetes had a cesarean rate of 33%, which was higher than that of untreated glucose-intolerant gravidas. These findings supported earlier recommendations of the US Preventive Services Task Force[21] that screening for glucose intolerance in pregnancy should be abandoned because of a lack of demonstrated maternal or fetal benefit. The report suggested that a scientifically rigorous randomized clinical trial demonstrating perinatal benefit was required to justify a screening program.

In 2005, Crowther *et al*[22] conducted a double blind, randomized trial of 1000 gravidas who were first identified by diabetes risk factors or by a 50-g, 1-hour glucose challenge (≥7.8 mmol/L [140 mg/dL]), and then diagnosed as GDM between 24 and 34 weeks of gestation by a 75-g, 2-hour GTT (WHO criteria: fasting plasma glucose value of <7.8 mmol/L [<140 mg/dL]) and 2-hour post-load value of 7.8–11 mmol/L (140–198 mg/dL). Thus, the trial effectively excluded patients with significant degrees of glucose intolerance. Gravidas were randomized to intervention (diet counseling, glucose monitoring instruction, four-times daily glucose testing, and insulin treatment for repetitive values of over 5.5 mmol/L [99 mg/dL] fasting and 7.0 mmol/L [126 mg/dL] 2 hours after meals) or to routine prenatal care. Prenatal care in the intervention group was that usually provided to women with GDM at each care site. Both the patients in the non-intervention group and their caregivers were blinded as to their having gestational diabetes. Despite the enrollment of only patients with mild glucose intolerance, 1% of offspring in the intervention group *versus* 4% of controls sustained serious perinatal outcomes (death, shoulder dystocia, fracture, or nerve palsy), a relative risk, adjusted for maternal age, race or ethnic group, and parity, of 0.33, but without a statistically significant difference in cesarean delivery rates (31% and 32%, respectively). There were five perinatal deaths among the controls, but none in those given diabetes care. This finding of efficacious pregnancy intervention among those with mild glucose intolerance changed the debate from that of whether screening for maternal glucose intolerance is justified to one addressing the best diagnostic threshold to be employed.

60 **Chapter 6**

DIAGNOSTIC CRITERIA FOR MATERNAL HYPERGLYCEMIA

As noted above, O'Sullivan *et al*[4] employed the diabetogenic effect of pregnancy as a condition to predict later diabetes in women. They chose statistical diagnostic limits of greater than or equal to 2 SD above mean glucose values from a 100-g, 3-hour OGTT. O'Sullivan's studies employed the Somogyi–Nelson method that identified other reducing substances in addition to glucose. As a result, glucose concentrations were elevated by approximately 0.28 mmol/L (5 mg/dL) over that determined by the more specific enzyme methods, now employed universally. Further, O'Sullivan measured glucose in venous whole blood; measurements in plasma being approximately 14% higher. Subsequent studies have confirmed that more recent translation of O'Sullivan's data accurately reflect his measures using glucose oxidase methods in venous plasma.[20,23]

The ADA 100-g, 3-hour OGTT, a transliteration of O'Sullivan's original test to modern laboratory values, is most commonly employed in the US. In 2003–4, it identified GDM among 4.2% of gravidas.[24] Perinatal mortality risk among pregnancies with GDM (ADA criteria) remains at roughly twice that of pregnancies without diabetes. Recent reports of the prevalence of pre-eclampsia or pregnancy-associated hypertension among gravidas with GDM using ADA criteria have ranged widely. However, a summary of 10 reports of risk of these disorders in pregnancy with *versus* without GDM observed an overall increased risk of hypertensive disorders of only 8% among the total of over 4000 pregnancies with GDM.[25]

In 1991, Lind *et al* reported GTTs in 1009 unselected gravidas at more than 16 weeks of gestation.[26] They proposed that values of 2 SD above the mean at fasting, 1 and 2 hours after a 75-g oral load (respectively 7, 11, and 9 mmol/L [126, 198, and 162 mg/dL]) be used for diagnostic thresholds; and that an elevated 2-hour and either an elevated fasting or 1-hour value be required to diagnose GDM. The use of these thresholds resulted in an incidence estimate of 1.2%, approximately one-third of that for the modified O'Sullivan criteria. Correlation with perinatal morbidity was not provided.

Outside the US, a 75-g, 2-hour OGTT adopted by the WHO[2] has been most commonly used to diagnose gestational diabetes. The test uses the same criteria to define gestational diabetes as are used to define impaired glucose tolerance in non-pregnant women, based on their association with diabetes-related morbidity. An abnormal test result requires only one abnormal value (Table 6.1).

As noted above, most testing in the US has been adapted from the O'Sullivan protocol, in which a 50-g, 1-hour screening test is applied without respect to time of day or time since the most recent meal, medications or exercise, but with a threshold value set sufficiently low (7.2–7.8 mmol/L [130–140 mg/dL]) to identify, respectively, between 94% and 91% of glucose-intolerant gravidas.[27]

Comparison of the two tests has not been sufficiently examined. Weiss *et al*[28] performed a randomized, crossover trial of 75-g and 100-g GTTs in mid-pregnancy. They showed that the 100-g, 1- and 2-hour values were, respectively, 0.9 mmol/L (16 mg/dL) and 0.5 mmol/L (9 mg/dL) higher than after a 75-g load.

A Brazilian study of the agreement between the ADA and WHO 75-g tests was carried out among 4977 gravidas enrolled between 1991 and 1995. The authors required that two of the three ADA threshold values be met to identify gravidas as meeting ADA criteria but only one of the WHO test thresholds was required for diagnosis. The proportion of subjects meeting these criteria was 2.4% and 7.2%, respectively.[29] Test function was adjusted for study center, ethnicity, neonatal sex, maternal height, age, prepregnancy BMI, and weight gain up to the time of study enrollment. Seventy-three percent of those meeting the WHO criteria were not identified by the ADA test and 22% of those meeting the ADA criteria were not identified by WHO standards. Both tests appeared to identify women who had increased risk ratios for macrosomia (1.29 and 1.45), pre-eclampsia (2.28 and 1.94), and perinatal mortality (3.10 and 1.59) However, the ADA risk ratio for macrosomia and the WHO risk ratio for perinatal mortality failed to achieve statistical significance, perhaps due to the relatively small study sample.

The limited available studies demonstrate that the tests' different oral glucose loads, threshold values, and number of thresholds required for diagnosis make a simple comparison between tests unrealistic. In 2001, the ADA Professional Practice Committee recommended use of the same threshold criteria for the fasting, 1- and 2-hour postprandial values for a 75-g, 2-hour OGTT for the diagnosis of gestational diabetes, with two abnormal values required for diagnosis.[5,6]

ALTERNATIVE CARBOHYDRATE CHALLENGE TESTS

The high osmolar concentration of simple glucose preparations conspire with the common gastrointestinal symptoms of pregnancy to cause nausea, abdominal discomfort, and occasional vomiting that compromises patient compliance and test reliability. To address this problem several alternative carbohydrate challenge tests have been proposed.

Oral glucose polymers

Reece et al[30] employed a commercially available glucose polymer containing 3% glucose, 7% maltose, 55% maltotriose, and overall 85% polysaccharides, with one-fifth the osmotic load of generally employed simple glucose solutions. Compared with the simple glucose solution, they demonstrated correlation with the 1-hour post 50-g load (k = 0.62) and the value 3 hours after the 100-g load (k = 0.45). However, data from this and other trials suggest that maternal glycemic response to an oral glucose polymer challenge may be sufficiently low so as to reduce screening and diagnostic sensitivity.

Breakfast tolerance tests

Chastang et al[31] performed the current ADA screening and GTT protocol and glucose measurements during fasting and 2 hours after a "usual breakfast" containing at least 25 g of carbohydrate among 354 gravidas. For the latter test, GDM was diagnosed if the fasting value was greater than or equal to 5 mmol/L (≥90 mg/dL) and the postprandial value greater than or equal to 6.7 mmol/L (≥120 mg/dL). Macrosomia was diagnosed in 14% of offspring. The breakfast test demonstrated sensitivity of 47% for fetal macrosomia at a 68% specificity compared to values of 16% and 80%, respectively, for the GTT. Though as yet not sufficiently standardized, a mixed nutrient meal is usually better tolerated, has been shown to elicit a more robust insulin response, and may be a more physiologic measure of maternal hyperglycemia and subsequent fetal macrosomia.

Intravenous glucose tolerance testing

OGTT engages the complex physiology of normal enteral feeding, and therefore probably correlates best with the effects of maternal glucose intolerance on fetal environment following meals. However, for reasons of gastric distress, inadequate patient compliance with the test protocol or because of alterations in gastric emptying and enteric hormonal responses due to Roux-en-Y or other gastric surgeries to reduce morbid obesity, oral glucose testing may not be feasible or appropriate. Silverstone

et al[32] adapted a 25-g intravenous glucose tolerance test (IVGTT) to pregnancy.

The test response is the rate of disappearance of glucose from the peripheral circulation:

$$\log_e y = \log_e A - kt$$

where y is the plasma glucose concentration, A is the y intercept and t is the elapsed time. The slope, k, can be computed as:

$$k = (\log_e A - \log_e B)/(\text{time B} - \text{time A}) \times 100$$

indicating that the higher the value of k the more rapid the disappearance of peripheral plasma glucose, the greater the peripheral insulin sensitivity and, by inference, the more glucose tolerant the patient. Posner et al[33] has provided a table that allows computation of the k value from the 10- and 60-minute postinfusion plasma glucose values. Silverstone et al found that the lower limit of the k value (mean − 2 SD) was 1.37 in the first, 1.18 in the second, and 1.13 in the third trimester.[32] O'Sullivan et al[34] observed a mean third-trimester k value of 2.02 and a postpartum mean value of 2.53. However, studies of IVGTTs in pregnancy have not examined the association of k values with maternal glycemic response to mixed nutrient meals or perinatal morbidity.

Other analytes associated with maternal hyperglycemia

Glycated proteins have the potential for serving as a marker for maternal hyperglycemia useful in identifying glucose-intolerant pregnancies at risk for diabetes-related perinatal morbidity. Glycation is the slow, almost irreversible, binding of a phosphorylated sugar to a protein. Binding of fructose to plasma proteins and glucose to hemoglobin (by several methods) have both been found to correlate with glucose among frank diabetic patients. Some studies have shown that hemoglobin A1c (HbA1c) glycation product concentrations can differentiate normal patients from those with gestational diabetes. Most, however, have failed to show sufficient sensitivity for identifying GDM at acceptable test specificity. Using an HbA1c threshold of 6.8%, for example, among unselected gravidas, Cousins et al[35] were able to achieve a sensitivity for GDM (ADA criteria) of 80% only at an unacceptably low specificity of 57%. Another glycated protein product, fructosamine, has been found to reflect chronic hyperglycemia, but, like HbA1c, lacked sufficient discriminatory power to be useful as a screening or diagnostic test for glucose intolerance. Among other investigators, Nasrat et al[36] found that among unselected gravidas, second- and third-trimester fructosamine values correlated poorly with fasting glucose values, identifying only 50% of GDM cases at a threshold at the 90th centile.

LaPolla et al[37] performed 50-g glucose challenge tests (GCTs) on 758 gravidas screened at 24–27 weeks of gestation and 100-g GTTs on those with abnormal GCTs. Macrosomia and ponderal index at birth did not differ among the four groups (negative GCT, positive GCT, one or two or more elevated GTT values). HbA1c values correlated with maternal glucose intolerance grouping. Logistic regression identified maternal GCT plasma glucose as the only independent correlate with macrosomia and ponderal index of greater than or equal to 2.85. The authors concluded that HbA1c does not predict fetal overgrowth in a screened obstetric population.

TESTING CONDITIONS

The glycemic stimulus obtained with oral testing is a function of the rapidity of gastric emptying and enteric endocrine responses, themselves a function of nutrients in the upper gastrointestinal track. A cross-sectional case series among unselected mid-pregnancy gravidas by Berkus et al[38] examined the effect of the interval between the last meal and administration of the 50-g glucose challenge 1-hour glucose value. They demonstrated a direct association between time interval and insulin response, but no measurable difference in glycemic response when the 50-g glucose challenge was ingested within 3 hours of the last meal. However, somewhat different findings were reported in a randomized cross-over trial, in which the impact of a mixed nutrient meal 1 hour prior to a 50-g OGT was examined separately in gravidas confirmed with and without gestational diabetes.[39] Little effect of the preceding diet was found among non-diabetic gravidas. In contrast, fasting patients with GDM had greater 1-hour post 50-g glucose load values than those obtained from the same subjects when they had eaten a 600 kcal mixed nutrient meal 1 hour prior to glucose load (9.7 mmol/L vs 8.6 mmol/L [173.9 mg/dL vs 154.9 mg/dL]; p = 0.01). These studies did not investigate sequential intervals between meals and glucose ingestion, nor the effect of preceding meals on glycemic response among those with very mild degrees of glucose intolerance.

EVIDENCE-BASED DIAGNOSTIC GLYCEMIC THRESHOLDS AND THERAPEUTIC INTERVENTIONS

The literature regarding testing thresholds has been flawed in several respects, including clear definition of groups studied, conditions of testing, choice of biologic and medical outcomes of interest, and, most saliently, failure to blind investigators, subjects, and caregivers to patient glycemic test data. Until recently,[40] no study has examined the association of mild degrees of maternal glucose intolerance with fetal outcome among a large number of gravidas in multiple racial and ethnic groups and geographic settings. Further, no large study has examined this association by employing protocols that insure that glucose tolerance status remains unknown to investigators and caregivers during the observation period. The likelihood of a bias in subject recruitment, inadequately defined (or inconsistently applied) testing and assessment protocols, confounding by treatment intervention and knowledge of glucose tolerance status by those examining pregnancy outcomes have significantly limited interpretation and generalizability of study findings. Finally, almost all studies have selected a priori screening or diagnostic thresholds, so that an assessment of the most appropriate threshold or thresholds could not be addressed.

Crowther et al's recent randomized trial of diagnosis and intervention in pregnancies with GDM (WHO criteria) established that dietary counseling, glucose surveillance, and insulin treatment improves outcome in the studied population whose glucose intolerance met WHO criteria, but did not investigate the diagnostic threshold of mild maternal glucose intolerance that would identify those who benefit from these interventions.[22] Consequently, the US Preventive Services Task Force (USPSTF) report in 2008 concluded that "current evidence is insufficient to assess the balance of benefits and harms of screening for gestational diabetes mellitus, either before or after 24 weeks' gestation".[41] Further, its authors noted that "the literature is limited by lack of a consistent standard for screening or diagnosis of gestational diabetes".[42] However, subsequent to the publication of the USPSTF report, another randomized, blinded multicenter study of the treatment of mild glucose intolerance in the US[1] found improvement in maternal and perinatal outcomes similar to those reported in Crowther's[22] study. Perhaps this reaffirmation of the benefits of treatment of mild gestational glucose intolerance will be sufficient to achieve recognition of the benefits of its treatment by the USPSTF and other bodies which set standards for clinical practice.

The limited understanding of the association of mild degrees of maternal glucose intolerance and unfavorable perinatal outcome was the rationale for the Hyperglycemia and Adverse Pregnancy Outcome (HAPO) study.

Its initial findings have recently been published.[40] This study has the following attributes that will uniquely address many of the above questions:

- Observational cohort study involving over 25 000 gravidas in nine countries
- 75-g OGTT (fasting, 1 and 2 hours) at 24–32 weeks of gestation
- Investigators, subjects, and caregivers were blinded to test results, except in subjects with fasting values greater than 5.8 mmol/L (>105 mg/dL) or 2-hour values greater than 11.1 mmol/L (>200 mg/dL)
- Outcomes included absolute and age-relative birthweights, primary cesarean delivery, cord serum c-peptide, protocol-driven neonatal glucose and bilirubin levels, and clinical neonatal hypoglycemia.

This study has identified a robust correlation between all three maternal GTT values below those meeting the study's exclusion criteria for diabetes, and absolute and relative birthweight and protocol-driven neonatal c-peptide and glucose values. These data are presently being examined to determine the best test glucose thresholds to be used for imposition of maternal glucose surveillance and intervention during pregnancy.

CONCLUSIONS

Since their development in the 1960s, the criteria used to define hyperglycemia first diagnosed during pregnancy have been, in most instances, neither uniform nor comparable. Central to this conundrum has been the lack of definitive evidence of a relationship between different degrees of glucose intolerance and clinically important maternal and perinatal outcomes. Further confounding the justification for establishing such criteria was the lack of evidence of efficacy of treatment of women identified as having gestational diabetes. In recent years, a controlled, double-blinded study did demonstrate that treatment of gestational diabetes does avert some perinatal and maternal adverse outcomes. In another large, multinational study, the nature of the quantitative relationship between levels of maternal glycemia and adverse maternal and perinatal outcomes was demonstrated to be progressive and continuous. It is hoped that the latter study will provide the basis for international consensus for the diagnostic criteria defining glucose intolerance in pregnancy. Once this consensus is achieved, studies may be designed to evaluate the effectiveness of different interventions on women whose diagnosis of gestational glucose intolerance is uniform, and whose results may therefore be universally applied.

REFERENCES

1 National Diabetes Data Group. Classification and diagnosis of diabetes mellitus and other categories of glucose intolerance. *Diabetes* 1979;**28**:1039–57.
2 World Health Organization. *WHO Consultation: Definition, Diagnosis and Classification of Diabetes Mellitus and Its Complications: Report of a WHO Consultation. Part 1: Diagnosis and Classification of Diabetes Mellitus.* WHO/NCD/NCS/99.2. Geneva: WHO, 1999.
3 American Diabetes Association. Gestational diabetes mellitus. *Diabetes Care* 2009;**32**:S62–7.
4 O'Sullivan JB, Mahan CM. Criteria for the oral glucose tolerance test in pregnancy. *Diabetes* 1964;**13**:278–85.
5 American Diabetes Association. Gestational diabetes mellitus. *Diabetes Care* 2000;**23** (Suppl 1):S77–9.
6 Professional Practice Subcommittee, American Diabetes Association. Clinical Practice Recommendations. *Diabetes Care* 2001;**2** (Suppl 1):S5–S10.
7 Karlsson K, Kjellmer I. The outcome of diabetic pregnancies in relation to the mother's blood sugar level. *Am J Obstet Gynecol* 1972;**112**:313–20.
8 O'Sullivan JB, Charles D, Mahan CM, *et al.* Gestational diabetes and perinatal mortality rate. *Am J Obstet Gynecol* 1973;**116**:901–4.
9 Aberg A, Rydhstrdöm H, Källén B, Källén K. Impaired glucose tolerance during pregnancy is associated with increased fetal mortality in preceding sibs. *Acta Obstet Gynecol Scand* 1997;**76**:212–7.
10 Kristensen J, Vestergaard M, Wisborg K, Kesmodel U, Secher NJ. Pre-pregnancy weight and the risk of stillbirth and neonatal death. *BJOG* 2005;**112**:403–8.
11 Conde-Agudelo A, Belizán JM, Díaz-Rossello JL. Epidemiology of fetal death in Latin America. *Acta Obstet Gynecol Scand* 2000;**79**:371–8.
12 Beischer NA, Wein P, Sheedy MT, *et al.* Identification and treatment of women with hyperglycaemia diagnosed during pregnancy can significantly reduce perinatal mortality rates. *Aust N Z J Obstet Gynaecol* 1996;**36**:239–47.
13 Dandrow RV, O'Sullivan JB. Obstetric hazards of gestational diabetes. *Am J Obstet Gynecol* 1966;**96**:1144–7.
14 Coustan DR, Imarah J. Prophylactic insulin treatment of gestational diabetes. *Am J Obstet Gynecol* 1984;**150**:836–42.
15 O'Sullivan JB, Gellis SS, Dandrwo RV, *et al.* The potential diabetic and her treatment in pregnancy. *Obstet Gynecol* 1966;**17**:683–9.
16 Naylor CD, Sermer M, Chen E, *et al.* Cesarean delivery in relation to birth weight and gestational glucose intolerance: pathophysiology or practice style? *JAMA* 1996;**275**:1165–70.
17 Vohr BR, McGarvey ST. Growth patterns of large-for-gestational-age and appropriate-for-gestational-age infants of gestational diabetic mothers and control mothers at age 1 year. *Diabetes Care* 1997;**20**:1066–72.

18 Boney CM, Verma A, Tucker R, Vohr BR. Metabolic syndrome in childhood: association with birth weight, maternal obesity, and gestational diabetes mellitus. *Pediatrics* 2005;**115**:e290–6.

19 Sermer M, Naylor CD, Farine D, *et al.* The Toronto Tri-Hospital Gestational Diabetes Project. A preliminary review. *Diabetes Care* 1998;**21** (Suppl 2):B33–42.

20 Carpenter MW, Coustan DR. Criteria for screening tests for gestational diabetes. *Am J Obstet Gynecol* 1982;**144**:768–73.

21 Screening for diabetes mellitus. In: *United States Preventive Services Task Force Guide to Clinical Preventive Services*, 2nd edn. Baltimore: Williams & Wilkins, 1996:193–208.

22 Crowther CA, Hiller JE, Moss JR, McPhee AJ, Jeffries WS, Robinson JS. Australian Carbohydrate Intolerance Study in Pregnant Women (ACHOIS) Trial Group. Effect of treatment of gestational diabetes mellitus on pregnancy outcomes. *N Engl J Med* 2005;**352**:2477–86.

23 Sacks, DA, Abu-Fadil S, Greenspoon JS, *et al.* Do the current standards for glucose tolerance testing in pregnancy represent a valid conversion of O'Sullivan's original criteria? *Am J Obstet Gynecol* 1989;**161**:638–41.

24 Getahun D, Nath C, Ananth CV, *et al.* Gestational diabetes in the United States: temporal trends 1989 through 2004. *Am J Obstet Gynecol* 2008;**198**:525.e1–5.

25 Cousins L. Obstetric complications. In: Reece EA, Coustan DR (eds). *Diabetes Mellitus in Women*, 3rd edn. 2004. Philadelphia: Lippincott Williams & Wilkins, 2004: 351–62.

26 Lind T, Phillips PR. Influence of pregnancy on the 75-g OGTT. A prospective multicenter study. The Diabetic Pregnancy Study Group of the European Association for the Study of Diabetes. *Diabetes* 1991;**40** (Suppl 2):8–13.

27 Bonomo M, Gandini ML, Mastropasqua A, *et al.* Which cutoff level should be used in screening for glucose intolerance in pregnancy? *Am J Obstet Gynecol* 1998;**179**:179–85.

28 Weiss PAM, Haeusler M, Kainer F, *et al.* Toward universal criteria for gestational diabetes: relationships between seventy-five and one hundred gram glucose loads and between capillary and venous glucose concentrations. *Am J Obstet Gynecol* 1998;**178**:830–5.

29 Schmidt MI, Duncan BB, Reichelt AJ, *et al.* Gestational diabetes mellitus diagnosed with a 2-h 75-g oral glucose tolerance test and adverse pregnancy outcomes. *Diabetes Care* 2001;**24**:1151–5.

30 Reece EA, Gabrielli S, Abdalla M, *et al.* Diagnosis of gestational diabetes by the use of a glucose polymer. *Am J Obstet Gynecol* 1989;**160**:383–4.

31 Chastang N, Hartemann-Heurtier A, Sachon C, *et al.* Comparison of two diagnostic tests for gestational diabetes in predicting macrosomia. *Diabetes Metab* 2003;**2**:139–44.

32 Silverstone FA, Solomons E, Rubricius J. The rapid intravenous glucose tolerance test in pregnancy. *J Clin Invest* 1961;**40**:2180–9.

33 Posner NA, Silverstone FA, Brewer J, *et al.* Simplifying the intravenous glucose tolerance test. *J Reprod Med* 1982;**27**:633–8.

34 O'Sullivan JB, Snyder PH, Sporer AC, *et al.* Intravenous glucose tolerance test and its modification by pregnancy. *J Clin Endocrinol Metab* 1970;**31**:33–7.

35 Cousins L, Dattel BJ, Hollingsworth DR, *et al.* Glycosylated hemoglobin as a screening test for carbohydrate tolerance in pregnancy. *Am J Obstet Gynecol* 1984;**150**:455–60.

36 Nasrat HA, Ajabnoor MA, Ardawi MS. Fructosamine as a screening-test for gestational diabetes mellitus: a reappraisal. *Int J Gynaecol Obstet* 1991;**34**:27–33.

37 Lapolla A, Dalfrà MG, Bonomo M, *et al.* Can plasma glucose and HbA1c predict fetal growth in mothers with different glucose tolerance levels? *Diabetes Res Clin Pract* 2007;**77**:465–70.

38 Berkus MD, Stern MP, Mitchell BD, *et al.* Does fasting interval affect the glucose challenge test? *Am J Obstet Gynecol* 1990;**163**:1812–17.

39 Coustan DR, Widness JA, Carpenter MW, *et al.* Should the 50 gram one hour screening test for gestational diabetes be administered in the fasting or fed state? *Am J Obstet Gynecol* 1986;**154**:1031–5.

40 HAPO Study Cooperative Research Group, Metzger BE, Lowe LP, *et al.* Hyperglycemia and adverse pregnancy outcomes. *N Engl J Med* 2008;**358**:2061–3.

41 U.S. Preventive Services Task Force. Screening for gestational diabetes mellitus: U.S. Preventive Services Task Force recommendation statement. *Ann Intern Med* 2008;**148**: 759–65.

42 Hillier TA, Vesco KK, Pedula KL, *et al.* Screening for gestational diabetes mellitus: a systematic review for the U.S. Preventive Services Task Force. *Ann Intern Med* 2008;**148**: 766–75.

43 Landon MB SC, Spony CY, Thom E, *et al.* A multicenter randomized trial of treatment for mild gestational diabetes. *N Engl J Med* 2009;**361**:1339–48.

7 Rationale for treatment of hyperglycemia in pregnancy

Robert Fraser

Academic Unit of Reproductive and Developmental Medicine, University of Sheffield, Sheffield, UK

PRACTICE POINTS
- Modern management of gestational diabetes mellitus (GDM) in pregnancy is designed to reduce perinatal morbidity.
- All women with GDM should be given appropriate professional dietary advice, as soon as possible after the diagnosis.
- Insulin remains the mainstay of hypoglycemic therapy, but the short-acting sulfonylureas and the biguanide metformin might have an increasingly important role in the future in GDM management.

CASE HISTORY

Mrs VR, 34 years of age, had two previous uncomplicated pregnancies 12 and 6 years earlier. The first pregnancy resulted in a normal vaginal delivery of a healthy female infant weighing 3.4 kg at 40 weeks of gestation. The second pregnancy also delivered at term but on this occasion the infant was a healthy male weighing 4.8 kg. The birthweight centiles were therefore 60% and above 90%. In her most recent pregnancy, a 75-g OGTT screening was performed at 28 weeks of gestation on the grounds of obesity (body mass index [BMI] 32 kg/m^2) and her previous macrosomic infant. The fasting plasma glucose level was 6.2 mmol/L (112 mg/dL) and the 2-hour value 10.1 mmol/L (192 mg/dL), confirming a diagnosis of GDM.

She was given standard dietary advice, but despite this her mean fasting and postprandial glucose levels on home testing were 6.3 mmol/L (113 mg/dL) and the 1-hour postprandial measure was at a mean of 12.0 mmol/L (216 mg/dL). Insulin therapy was commenced at 31 weeks to achieve target glucose levels of less than 5.0 mmol/L (90 mg/dL) fasting and less than 7.8 mmol/L (140 mg/dL) 1-hour postprandial. Serial

ultrasound scans of head circumference at 31, 33, 35, and 37 weeks were all at the 75th centile, but the abdominal circumferences were on the 97th centile at 31 and 33 weeks, and on the 90th centile at 35 and 37 weeks. This suggests a positive response to the insulin prescription in preventing a recurrence of fetal overgrowth. The infant was delivered following induction of labour at 38 weeks of gestation, and was at 3.8 kg, the 90th centile for gestational age, and had no neonatal morbidity. This case illustrates a successful use of GDM screening and a positive response to targeted insulin therapy.

- What evidence is there for adverse effects on the fetus of hyperglycemia in the second half of pregnancy?
- What evidence is there for the modification of these adverse effects by treatment aimed at reducing hyperglycemia?
- What are the roles of diet therapy, insulin, and/or oral hypoglycemic agents in the control of hyperglycemia?

BACKGROUND

The adverse effects of hyperglycemia on the fetus have been recognized since women with diabetes first began to survive and reproduce. Very high rates of late pregnancy fetal loss, and excessive fetal growth were recognized several years ago. In the observational study of Karlsson and Kjellmer, for instance, evidence appeared to suggest that perinatal mortality, if not morbidity, could be mediated by impaired maternal glycemic control.[1] The recognition that similar risks of increased perinatal mortality and morbidity were present in gestational diabetes really started with the studies of O'Sullivan in Boston.

In the late 1950s, O'Sullivan and his colleagues identified a normal range for the 100-g oral glucose tolerance test (OGTT) in pregnancy, which is the basis for screening criteria still used commonly in the US today. In a series of pioneering experiments, they established by randomized controlled trial that untreated GDM was associated with an excess of perinatal mortality and fetal macrosomia. They randomized women with GDM to treatment with prophylactic insulin (20 U of isophane, 10 U of regular insulin) each morning, or no treatment, and compared them with a non-diabetic control group. Insulin treatment resulted in a non-significant trend to lower perinatal mortality: treated 4 of 111 (3.6%); untreated 10 of 118 (8.5%). Those most at risk of perinatal loss were further identified by subgroup analysis as principally women over the age of 25 years and overweight for height. There was a significant reduction in macrosomia (birthweight >4.0 kg) at birth from 13.1% in the untreated group to 4.3% in the insulin-treated group.[2]

It became practice for treatment with prophylactic insulin to be offered. After this practice was evaluated by such as Gabbe *et al*,[3] it was reported that the recognition and treatment of gestational diabetes was in fact associated with a *lower* perinatal mortality than that of the hospital population. Further uncontrolled studies of insulin therapy offered prophylactically by Coustan and colleagues[4] in the US suggested that birthweight was very sensitive to the regime of once-daily prophylactic insulin, but women managed solely on dietary regimes had an expectation of birthweight similar to women with GDM who were untreated. Unfortunately these studies were observational rather than prospective controlled trials and it is likely that selection bias influenced the reported outcomes.

One group working in Italy, using the US diagnostic criteria, identified an apparent increase in the frequency of neonatal complications, including macrosomia, congenital abnormalities, perinatal mortality, and prematurity, as well as maternal complications such as pre-eclampsia and cesarean section in women who had a normal 100-g OGTT but who had intermediate levels of 2-hour plasma glucose within the "normal range". This group identified 16% of their population as being at increased risk of typical diabetes-related morbidity rather than the expected 3–4%.[5] Further studies suggested that one abnormal value rather than two could be associated with an adverse outcome of pregnancy.[6]

In the late 1980s and early 1990s, the idea became more widespread that the adoption of these diagnostic criteria of impaired glucose tolerance using the World Health Organization (WHO) criteria or one abnormal value using the National Diabetes Data Group (NDDG) crite-

ria might very well be over-diagnosing non-existent medical problems and involving women in potentially dangerous therapeutic intervention programs, and at the same time labeling them as having a high-risk pregnancy when in fact they did not.[7] On the other hand, there was evidence that rates of macrosomia, pre-eclampsia, and cesarean section rose in women with milder degrees of abnormal glucose tolerance in a dose–response manner.[8] This was clearly an unsatisfactory situation and in response three large-scale trials were established, the first to identify the range of adverse outcomes which might be associated with untreated mild gestational diabetes (the Hyperglycemia and Adverse Perinatal Outcome [HAPO] trial). Two double blind studies, one performed principally in Australia (Australian Carbohydrate Intolerance Study in Pregnant Women [ACHOIS])[9] and one in the US (the Maternal Fetal Medicine Units [MFMU] network randomized controlled trial), were designed to identify any adverse outcomes of untreated mild GDM, but also to evaluate any benefit of treatment if adverse outcomes were present in the untreated groups.

EVIDENCE FOR TREATMENT: INTERVENTION TRIALS

The results of the HAPO trial have been discussed in chapter 6 and suggest that in untreated women with mild gestational diabetes there is an increase in each of the primary study outcomes associated with increasing fasting glucose levels and increasing 1- and/or 2-hour glucose levels. These primary outcomes were cesarean delivery, increased birthweight, neonatal hypoglycemia, and fetal hyperinsulinism, detected by cord blood c-peptide measurements. The HAPO study is an observational study and therefore cannot be used to produce guidance on treatment, but it can certainly relate to appropriate cut-offs for the interpretation of glucose tolerance testing in pregnancy.

ACHOIS trial

The ACHOIS trial is the first reported trial of treatment of gestational diabetes with a double blind design in which half the women who were randomized (n = 510) were not told that they had impaired glucose tolerance/gestational diabetes, nor were their medical attendants aware of this. The headline findings of this trial were that identification and treatment of gestational diabetes was associated with a relative risk of 0.33 (95% CI 0.14–0.75) of serious perinatal complications taken as a composite measure falling from 23 of 510 (4%) to 7 of 490 (1%). Induction of labor was more common in the intervention group as many units had a policy of elective induction with a diagnosis of gestational diabetes. The proportion of large for gestational age babies was 68 of 490 (13%) in the treated group and 115 of 510 (22%) in the routine care group (RR 0.62, 95% CI 0.47–0.81). Cesarean delivery rates were identical in the two groups.

The study included various measures of psychologic well-being to determine if patients' knowledge of their diagnosis of gestational diabetes leads to adverse outcomes. In fact, there was a general improvement in mood and well-being in the treated group, with a halving in the incidence of postnatal depression: 23 of 490 (8%) *versus* 50 of 510 (17%) (RR 0.46, 95% CI 0.29–0.73).

The ACHOIS trial was subjected to a certain amount of criticism, not least because the total incidence of adverse perinatal outcomes was that which was expected when combining the treated and untreated groups. This raised the possibility that the differences seen were a chance finding. It is more likely that this general benefit was seen as a result of a Hawthorne effect.[10] The most likely explanation for the low rate of complications overall was that the median 2-hour value in the women randomized in the ACHOIS trial was at the low end of the impaired range at 8.6 mmol/L (155 mg/dL). It was, however, a well-conducted trial with a positive endpoint, suggesting that treatment in mild gestational diabetes is beneficial and should be recommended.

MFMU Network Trial

The recently reported MFMU trial has a similar double-blind methodology to the ACHOIS trial,[11] but uses different diagnostic criteria for mild gestational diabetes. These were a fasting glucose level of less than 5.3 mmol/L (<95 mg/dL) and after a 100-g load two or more hourly glucose measurements above the following thresholds: 1 hour 10.0 mmol/L (180 mg/dL); 2 hours 8.6 mmol/L (155 mg/dL); and 3 hours 7.8 mmol/L (140 mg/dL). The primary endpoint was a composite outcome of features associated with maternal hyperglycemia, which included perinatal death, neonatal hypoglycemia, hyperbilirubinemia, hyperinsulinemia, and birth trauma. There was no significant difference in this composite primary outcome (treated group n = 485, 149 of 460 [32.4%]; control group n = 473, 163 of 440 [37.0%]; RR 0.87 [97% CI 0.72–1.07]; p = 0.14). The study cohorts included no perinatal deaths. The study did, however, report significant reductions in a series of important secondary out-

comes, mean birthweight was approximately 100 g less in the treatment group and the number of large for gestational age infants was significantly reduced in the treatment group: 34 of 477 (7.1%) compared to 66 of 454 (14.5%) in the control group; RR 0.49 (97% CI 0.32–0.76); p < 0.001. Cesarean delivery was significantly reduced (26.9% in the treatment group compared to 33.8% in the control group) and shoulder dystocia was also significantly reduced (7 [1.5%] versus 18 [4%], respectively; RR 0.37 [97% CI 0.14–0.97]; p 0.02).

In both this study and the ACHOIS trial reported above there was a significant reduction in the frequency of pre-eclampsia.

Taken together these two important studies suggest that treatment of mild GDM is likely to improve the outcome of pregnancy to an extent to make it worthwhile.

TIMING OF INTERVENTION

Gestational diabetes is a disorder of the second half of pregnancy in the majority of cases, and probably for most women only the third trimester. The endocrine-induced insulin resistance (the inverse of insulin sensitivity) of pregnancy, which would tip susceptible women over into gestational diabetes, is established by about 26 weeks in most women (Fig. 7.1).

It is the case, however, that insulin sensitivity in pregnancy can be manipulated both up and down by dietary choices, and in those women who are considered susceptible to gestational diabetes, particularly those with pre-existing obesity, the adoption of a healthy eating pattern from early pregnancy may be prophylactic against gestational diabetes later in non-diabetic women. We and others have shown that a high carbohydrate, low glycemic index (GI) diet is associated with enhanced insulin sensitivity in later pregnancy.[12] Such a dietary approach has no known adverse effects, and when applied by the DIAGEST group of Romon and colleagues (Table 7.1),[13] the percentage of large for gestational age babies in women with gestational diabetes managed on diet is inversely proportional to the quintile of carbohydrate intake. A further theoretical advantage of the low GI diet is the abolition of relative ketonemia seen in late pregnancy on a relatively high GI diet (Fig. 7.2). This is important because of the continuing concern that maternal ketonemia in late pregnancy might be capable of inducing neurodevelopmental handicap, including a lowering of IQ.[14]

In contrast, one non-randomized cohort study reported lower requirements for insulin, and lower rates

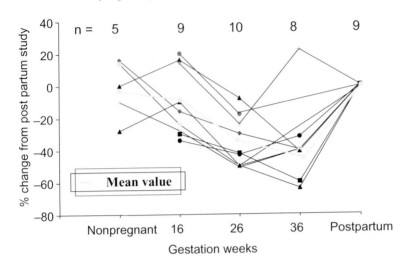

Insulin sensitivity of individual subjects throughout pregnancy expressed as % of postnatal study

Fig. 7.1 Insulin sensitivity of individual subjects and mean throughout pregnancy expressed as a percentage of postnatal study. Negative percentage change represents increasing insulin resistance. (Modified from Stanley et al. with permission from *Br J Obstet Gynaecol* 1998;105:756–9.)

Table 7.1 Proportions of large for gestational age (LGA) and small for gestational age (SGA) infants by quintiles of maternal habitual carbohydrate intake in gestational diabetes. (Modified from Romon et al[13].)

Maternal habitual carbohydrate intake (g)	<173	173–186	186–211	211–243	>243
LGA	5 (37%)	2 (12%)	4 (25%)	0 (0%)	0 (0%)
SGA	0 (0%)	0 (0%)	2 (13%)	0 (0%)	1 (6%)

of cesarean sections and newborn macrosomia with a low carbohydrate regime.[15]

STRUCTURED EDUCATION PROGRAMS

Structured education programs, such as DAFNE (Dose Adjustment For Normal Eating), which are established in the management of Type 1 diabetes, are now becoming more widely used in Type 2 diabetes. Although no appropriate studies have been performed in pregnancy, it might be assumed that structured education programs with a component of dietary management would be appropriate as a starting point for therapy in newly diagnosed gestational diabetes. Such programs have been associated with statistically significant reductions in Type 2 diabetes in percentage hemoglobin A1c (HbA1c) and include X-PERT[16] and DESMOND.[17]

In all events the presence of a trained dietitian is necessary in the multidisciplinary team, providing care for both short- and long-term lifestyle advice for this vulner-

able group, and in the short term helping to avoid the need for insulin or hypoglycemic therapy.

METHODS OF TREATMENT

Insulin regimes

In a study addressed to the wisdom of the American practice (see above) of recommending prophylactic insulin to everyone with a diagnosis of gestational diabetes, Persson and colleagues in Sweden performed a randomized trial in 200 women with impaired glucose tolerance.[18] At the time of entry, all patients were given dietary instructions by a dietitian to take a diet containing 50% of calories from carbohydrate, 20% from protein, and 30% from fat. The diet alone group was given supplementary insulin during the period of follow-up in the second half of pregnancy if the fasting blood glucose exceeded 7 mmol/L (126 mg/dL) or the 1-hour postprandial blood glucose exceeded 9 mmol/L

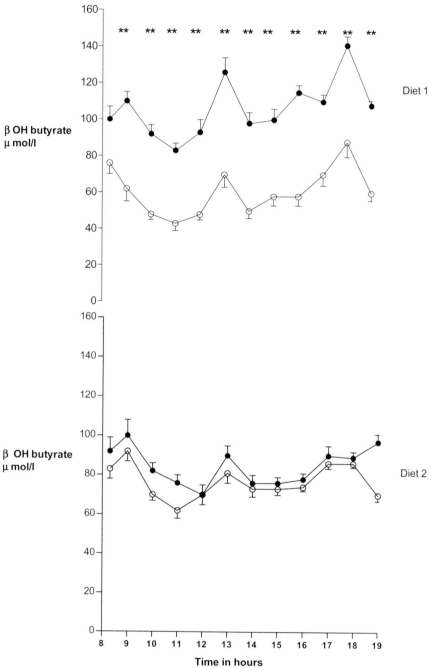

Fig. 7.2 β-Hydroxybutyrate levels in a cross-over study of pregnant subjects (●) and non-pregnant subjects (○) showing the abolition of pregnancy-induced relative ketonemia by an isocaloric low glycemic index (Diet 2) compared with a regular diet (Diet 1). ** statistically significant difference p < 0.01 (Adapted from Fraser *et al.* with permission[12])

Table 7.2 Perinatal outcomes in a randomised trial of diet alone versus diet and routine insulin in the management of gestational diabetes mellitus. (Modified from Persson *et al*[18].)

	Diet (n = 105)	Diet and insulin (n = 97)	Statistical difference
Size at birth			
Mean birthweight (g)	3560	3630	NS
SGA	3	0	NS
Appropriate for gestational age	88	86	NS
LGA	14	11	NS
Triceps skinfold thickness (mm)	5.1	4.9	NS
Neonatal morbidity			
Respiratory distress	9	15	NS
Hypoglycemia	13	18	NS
Hyperbilirubinemia	6	8	NS
Polycythemia	5	6	NS

LGA, large for gestational age; SGA, small for gestational age

(162 mg/dL) on at least three occasions during a period of 7 days. The group on routine insulin with diet were prescribed 8–12 IU/day of rapid or intermediate acting insulin and doses were adjusted to attempt to maintain fasting glucose below 5 mmol/L (90 mg/dL) and 1-hour postprandial values below 6.5 mmol/L (117 mg/dL). Fifteen patients (14%) in the diet-treated group required insulin. The important maternal and infant outcomes are summarized in Table 7.2, and it can be seen that birthweights were not significantly different nor was there an excess of large for gestational age infants in the diet-treated group. Measurements were made of the c-peptide levels in cord blood as an index of metabolic perturbation and there was no difference between the two groups. The conclusion of this important study, which has not been superseded, is that there is no obvious benefit to routine hypoglycemic therapy in gestational diabetes if diet therapy is capable of maintaining blood glucose profiles within the targeted range. The likelihood of a woman with gestational diabetes requiring additional hypoglycemic therapy is about 15%.

A refinement of the selection of women for insulin treatment using ultrasound parameters of fetal growth has been reported in two distinct studies. The study of Buchanan and colleagues[19] randomized women with gestational diabetes who had a fasting plasma glucose on a glucose tolerance test, less than 5.8 mmol/L (105 mg/dL) and a fetal abdominal circumference above the 75th centile for gestational age between 29 and 33 weeks of gestation. Subjects were randomized to either diet or diet plus twice-daily insulin using glycemic targets premeal of less than 5.8 mmol/L (<104 mg/dL) of glucose and 2 hours postmeal of less than 6.7 mmol/L (<120 mg/dL) of glucose. Mean birthweights in the insulin-treated *versus* diet-treated groups were 3.64 *versus* 3.87 kg, and the prevalence of large for gestational infants was 13% *versus* 45%, respectively, which was statistically significant.

The second study of Kjos and colleagues[20] had a different design in which 98 women with gestational diabetes and a fasting plasma glucose of 5.8–6.7 mmol/L (105–120 mg/dL) were randomized to a standard group, who all received insulin treatment, and an experimental group, who only received insulin if their fasting plasma glucose exceeded 6.7 mmol/L (120 mg/dL) or the ultrasound measured abdominal circumference in any 4-week period was above the 70th centile. In this study maternal and perinatal outcomes were not significantly different, although there was an unexplained reduction in the cesarean section rate in the insulin-treated group. Thirty of 49 women in the experimental group ended up on insulin before delivery but this was interpreted as a 38% reduction in the number of patients who required insulin therapy. This reduction could be achieved without any increase in maternal or perinatal morbidity.

Treatment targets

One randomized controlled trial in GDM has been published looking at the timing of blood glucose monitoring in relation to insulin therapy.[21] This study involved 66 women with gestational diabetes who were judged to require insulin therapy based on fasting plasma glucose levels of ≥5.9 mmol/L (105 mg/dL) or 1-hour postprandial glucose levels of ≥7.8 mmol/L (140 mg/dL) despite diet therapy. Randomization was to the timing schedule of blood glucose measurements as a guide to therapy. In one

Table 7.3 Pregnancy outcomes in a randomized controlled trial comparing preprandial and postprandial blood glucose monitoring in women with gestational diabetes. (Modified from de Veciana et al[21].)

	Preprandial (n = 33)	Postprandial (n = 33)	RR (95% CI)	p value
Target control met (%)	86.0 ± 4.1	88.0 ± 5.2		
Insulin dose (U/day)	76.8 ± 21.4	100.4 ± 29.5		0.003
Final HbA1c (%)	8.1 ± 2.2	6.5 ± 1.4		0.007
Maternal outcomes				
Pre-eclampsia	2 (6%)	2 (6%)		NS
GA at delivery (weeks)	37.6 ± 3.8	37.9 ± 1.4		NS
CS	13 (39%)	8 (24%)		NS
3° or 4° tear	8 (24%)	3 (9%)		NS
Neonatal outcomes				
Birthweight (g)	3848 ± 434	3469 ± 668		0.01
LGA	14 (42%)	4 (12%)	3.5 (1.3–9.5)	0.01
SGA	0	1 (3%)		NS
Shoulder dystocia	6 (18%)	1 (3%)		NS
Hypoglycemia (<1.6 mmol/L [29 mg/dL])	7 (21%)	1 (3%)	7.0 (0.9–53.8)	NS

CS, cesarean section; LGA, large for gestational age; SGA, small for gestational age

group glucose was measured preprandially with a target of 3.3–5.0 mmol/L (60–90 mg/dL) and in the second group, glucose was measured postprandially 1 hour after a meal with a target of less than 7.8 mmol/L (140 mg/dL).

The results are summarized in Table 7.3, and it can be seen that the majority of women met their target control but the insulin dose was 25% higher in the postprandial than the preprandial group, and this was associated with a significantly lower final HbA1c, a lower birthweight, and a lower frequency of large for gestational age babies. There were non-significant trends to high rates of shoulder dystocia and neonatal hypoglycemia in the preprandial group, but the trial was obviously limited by relatively small numbers. It does seem clear, however, that postprandial targets will produce a better outcome than preprandial targets, but involve significantly higher daily insulin doses.

Oral hypoglycemic drugs

Whilst diet alone is obviously effective in the prevention of perinatal morbidity and mortality, insulin regimes will be required by about 15% of women with GDM. Insulin is not without risks, however, and recent randomized controlled trials have addressed the value of oral hypoglycemic agents, including glyburide and metformin, as alternatives to insulin. Oral treatment may be more acceptable to women than self-injection with insulin.

One large randomized controlled trial has been published[22] in which 404 women with gestational diabetes were randomized to glyburide at a dose of 2.5 mg daily, rising to 20 mg daily, or insulin 0.7 U/kg, both adjusted weekly. Glyburide is a short-acting sulfonylurea (marketed as Glibenclamide in some countries). Glycemic targets were a fasting blood glucose concentration of 3.4–5.0 mmol/L (60–90 mg/dL), a preprandial blood glucose concentration of 4.5–5.3 mmol/L (80–95 mg/dL), and a postprandial blood glucose concentration at 2 hours after a meal of less than 6.7 mmol/L (120 mg/dL). The glyburide dose was adjusted upwards but the 20-mg dose failed to maintain glycemic targets in eight women (4%). This small group of women were switched to insulin therapy but remained in the original group for analysis. There were no significant differences in percentage HbA1c in the third trimester, nor in the proportion of large for gestational age babies or the cord insulin level, and nor was there any difference in the proportion of infants with respiratory distress syndrome (8% *versus* 6%), hypoglycemia requiring intravenous dextrose (14% *versus* 11%) or neonatal unit admissions (6% *versus* 7%). Glyburide was not detected in the cord serum of any infant. This study suggests that there is likely to be a significant place for oral hypoglycemic drugs, including the sulfonylureas. Such treatment would theoretically have considerable advantages over insulin in terms of convenience and safety. Sulfonylureas, however, have their beneficial

Table 7.4 Neonatal complications in the MiG study. (Modified from Rowan *et al*[23].)

Outcome	Metformin group (n = 363) (% (n))	Insulin group (n = 370) (% (n))	Relative risk (95% CI)	p value
Recurrent blood glucose level <2.6 mmol/L [<47 mg/dL]	15.2 (55)	18.6 (69)	0.81 (0.59–1.12)	0.21
Respiratory distress	3.3 (12)	4.3 (16)	0.76 (0.37–1.59)	0.47
Birth trauma	4.4 (16)	4.6 (17)	0.96 (0.49–1.87)	0.90
5-Min Apgar score <7	0.8 (3)	0.3 (1)	3.06 (0.32–29.26)	0.37
Preterm birth (<37 weeks of gestation)	12.1 (44)	7.6 (28)	1.60 (1.02–2.52)	0.04
>24 h stay in neonatal intensive care unit	12.7 (46)	12.2 (45)	1.04 (0.71–1.53)	0.83

effects by enhancing insulin secretion, and like insulin might be the cause of excessive fat retention after pregnancy, especially in overweight or obese women.

Metformin

A randomized study (the MiG study) on a similar basis, using the biguanide metformin rather than a sulfonylurea, has recently been reported.[23] Metformin would have some theoretical advantages over sulfonylurea, in particular in women with Type 2 diabetes who are overweight at the onset of gestation. In the study, 363 women were randomized to receive metformin and 370 randomized to receive insulin, after exclusions. Randomization took place after lifestyle intervention and dietary advice left women with persisting fasting capillary blood glucose levels greater than 5.4 mmol/L (>97 mg/dL) or more than one 2-hour postprandial glucose level greater than 6.7 mmol/L (>121 mg/dL).

In the metformin arm of the MiG study, 195 subjects received metformin alone, although nine of these subjects stopped taking it before delivery. One hundred and sixty-eight subjects randomized to metformin required supplementary insulin when the glycemic targets were not maintained despite the maximum metformin dose of 2500 mg/day. All but 18 of these women continued metformin with supplementary insulin. There were no significant baseline characteristic differences between the metformin and the insulin groups. The neonatal outcomes are summarized in Table 7.4. There was no excess of neonatal hypoglycemia in the metformin group nor of respiratory distress syndrome, birth trauma, or low Apgar scores. There were no significant differences in rates of birthweight below the 10th or above the 90th centile or in any of the neonatal anthropometry measurements undertaken, including multiple skinfold thicknesses and pon-

deral index. Cord blood serum insulin concentrations were slightly higher in the metformin arm infants but this difference was not statistically significant.

It would therefore seem that there is a place for the use of metformin in the management of gestational diabetes, but that up to 46% of women treated with metformin will require supplementary insulin to maintain reasonable glycemic targets.

The secondary outcome of this study, which is probably of greatest long-term interest in relation to mother's health and prevention of future gestational diabetes or indeed Type 2 diabetes in later life, is the net weight change in the two groups. The loss of weight from enrolment to the postpartum visit was 8.1 ± 5.1 kg in the metformin group and 6.9 ± 5.3 kg in the insulin group, and this difference was highly significant (p = 0.006).

FUTURE RESEARCH

Although there is a place for surrogate measurements of beneficial outcomes of treatment of gestational diabetes, such as birthweight and shoulder dystocia, it is the case that an objective measure of long-term metabolic perturbation of the fetus is reflected in the insulin levels circulating in the fetus, which are directly proportional to the insulin levels in the amniotic fluid. Fig. 7.3 from our own laboratory shows distribution of amniotic fluid insulin at delivery, usually by cesarean section, in 45 women with normal glucose tolerance compared to a group with treated gestational diabetes and a group with treated Type 1 and Type 2 diabetes. It can be seen that despite our practice of glycemic target-oriented therapy accompanied by intensification of insulin therapy with ultrasound evidence of incipient fetal macrosomia, still at least a third of newborns of women with gestational diabetes

Amniotic Fluid Insulin at Delivery

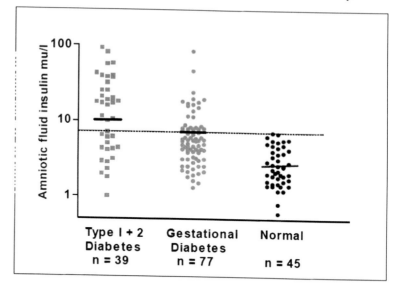

Fig. 7.3 Amniotic fluid (AF) insulin levels at delivery in cohorts of women with pre-existing diabetes, GDM, and normal glucose tolerance. AF insulin above the normal range suggests the extent of metabolic perturbation experienced by the fetus (Fraser R, Bruce C, unpublished observations).

have amniotic fluid insulin levels above the upper limit of the normal distribution. This almost certainly explains the continuing morbidity seen in such cases and represents a therapeutic target which can be addressed by enhanced maternal diabetic control, either with diet and insulin or oral hypoglycemics. Weiss *et al* reported a small number of women who had serial amniocentesis performed and, when their liquor insulin levels were above the normal range, intensification of insulin therapy was applied. In each case reported, fetal insulinization appeared to be corrected and the authors report no typical fetal morbidity in their series.[24]

One randomized study has been reported in which 123 women were managed either on the basis of mean blood glucose or mean blood glucose with enhanced insulin therapy if amniocentesis revealed fetal hyperinsulinemia. The test was performed between the 28th and 32nd week of pregnancy. There were significant reductions in the proportion of large for gestational age babies and the frequency of neonatal hypoglycemia in this study.[25]

CONCLUSIONS

There is good quality evidence that treatment of relative hyperglycemia in pregnancy is associated with an improved short-term outcome for the newborn infant. Whilst insulin remains the mainstay of treatment, par-

ticularly in those with pre-existing diabetes, the importance of good quality dietary advice and the potential role of oral hypoglycemic drugs will be increasingly important for the treatment of hyperglycemia in gestational diabetes.

REFERENCES

1 Karlsson K, Kjellmer I. The outcome of diabetic pregnancies in relation to the mother's blood sugar levels. *Am J Obstet Gynecol* 1972;**112**:213–20.

2 O'Sullivan JB. Prospective study of gestational diabetes and its treatment. In: Sutherland HW, Stowers JM (eds). *Carbohydrate Metabolism in Pregnancy and the Newborn.* Edinburgh: Churchill Livingstone, 1975:195–204.

3 Gabbe SG, Mestman JH, Freeman RK, Anderson GV, Lowensohn RI. Managaement and outcome of Class A diabetes mellitus. *Am J Obstet Gynecol* 1977;**127**:465–9.

4 Coustan DR, Lewis SB. Insulin therapy for gestational diabetes. *Obstet Gynecol* 1978;**51**:306–10.

5 Tallarigo L, Giampietro O, Penno G, Miccoli R, Gregori G, Navalesi R. Relation of glucose tolerance to complications of pregnancy in nondiabetic women. *N Engl J Med* 1986; **315**:989–92.

6 Langer O, Anyaebunam A, Brustman L, Divons M. Management of women with one abnormal oral glucose tolerance value reduces adverse outcome in pregnancy. *Am J Obstet Gynecol* 1989;**61**:593–99.

7 Ales KL, Santini DL. Should all pregnant women be screened for gestational glucose intolerance. *Lancet* 1989;**1**:1187–91.

8 Sermer M, Naylor DC, Gare DJ, *et al.* Impact of increasing carbohydrate intolerance on maternal-fetal outcomes in 3637 women with gestational diabetes: The Toronto tri-hospital gestational diabetes project. *Am J Obstet Gynceol* 1995;**173**:146–56.

9 Crowther CA, Hiller JE, Moss JR, McPhee AJ, Jeffries WS, Robinson JS. Effect of treatment of gestational diabetes on pregnancy outcomes. *N Engl J Med* 2005;**352**:2477–86.

10 Roethlis-Berger FJ, Dickinson WJ. *Management and the Worker: An Account of a Research Programme Conducted by the Western Electric Company, Hawthorne Works, Chicago.* Cambridge: Havard University Press, 1939.

11 Landon MB, Spong CY, Thom E, *et al.* A multicenter, randomised trial of treatment for mild gestational diabetes. *N Engl J Med* 2009;**361**:1339–48.

12 Fraser RB, Ford FA, Lawrence GF. Insulin sensitivity in third trimester pregnancy: A randomised study of dietary effects. *Br J Obstet Gynaecol* 1988;**95**:223–9.

13 Romon M, Nuttens MC, Vambergue A, *et al.* Higher carbohydrate intake is associated with decreased incidence of newborn macrosomia in women with gestational diabetes. *J Am Dietet Assoc* 2001;**101**:897–902.

14 Rizzo TA, Metzger BE, Burns WJ, Burns K. Correlations between antepartum maternal metabolism and intelligence of offspring. *N Engl J Med* 1991;**325**:911–16.

15 Major CA, Henry J, De Veciana M, Morgan MA. The effects of carbohydrate restriction in patients with diet controlled gestational diabetes. *Obstet Gynecol* 1998;**91**:600–4.

16 Deakin TA, Cade JE, Williams R, Greenwood DC. Structured patient education: the diabetes X-PERT programme makes a difference. *Diabet Med* 2006;**23**:933–4.

17 Skinner TC, Carey ME, Cradock S, *et al.* Diabetes education and self-management for ongoing and newly diagnosed (DESMOND): process modelling of pilot study. *Patient Educ Counsel* 2006;**64**:369–77.

18 Persson B, Stangenberg M, Hansson U, Nordlander E. Gestational Diabetes Mellitus (GDM) Comparative evaluation of two treatment regimens, diet versus insulin and diet. *Diabetes* 1985;**34** (Suppl 2):101–5.

19 Buchanan TA, Kjos S, Montoro MN, *et al.* Use of fetal ultrasound to select metabolic therapy for pregnancies complicated by mild gestational diabetes. *Diabetes Care* 1994;**17**:275–83.

20 Kjos SL, Schaefer-Graf U, Sardesi S, *et al.* A randomised controlled trial using glycemic plus fetal ultrasound parameters versus glycemic parameters to determine insulin therapy in gestational diabetes with fasting hyperglycemia. *Diabetes Care* 2001;**24**:1904–10.

21 de Veciana M, Major CA, Morgan MA, *et al.* Postprandial versus preprandial blood glucose monitoring in women with gestational diabetes mellitus requiring insulin therapy. *N Engl J Med* 1995;**333**:1237–41.

22 Langer O, Conway DL, Berkus MD, Xenakis EMJ, Gonzales O. A comparison of Glyburide and insulin in women with gestational diabetes mellitus. *N Engl J Med* 2000;**343**:1134–8.

23 Rowan JA, Hague WM, Gao W, Battin MR, Moore MP. Metformin versus insulin for the treatment of gestational diabetes. *N Engl J Med* 2008;**358**:2003–15.

24 Weiss PAM, Hofman HM, Winter RR, Lichtenegger W, Pürstner P, Haas J. Diagnosis and treatment of gestational diabetes according to amniotic fluid insulin levels. *Arch Gynecol* 1986;**239**:81–91.

25 Hopp H, Vollert W, Ragosch V, *et al.* indication and results of insulin therapy for gestational diabetes mellitus. *J Perinat Med* 1996;**24**:521–30.

Section 3

Prepregnancy and pregnancy care

8 Prepregnancy care for Type 1 and Type 2 diabetes

Rosemary C. Temple

Elsie Bertram Diabetes Centre, Norfolk and Norwich University Hospital NHS Trust, Norwich, Norfolk, UK

PRACTICE POINTS

- Prepregnancy care is the additional support needed to prepare a woman with diabetes for pregnancy and should begin at least 6 months before pregnancy. A principle goal is to advise and support the woman to achieve optimization of glycemic control before conception.
- Prepregnancy care for women with Type 1 diabetes is associated with improved glycemic control in early pregnancy and a three-fold reduction in the risk of major congenital malformations in the offspring.
- Pregnancy outcomes for women with Type 2 diabetes are the same or worse as those for women Type 1 diabetes. However, women with Type 2 diabetes are less likely to receive formal prepregnancy care.
- Preconception counseling includes discussion with the patient about future plans for pregnancy, contraceptive advice, education about the increased risks associated with unplanned pregnancies, and advice on how to access prepregnancy care.
- Prepregnancy care also includes commencement of folic acid supplements, discontinuation of oral medications that have teratogenic potential, such as statins and ACE inhibitors, smoking cessation, and dietary input to encourage a healthy weight before pregnancy.

CASE HISTORY

Mary, a 25-year-old, was delighted to find she was expecting a second baby. Her first pregnancy had been complicated by gestational diabetes for which she was treated with diet from 20 weeks until delivery. Despite advice to lose weight, she had become depressed following the pregnancy and gained 9 kg. Two years later she had been diagnosed with Type 2 diabetes. She found it difficult to

keep to the recommended diet and required metformin and gliclazide to keep her blood glucose controlled. Recently she had been started on treatment for hypertension.

She was 9 weeks' pregnant. Her doctor referred her urgently to the diabetic antenatal clinic where she was shocked to discover she would need insulin treatment during her pregnancy. Her hemoglobin A1c (HbA1c) at booking was 8.4%. She commenced twice-daily insulin injections and discontinued her metformin and gliclazide. Her blood pressure medication was changed and she was prescribed folic acid tablets. Her 20-week fetal echocardiogram showed a ventricular septal defect. After 20 weeks, her diabetes became more difficult to control and she was changed to four insulin injections daily. When her blood pressure increased at 28 weeks, a second oral antihypertensive medication was added. Development of pre-eclampsia led to an emergency cesarean section at 35 weeks. The baby was admitted to the neonatal intensive care unit for treatment of hypoglycemia. The latter led to difficulties establishing breastfeeding. She was informed that the baby would require surgery later to correct the cardiac defect.

- How effective is prepregnancy care in reducing risks of complications in women with diabetes?
- What evidence is there for prepregnancy care in women with Type 2 diabetes?
- What should preconception counseling include?
- Why do women not access prepregnancy care?
- Is prepregnancy care cost-effective?

BACKGROUND

Prepregnancy care for women with diabetes was introduced over 30 years ago and is associated with improved pregnancy outcomes. However, overall pregnancy outcomes remain very poor for women with diabetes with only a third receiving prepregnancy care. Worldwide, Type 2 diabetes is the most common type of diabetes to complicate pregnancy. Women with Type 2 diabetes are more likely to enter pregnancy with obesity and taking potentially teratogenic medications. It is therefore essential that all healthcare professionals delivering diabetes care to reproductive-age women and female adolescents understand the importance of prepregnancy care and are able to provide preconception counseling at routine consultations with women of reproductive age.

HISTORY OF PREPREGNANCY CARE

Molsted-Pedersen first described in 1964 the high incidence of congenital malformations in infants of diabetic women, with 6.4% having a malformation compared to 2.1% of those born to women without diabetes.[1] Hyperglycemia was proposed as a possible mechanism with both animal and human studies supporting this hypothesis.[2,3] However, the concept of prepregnancy care for women with diabetes to decrease the incidence of fetal malformations was developed after Pedersen observed the relationship between maternal hyperglycemia and the development of fetal anomalies. He noted that, "the occurrence of hypoglycemic reactions and insulin coma during the first trimester was low in mothers with malformed infants indicating a positive relationship between maternal hyperglycemia early in pregnancy and the development of fetal malformations".[4]

Judith Steel established a prepregnancy clinic in Edinburgh in 1976.[5] The aims of her prepregnancy clinic included:
• Assessment of patients for complications of diabetes
• Explanation of the importance of good glucose control at all stages of pregnancy, and to improve cooperation and motivation
• Optimization of diabetic control at the time of conception
• Encouragement of women to book early for antenatal care.

EFFECTIVENESS OF PREPREGNANCY CARE

Prepregnancy care and congenital malformations

Fuhrmann's study of 420 women with Type 1 diabetes[6] showed that preconception optimization of maternal blood glucose was associated with a significant reduction in congenital malformations. In this study, intensification of glucose control included regular hospital admissions before and during pregnancy, and patients being seen twice weekly. He found a malformation rate of 0.8% in the group that had established preconception glycemic control compared to 7.5% in the control group. Later studies confirmed the effectiveness of prepregnancy care in reducing the risk of malformations (Table 8.1).[5,7–14] A meta-analysis of 14 studies of prepregnancy care, which included 1192 offspring of mothers who received prepregnancy care and 1459 offspring of mothers who did not, showed that lack of prepregnancy care was

Table 8.1 Prepregnancy care (PPC) and congenital malformations in Type 1 diabetes. (Data from references 5–14.)

Author	Year	PPC		No PPC	
		Number	Malformations (%)	Number	Malformations (%)
Fuhrmann et al[6]	1983	128	0.8	292	7.5
Goldman et al[7]	1986	44	0	31	9.7
Mills et al[8]	1988	347	4.9	279	9.0
Kitzmiller et al[9]	1991	84	1.2	110	10.9
Rosenn et al[10]	1991	28	0	71	1.4
Cousins[11]	1991	27	0	347	6.6
Drury & Doddridge[12]	1992	100	1.0	244	4.1
Willhoitte et al[13]	1993	62	1.6	123	6.5
Steel[5]	1994	196	1.5	117	12.0
Temple et al[14]	2006	110	1.8	180	6.1

Table 8.2 Prepregnancy care (PPC) and pregnancy outcomes in women with Type 1 diabetes. (Data from Temple *et al*[14].)

	PPC (n = 110)	No PPC (n = 180)	p value
Pregnancy complications			
Delivery <34 weeks (%)	5.0	14.2	0.02
Macrosomia (%)	44.0	43.4	NS
Pre-eclampsia (%)	13.1	12.7	NS
Pregnancy outcome[†]			
Spontaneous abortion	6 (5.7)	22 (14.0)	0.056
Malformation	2 (1.8)	11 (6.1)	0.065
Stillbirth	1	4	
Neonatal death	0	2	
Adverse outcome[*]	3 (2.9)	16 (10.2)	0.026

†Pregnancy outcomes are given as number (%) with percentages expressed as % of total number of pregnancies
*Adverse outcomes include congenital malformations, stillbirths and neonatal deaths

associated with a three-fold increase in the risk of major congenital malformation.[15]

Prepregnancy care and spontaneous abortions

Studies have shown that the risk of spontaneous abortion is increased three- to four-fold in women with poor glycemic control in early pregnancy.[16,17]

One early study showed that prepregnancy care is associated with a reduced risk of spontaneous abortion (8.4% compared to 28%).[18] A further study reported that prepregnancy care was associated with a strong trend towards a significant reduction in risk of spontaneous abortion (5.7% compared to 14.0%) (Table 8.2).[14]

Prepregnancy care and perinatal morbidity

There are few data on the effect of prepregnancy care on perinatal morbidity or obstetric complications. A study in Type 1 diabetes showed prepregnancy care was associated with a non-significant reduction in neonatal care admissions (17% *vs* 34%).[19] Further research in 290 women with Type 1 diabetes showed that prepregnancy care was associated with a significant reduction in delivery before 34 weeks of gestation (5.0% *vs* 14.2%).[14]

Some authors have suggested a link between early glycemic control and risks of macrosomia and pre-eclampsia.[20,21] However, a recent study showed no relationship between prepregnancy care and risk of macrosomia or pre-eclampsia, suggesting that these

complications are related to glycemic control in later rather than early pregnancy (Table 8.2).[14]

Prepregnancy care in Type 2 diabetes

A small number of studies of prepregnancy care and malformation have included women with Type 2 diabetes, but there have been no studies of Type 2 diabetes as a separate group.[11,13]

One study of 389 women with Type 1 diabetes and 146 women with Type 2 diabetes showed outcomes were significantly poorer in women with Type 2 diabetes, with a four-fold increase in risk of major malformation. The women with Type 2 diabetes, compared to the women with Type 1 diabetes, were less likely to have received any prepregnancy care (28.7 *vs* 40.5%).[22]

UK CONFIDENTIAL ENQUIRY INTO MATERNAL AND CHILD HEALTH

The 2002–2003 UK Confidential Enquiry into Maternal and Child Health (CEMACH) report has confirmed how poor pregnancy outcomes remain for women with diabetes.[23–25] It described 2767 pregnancies in women with Type 1 diabetes and 1041 pregnancies in women with Type 2 diabetes. There was an almost four-fold increase in risk of malformations of the nervous and cardiovascular systems. The study included a confidential enquiry of 222 pregnancies with a poor outcome (death of baby between 20 weeks of gestation and 28 days after delivery or major congenital anomaly), 220 control cases with a good outcome, and also a further 79 cases in women with Type 2 diabetes with a good pregnancy outcome. Its conclusions, in relation to prepregnancy care, are summarized.

1 Only 17% of the units provided multidisciplinary prepregnancy care for women with diabetes.
2 62% of women with Type 1 diabetes and 75% of women with Type 2 diabetes had *no* evidence of prepregnancy counseling.
3 68% of women had *no* record of discussion of contraception.
4 73% of women were defined as having substandard preconception care.
5 63% of women had *no* test of glycemia in the 6 months before pregnancy.
6 65% of women with Type 1 diabetes and 51% women with Type 2 diabetes had an HbA1c above 7% at the end of the first trimester.
7 Suboptimal preconception care was associated with a five-fold increased risk of poor pregnancy outcome (defined as death of the baby after 20 weeks until 28 days following delivery or a major congenital malformation).
8 The CEMACH report concluded that preconception services across the UK are "fragmented and ineffective" and thus not meeting the needs of women with diabetes.

WHY DO WOMEN NOT ATTEND FOR PREPREGNANCY CARE?

The CEMACH study showed only a third of women attended for prepregnancy care. In contrast, a nationwide study from the Netherlands showed that 70% women with Type 1 diabetes planned their pregnancies.[26]

The differences between women who do or do not attend for prepregnancy care have been well-documented (Table 8.3).[27,28] In particular, many women with Type 2 diabetes have often received little or no preconception counseling and no prepregnancy care.[24]

There are no simple solutions to increasing the utilization of prepregnancy care, but the following recommendations may be useful when developing a prepregnancy service.

1 Education of all healthcare professionals involved with reproductive-age women and adolescents who have diabetes about the importance of preconception counseling and prepregnancy care.
2 Preconception counseling to be given to, and documented for, all women with Type 1 and Type 2 diabetes, on a regular basis.

Table 8.3 Differences between women with diabetes who plan their pregnancy and have prepregnancy care and women who do not.[27,28] Factors which may be improved by positive interactions between the provider and his/her patient are shown in bold.

Pregnancy planned	Pregnancy unplanned
Higher socioeconomic status	Lower socioeconomic status
Higher level of education	Lower level of education
Married or stable relationship	Unmarried or no supportive partner
More likely to have Type 1 diabetes	Less likely to have Type 1 diabetes
Employed	Unemployed
Older	Younger
European, white	Belonging to ethnic minority group
Non-smoker	Smoker
Positive relationship with healthcare team	**Negative relationship with healthcare team**
Positive preconception advice	**Discouraged from pregnancy**

3 There should be easy access to prepregnancy care for all women with diabetes.
4 Positive information about pregnancy should be given as far as possible to encourage a partnership between the woman and her diabetic team.
5 Risks must be explained but the woman's wishes must also be respected and supported.
6 Blood glucose targets should be individualized and agreed upon in consultation with the woman and her partner.

COMPONENTS OF A PREPREGNANCY SERVICE

There are two separate major components to prepregnancy care:
- *Preconception counseling*, which involves discussion and education
- *Prepregnancy care*, which involves planning a pregnancy in conjunction with healthcare professionals.

Preconception counseling

Preconception counseling is the education of, and the discussion with, women of reproductive age about pregnancy and contraception. It is an essential component of every consultation in primary and/or specialist care.

- Preconception counseling is complex and not something that can be given in 2 minutes, on just one occasion, at the end of a routine diabetes consultation. It is the responsibility of *all* healthcare professionals delivering diabetes care to deliver preconception counseling.
- Discussion about future pregnancy plans.
- Education about what prepregnancy care is and how this can improve pregnancy outcomes.
- Education about increased risks of poor pregnancy outcome with poor glycemic control before and during early pregnancy.
- Advice about how to access prepregnancy care, including contact details for self-referral to the prepregnancy care team.
- Education of women with Type 2 diabetes about stopping oral hypoglycemic agents prior to conception and possible need for insulin before and/or during pregnancy.
- Documentation about use of and provision of contraception, and advise about contraception. This may involve a discussion of different types of contraception and how to obtain emergency contraception. It is important to emphasize the importance of continuing reliable contraception until optimization of glucose control has been achieved when planning a pregnancy.
- Education about necessity for commencement of folic acid supplements before pregnancy.
- Education about avoidance of statins, angiotensin-converting enzyme (ACE) inhibitors, and angiotensin-receptor blockers (ARBs) during pregnancy.
- Discussion about how diabetic complications may affect any future pregnancy.
- Information about the importance of urgent referral to a diabetic antenatal clinic should an unplanned pregnancy occur.
- Documentation of any discussion/education. In particular, preconception counseling should be documented at all annual reviews.

Prepregnancy care

Prepregnancy care is the additional care needed to prepare a woman with diabetes for pregnancy, and involves a close partnership between the woman and healthcare professionals. It includes optimization of glucose control, prescribing folic acid supplements, avoidance of potentially teratogenic medication, and discussion of maternal and fetal risks.

Prepregnancy care should ideally begin 6–12 months before a woman with diabetes embarks on a pregnancy. The time required depends on several factors, including current level of glycemic control and presence of diabetic complications.

A suggested care pathway is shown detailing the components of prepregnancy care (Table 8.4). It is preferable for prepregnancy care to be delivered by the multidisciplinary team who will care for the woman during her pregnancy, so that relationships between the patient and members of the team can be developed before the pregnancy begins. The use of a prepregnancy proforma may be useful for documentation of all the different aspects of prepregnancy care (Fig. 8.1). The proforma shown has been developed for use in 10 hospitals in one region of the UK, and has been found to be of great use when going through the many different aspects of care needed when delivering prepregnancy care.

When delivering prepregnancy care, it is important to always remember that it is a partnership between the healthcare professionals and the patient, and not a dictatorship.

Glycemic targets

Although glucose targets are suggested in the care pathway, it is important to individualize prepregnancy glycemic targets, aiming for the lowest HbA1c possible while avoiding severe hypoglycemia. Targets should be agreed upon in discussion with the patient and her family. Asking the woman how she perceives her glycemic control may give valuable insight as to how to best advise the patient to optimize her control.

Women with Type 1 diabetes should be encouraged to do up to seven blood glucose tests daily, including some night-time tests, and to record results in a home blood glucose monitoring diary. During the day, tests should be done on waking, before lunch, dinner, and bed, and 1 hour following the three main meals. Downloading glucose meters at clinic visits rather than relying on a patient's diary of results can be helpful to verify glucose monitoring. A printout of these results at each visit may assist the patient in understanding the rationale(s) for changes in insulin dose, diet distribution, or activity at given times

In occasional patients, continuous glucose monitoring systems can be extremely helpful, e.g. to identify erratic blood glucose levels in patients with a suboptimal HbA1c (Fig. 8.2).

Table 8.4 Prepregnancy care pathway for women with Type 1 or Type 2 diabetes.

At every visit, ask patient about plans for pregnancy within next 12 months	
Keen for pregnancy in next 12 months	No wish for pregnancy in next 12 months

Keen for pregnancy in next 12 months

Contraception
Document use of effective contraception
Continue contraception until optimum HbA1c achieved

Optimize glucose control
Aim for HbA1c as close to normal range as possible without significant
   hypoglycemia
Advise HGBM, 4–7 tests daily.
- Fasting glucose <5.6 mmol/L (<101 mg/dL)
- Pre-meal glucose <6 mmol/L (<108 mg/dL)
- Post-meals <7.8 mmol/L (<140 mg/dL)
Intensify insulin regime in T1 DM if needed, e.g. basal-bolus regime or
   insulin pump
Counsel about lack of data on use of long-acting insulin analogs in
   pregnancy
If Type 2 diabetes, stop oral agents and initiate insulin if suboptimal
   glucose control

Hypoglycemia
Educate about increased risk of hypos and loss of hypo awareness
   during pregnancy
Educate family about use of glucagon
Advise the patient she must test blood glucose before driving and must
   discontinue driving if she loses hypoglycemic awareness

Diet and exercise
Smoking and alcohol cessation advice
Consider education of carbohydrate counting
Emphasize consistent timing of meals and snacks
Consider recommendation of weight loss (see text)
Encourage regular exercise

Prescribe folic acid supplements
Supplemental dose may be 400 μg to 5 mg daily

Screening for diabetic complications
If retinopathy present, refer to ophthalmologist
If proteinuria present or reduced GFR, refer to nephrologist
Assess cardiac status and consider referral to cardiologist
Check thyroid function tests

Review other medication
Stop ACE inhibitors, ARBs, statins, diuretics
Treat hypertension with methyldopa or labetalol

Counsel about risks of diabetes and pregnancy
To fetus: miscarriage, malformation, stillbirth, neonatal death,
   macrosomia
To pregnancy: eclampsia, premature delivery, cesarean section
To mother: increased risk of severe hypos and DKA. Educate about sick
   day rules

Risks of retinopathy and nephropathy
Counsel about the risks of development or progression of retinopathy
   or nephropathy

Consider referral to obstetrician or perinatologist

No wish for pregnancy in next 12 months

Contraception
Document use of effective contraception

Document if preconception counseling (see text)
Continue regular review of glycemic control, screening
   every 12 months for diabetic complications,
   education on weight management and smoking
   cessation

HGBM, home glucose blood monitoring; DM, diabetes mellitus; GFR, glomerular filtration rate; ACE, angiotensin-converting enzyme; ARB, angiotensin-receptor blocker; DKA, diabetic ketoacidosis

EASIPOD
East Anglia Study Group
Improving Pregnancy Outcomes
in Diabetes

Submit by Email
Print Form
Reset Form

Patient name/code:

Date of Visit

Gravida   Parity   DOB (eg 31/1/1980):   Post code:

Type of diabetes:
- Type 1
- Type 2
- Other (specify)

Diabetes complications
- Retinopathy
- Neuropathy
- Nephropathy
- Vascular

Ethnicity
- Caucasian
- Afro-Caribbean
- Asian
- Other (please state)

Folic acid:
- None
- 400µg / day
- 5mg / day

Started:

Diabetes therapy:
- Diet alone
- Insulin
- Sulphonylurea
- Metformin
- Glitazone
- Other (specify)

Other therapy
- Statin
- ACE inhibitor
- Antidepressant
- Anti-epileptic
- Other

Insulin therapy :
- Pump
- Injections   Number

Total daily dose (Units)

Rubella immune:
- Yes
- No

Blood glucose monitoring:

Current HbA1c: Target HbA1c:

Weight (kg):   Height (m):   Contraception: Smoking:

Prepregnancy care health professionals seen:
- DSN/Educator
- Dietitian
- Obstetrician
- Other
- Midwife
- Physician
- Multidisciplinary team

Severe hypo in last 12 mths:
- Yes
- No

DKA in last 12 mths:
- Yes
- No

Comments

Risks discussed: (CEMACH figures)
- Hypoglycaemia / Warning signs change
- DKA
- Pre-eclampsia increased risk
- Caesarean delivery rate 66%
- Congenital malformation 2x greater risk
- Stillbirth 5x greater risk
- Perinatal death 3x greater risk
- Macrosomia risk 50%
- Premature delivery 3x greater risk
- Increased BMI

Follow-up prepregnancy visits

Date: HbA1c
Date: HbA1c
Date: HbA1c
Date: HbA1c
Date: HbA1c

Number of phone contacts:

Number of clinic visits:

Fig. 8.1 Prepregnancy proforma developed for use by 10 hospitals within a region of the UK. Educator includes diabetes specialist nurse or certified diabetes educator.

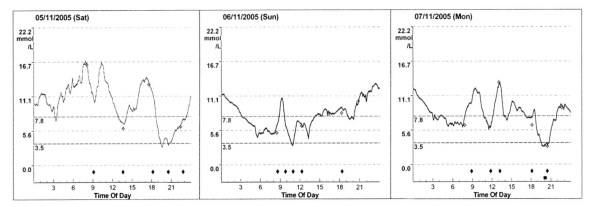

Fig. 8.2 Continuous glucose monitoring system reveals erratic blood glucose levels overnight and high postprandial peaks in a patient with Type 1 diabetes receiving prepregnancy care and managed with a basal and prandial insulin regime.

Discussing periconceptional glucose control and the risk of malformations with the patient

It is important to discuss the risk of malformations with the patient but also to be aware that giving "impossible" glycemic targets can discourage her from attending for prepregnancy care.[28]

Recent meta-analyses of studies of glycemic control and pregnancy outcome in Type 1 diabetes have shown that risks are reduced with any improvement in HbA1c. One meta-analysis of glycemic control and malformations showed a 0.4–0.6 relative risk reduction of congenital malformations for each 1% fall in HbA1c.[29] Another meta-analysis also showed a stepwise fall in risk with fall in HbA1c, with a 3% risk of malformation for a HbA1c of 6%, a 6% risk for an HbA1c of 9%, and a 12% risk for an HbA1c of 12%.[30]

A stepwise approach to reducing HbA1c may be helpful to women who are overwhelmed at the prospect of achieving an HbA1c of 6–7%. Women may be encouraged by knowing that each 1% reduction in HbA1c will improve their chance of having a healthy baby.

Hypoglycemia and hypoglycemic unawareness

This is mainly a problem for women with Type 1 diabetes. All women must be informed that they may lose their usual warning signs of hypoglycemia, and of the need to test their blood glucose before driving. Women should stop driving if they experience loss of hypoglycemic awareness. Family members should be instructed in the use of glucagon and glucogel. Although there is no human evidence to show hypoglycemia is damaging to the fetus, it is potentially harmful to the mother and can often limit the patient's success in achieving optimum glycemic control.

Several studies have shown a risk of severe hypoglycemia is most common in early pregnancy (Fig. 8.3). Evers and colleagues have shown that risk of severe hypoglycemia in the first trimester is increased in women with a lower HbA1c, increased duration of diabetes, and a history of hypoglycemia preceding pregnancy.[31] However, a recent study showed no increase in risk of severe hypoglycemia with prepregnancy care despite women with prepregnancy care having a lower HbA1c at booking.[14]

Differences between Type 1 and Type 2 diabetes

The factors contributing to poor outcome in Type 2 diabetes are complex and include suboptimal glucose control, obesity, potentially teratogenic drugs, older age, greater socioeconomic deprivation, and diverse ethnicity. Many of these can be improved with preconception care.

Obesity must be addressed with intensive dietary support to encourage an optimum body mass index (BMI). In the UK, the National Institute for Health and Clinical Excellence (NICE) guidelines on diabetes and pregnancy have recommended that women with a BMI above 27 should be given weight reduction advice prior to pregnancy.[32] This is in line with NICE guidance on obesity and results from several studies relating obesity to increased risk of malformations, macrosomia, and

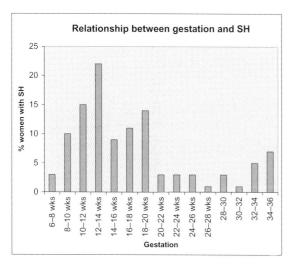

Fig. 8.3 Relationship between gestation and episodes of severe hypoglycemia (SH) in 81 women with Type 1 diabetes. The vertical axis shows the percentage of women who had at least one episode of severe hypoglycemia during the time period (Temple, unpublished data).

hypertensive disorders. Women must be advised of the increased risks of pregnancy with obesity, including maternal death, congenital malformations, and thromboembolic disorders. Treatment with orlistat, a lipase inhibitor, and sibutramine, a norepinephrine and serotonin reuptake inhibitor, have been shown to decrease weight in obese patients. Treatment with these drugs in the prepregnancy period may be considered to supplement medical nutritional therapy.

Unless the woman has polycystic ovary syndrome and the benefits of metformin outweigh the potential disadvantages, women with Type 2 diabetes should be transferred to insulin before pregnancy and oral hypoglycemic agents discontinued.

Folic acid supplements

Research has consistently shown that diabetes increases the risk of neural tube defects. It is therefore recommended that all women with diabetes take folic acid supplements when planning a pregnancy and continue this for the first 12 weeks. There are different recommendations on dose of folic acid supplements on either side of the Atlantic. In the UK, NICE guidelines recommend 5 mg daily, since this higher dose has been shown to reduce risk of neural tube defect in women who have a previous history of neural tube defect.[32] In the US,

current recommendation is for women to take folic acid 400 μg to 4 mg daily in the periconception period, the dose being dependent on whether there is a previous history of a neural tube defect.[33]

Diabetic complications

Generally patients can be reassured that pregnancy is not associated with an increased risk of microvascular complications.[34]

Retinopathy

Both pregnancy and intensification of glycemic control may increase risk of progression of retinopathy. It is therefore essential that retinal imaging is performed in the prepregnancy period and that any retinopathy be assessed and treated, if necessary, before initiation of tight glycemic control and conception. Women who have longer duration diabetes or whose retinopathy is present in early pregnancy are most at risk of deterioration in retinopathy during pregnancy.[35] Women must be advised of the need for regular ophthalmic assessment during pregnancy and of the risk of development or progression of retinopathy during pregnancy.

Renal disease

Women should have an assessment of renal function (e.g. urinalysis, serum creatinine, creatinine clearance, albumin-to-creatinine ratio, 24-hour protein) before conception. Pregnancy outcome is usually good in women with mild renal disease, but women need to be advised of the increased risk of deterioration of renal function and preeclampsia, both of which may well result in the need to deliver prematurely. These risks may be reduced with early and aggressive antihypertensive treatment.[36] Counseling about the risks for pregnancy in women with moderate to severe renal dysfunction must be done sensitively, and in women with more advanced renal dysfunction, pregnancy is contraindicated. Although the risk of complications in pregnancy is increased in women with renal transplantation, pregnancy is often associated with a good outcome. NICE recommends that women with an effective glomerular filtration rate below 45 ml/min should be seen in a joint consultation with a nephrologist before discontinuation of contraception.

Cardiovascular disease and hypertension

There is an increased risk of mortality in women who have diabetes and documented ischemic heart disease,[37] and such women should be referred for assessment by a cardiologist. They need to be counseled sensitively about the increased maternal risk with pregnancy. Severe ischemic heart disease is considered a major contraindication to pregnancy.

In women with pre-existing hypertension, strict blood pressure control should commence before pregnancy and use of ACE inhibitors, ARBs, and statins should all be discontinued. Women who conceive on ACE inhibitors are at increased risk of major congenital malformation.[38]

COST-EFFECTIVENESS OF PREPREGNANCY CARE

Several studies have established that prepregnancy care is cost-effective. One study used a combination of literature review, expert opinion, and surveys of medical care to estimate the costs and clinical consequences of prepregnancy care compared to no prepregnancy care. It was estimated that, from a combination of reduced antenatal care costs and fewer adverse maternal and neonatal outcomes, there was a saving of US$1.86 for each dollar spent.[39] A second study of 24 women with prepregnancy care and 74 women with no prepregnancy care found a net cost saving of US$34,000 per patient with prepregnancy care.[40] This was due to less hospitalization during pregnancy, a shorter stay following delivery, and both less intensity of and a shorter inpatient stay for the baby.

It is, however, important to remember both the enormous and immeasurable emotional cost to a woman of either "losing her baby" or having to care for a child with birth defect-related impairments. Such costs cannot be counted in financial terms.

FUTURE RESEARCH

The effectiveness of prepregnancy care on improving pregnancy outcomes in Type 1 diabetes is well-documented. In particular, a recent study has shown that "documentation of achievement of an optimal haemoglobin A1c prior to discontinuation of contraception" was the marker associated with the lowest risk of adverse outcome.[41]

However, there are many important areas for further study. It is essential we increase our understanding of why so few women who have diabetes and no barriers to obtaining preconception care will not access that care. This will require studies in different populations and will almost certainly also require in-depth interviews to deepen our understanding of this problem. With the obesity epidemic and rapid rise in Type 2 diabetes, it is important to study whether prepregnancy care in Type 2 diabetes is as effective, or possibly even more effective, than in Type 1 diabetes.

Prepregnancy care is one of the most effective ways to improve pregnancy outcomes in diabetes. Greater awareness both for women with diabetes and healthcare professionals is essential if we are to improve outcomes.

REFERENCES

1 Pedersen LM, Tygstrup I, Pedersen J. Congenital malformations in newborn infants of diabetic women. *Lancet* 1964;**1**:1124–6.

2 Karlsson K, Kjellemer I. The outcome of diabetic pregnancies in relation to the mother's blood sugar level. *Am J Obstet Gynecol* 1972;**112**:213–20.

3 Morii K, Watanabe G, Ingalls TH. Experimental diabetes in pregnant mice: prevention of congenital malformations in the offspring by insulin. *Diabetes* 1966;**15**:194–204.

4 Pedersen J. Congenital malformations. In: *The Pregnant Diabetic and her Newborn*, 2nd edn. Copenhagen: Munksgaard, 1977:196.

5 Steel JM. Personal experience of pre-pregnancy care in women with insulin-dependent diabetes. *Aust NZ J Obstet Gynaecol* 1994;**34**:135–9.

6 Fuhrmann K, Reiher H, Semmler K. Prevention of malformations in infants of insulin-dependent diabetic mothers. *Diabetes Care* 1983;**6**:219–23.

7 Goldman JA, Dicker D, Feldberg D, Yeshaya A, Samuel N, Karp M. Pregnancy outcome in patients with insulin-dependent diabetes mellitus with preconceptional diabetic control: A comparitive study. *Am J Obstet Gynaecol* 1986;**155**:293–7.

8 Mills JL, Knopp RH, Simpson JL, *et al.* Lack of relation of increased malformation rates in infants of diabetic mothers to glycaemic control during organogenesis. *N Engl J Med* 1988;**318**:671–6.

9 Kitzmiller JL, Gavin LA, Gin GD, Jovanovic-Peterson L, Main EK, Zigrang WD. Pre-conception care of diabetes: glycaemic control prevents congenital anomalies. *JAMA* 1991;**265**:731–6.

10 Rosenn B, Miodovnik M, Combs CA, Khoury J, Siddiqi TA. Pre-conception management of insulin dependent diabetes: improvements in pregnancy outcome. *Obstet Gynecol* 1991;**77**:846–9.

11 Cousins L. The California Diabetes and Pregnancy Programme: a statewide collaborative program for the preconception and prenatal care of diabetic women. *Ballieres Clin Obstet Gynecol* 1991;**5**:443–59.

12 Drury PL, Doddridge M. Pre-pregnancy clinics for diabetic women. *Lancet* 1992;**340**:919.

13 Willhoite MB, Bennert HW Jr, Palomaki GE, *et al.* The impact of pre-conception counselling on pregnancy outcomes. *Diabetes Care* 1993;**16**:450–5.

14 Temple RC, Aldridge VJ, Murphy HR. Prepregnancy care and pregnancy outcomes in women with type 1 diabetes. *Diabetes Care* 2006;**29**:1744–9.

15 Ray JG, O'Brien TE, Chan WS. Preconception care and the risk of congenital anomalies in the offspring of women with diabetes mellitus: a meta-analysis. *Q J Med* 2001;**94**:435–44.

16 Combs CA, Kitzmiller JL. Spontaneous abortion and congenital malformations in diabetes. *Ballieres Clin Obstet Gynaecol* 1991;**5**:315–31.

17 Temple R, Aldridge V, Greenwood R, Heyburn P, Sampson M, Stanley K. Association between outcome of pregnancy and glycaemic control in early pregnancy in type 1 diabetes: population based study. *BMJ* 2002;**325**:1275–6.

18 Dicker D, Feldberg D, Samuel N, Yeshaya A, Karp M, Goldman GA. Spontaneous abortions in patients with insulin-dependent diabetes mellitus: the effect of preconceptual diabetic control. *Am J Obstet Gynecol* 1988;**158**:1161–4.

19 Dunne FP, Brydon P, Smith T, Essex M, Nicholson H, Dunn J. Pre-conception diabetes care in insulin-dependent diabetes mellitus. *Q J Med* 1999;**92**:175–6.

20 Gold AE, Reilly R, Little J, Walker JD. The effect of glycaemic control in the pre-conception period and early pregnancy on birth weight in women with IDDM. *Diabetes Care* 1998;**21**:535–8.

21 Hanson U, Persson B. Epidemiology of pregnancy-induced hypertension and preeclampsia in type 1 (insulin-dependent) diabetic pregnancies in Sweden. *Acta Obstet Gynecol Scand* 1998;**77**:620–4.

22 Roland JM, Murphy HR, Ball V, Northcote-Wright J, Temple RC. The pregnancies of women with type 2 diabetes: poor outcomes but opportunities for improvement. *Diabet Med* 2005;**22**:1774–7.

23 Confidential Enquiry into Maternal and Child Health. *Maternity Services in 2002 for Women with Type 1 and Type 2 Diabetes, England, Wales and Northern Ireland.* London: RCOG Press, 2004.

24 Confidential Enquiry into Maternal and Child Health. *Pregnancy in Women with Type 1 and Type 2 Diabetes in 2002–3, England, Wales and Northern Ireland.* London: CEMACH, 2005.

25 Confidential Enquiry into Maternal and Child Health. *Diabetes in Pregnancy: Are We Providing the Best Care? Findings of a National Enquiry: England, Wales and Northern Ireland.* London: CEMACH, 2007.

26 Evers IM, de Valk HW, Visser GH. Risk of complications of pregnancy in women with type 1 diabetes: nationwide prospective study in the Netherlands. *BMJ* 2004;**328**:915.

27 Janz NK, Herman WH, Becker MP, *et al.* Diabetes and pregnancy: factors associated with seeking pre-conception care. *Diabetes Care* 1995;**18**:157–65.

28 Holing EV, Beyer CS, Brown ZA, Connell FA. Why don't women with diabetes plan their pregnancies? *Diabetes Care* 1998;**21**:889–95.

29 Inkster ME, Fahey TP, Donnan PT, Leese GP, Mires GJ, Murphy DJ. Poor glycated haemoglobin control and adverse pregnancy outcome in type 1 and type 2 diabetes: systematic review of observational studies. *BMC Pregnancy Childbirth* 2006;**6**:30–5.

30 Guerin A, Nisenbaum R, Ray JG. Use of maternal GHb concentration to estimate the risk of congenital anomalies in the offspring of women with prepregnancy diabetes. *Diabetes Care* 2007;**30**:1920–3.

31 Evers IM, ter Braak EW, de Valk HW, van Der Schoot B, Janssen N, Visser GH. Risk indicators predictive for severe hypoglycaemia during the first trimester of type 1 diabetic pregnancy. *Diabetes Care* 2002;**25**:554–9.

32 National Institute for Health and Clinical Excellence. *Diabetes in Pregnancy: Management of Diabetes and its Complications from Preconception to the Postnatal Period.* NICE Clincal Guideline 63, March 2008. www.nice.org.uk

33 American College of Obstetricians and Gynecologists. ACOG Practise Bulletin No. 44. Neural tube defects. *Obstet Gynecol* 2003;**102**:203–13.

34 Verier-Mine O, Chaturvedi N, Webb D, Fuller JH. Is pregnancy a risk factor for microvascular complications? The EURODIAB Prospective Complications Study. *Diabet Med* 2005;**22**:1503–9.

35 Temple RC, Aldridge VJ, Sampson MJ, Greenwood RH, Heyburn PJ, Glenn A. Impact of pregnancy on progression of retinopathy in Type 1 diabetes. *Diabet Med* 2001;**18**:573–7.

36 Nielsen LR, Muller C, Damm P, Mathiesen ER. Reduced prevalence of early preterm delivery in women with Type 1 diabetes and microalbuminuria-possible effect of early anti-hyprtensive treatment during pregnancy. *Diabet Med* 2006;**23**:426–31.

37 Bagg W, Henley PG. Pregnancy in women with diabetes and ischaemic heart disease. *Aust N Z Obstet Gynaecol* 1999;**39**:99–102.

38 Cooper WQ, Hermandez-Diaz S, Arbogast PG, *et al.* Major congenital malformations after first trimester exposure to ACE inhibitors. *N Engl J Med* 2005;**354**:2443–51.

39 Elixhauser A, Weschler JM, Kitzmiller JL, *et al.* Cost-benefit analysis of preconception care for women with established diabetes mellitus. *Diabetes Care* 1993;**16**:1146–57.

40 Herman WH, Janz NK, Becker MP, Charron-Prochownik. Diabetes and pregnancy. Preconception care, pregnancy outcomes, resource utilisation and costs. *J Reprod Med* 1999;**44**:33–8.

41 Pearson DWM, Kernaghan D, Lee R, Penney GC. The relationship between prepregnancy care and early pregnancy loss, major congenital anomaly and perinatal death in type 1 diabetes mellitus. *BJOG* 2007;**114**:104–7.

9 Provision of pregnancy care

Susan Quinn,[1] Gretta Kearney,[1] Nazia Arfin,[2] Kirsty Shaw[2] & Martin K. Rutter[2]

[1] St Mary's Hospital for Women and Children, Manchester, UK
[2] Manchester Diabetes Centre, Manchester, UK

PRACTICE POINTS

- There is a lack of international consensus regarding the management of diabetes in pregnancy.
- The UK 2007 Confidential Enquiry into Maternal and Child Health (CEMACH) indicated that the outcomes for women with diabetes in pregnancy are alarmingly poor.
- Across the UK the quality of care for these women with diabetes is patchy and suboptimal. In the US, lack of uniformity in the availability of healthcare services is an additional barrier to provision of adequate preconception care.
- A single international guideline, along with improvements in preconception care and the universal adoption of a multidisciplinary team approach, could transform the quality of care provided to these women.

CASE HISTORY

Emma is a 32-year-old primigravida who has a history of Type 1 diabetes dating back to the age of 5 years. Background retinopathy and proteinuria were first noted in her mid-20s. She smokes 20 cigarettes daily. She and her long-term partner are thinking about starting a family but have not discussed this with medical staff. When she attended her diabetes center for annual review her body mass index (BMI) was 28 kg/m^2 and HbA1c 9.3%. Her diabetes physician routinely reminded her of the importance of pregnancy planning, and the potential fetal complications should conception occur in association with poor glycemic control. She was also advised of the need to stop her lisinopril and simvastatin at least 2 months prior to conception, and of the value of folic acid 5 mg daily, and the importance of contraception.

Following referral to the local antenatal clinic, Emma met a diabetes specialist midwife who discussed the likely outcomes and risks of pregnancy, and the pros and cons of optimal glycemic control for mother and baby. The diabetes specialist dietitian updated her knowledge and skills on carbohydrate counting, and provided weight reduction and smoking cessation advice. She also had consultations with her diabetes physician and obstetrician.

Emma attended the diabetes center regularly over the next 6 months. Her progress was monitored by her diabetes specialist nurse and dietitian. After 4 months when her HbA1c was below 7% and with no significant hypoglycemia, her doctor advised her to stop contraception. Two months later a pregnancy test was positive and her care was immediately transferred back to the joint diabetes antenatal clinic. She was reviewed every 1–3 weeks at this clinic by the team, with phone call support between visits.

At 35 weeks of gestation Emma developed hypertension and proteinuria which progressed in severity over the following weeks, requiring induction at 37 weeks. After successful management of her diabetes during labor using a glucose/insulin infusion according to a standard protocol she delivered normally a healthy baby.

Following delivery, her physician reduced her subcutaneous insulin dosing to that approaching her prepregnancy insulin regime. At her 6-week postnatal review she had stopped breast feeding was given contraceptive advice and her angiotensin converting enzyme inhibitor (ACE-I) was restarted. She selected an intrauterine contraceptive device which was inserted at that visit. In addition, her statin was restarted. She was referred back to her diabetes center for ongoing diabetes care.

- Women with diabetes in pregnancy are a captive group, it is a time when women are motivated to learn new skills and optimize diabetic control. How can we provide ongoing seamless care after pregnancy to prepare them for future pregnancies and for long-term improvements in outcomes?

A Practical Manual of Diabetes in Pregnancy, 1st Edition.
Edited by David R. McCance, Michael Maresh & David A. Sacks.
© 2010 Blackwell Publishing

- How do we improve access to maternity care when women with pre-existing diabetes suspect they are pregnant?
- How can we deliver timely appropriate preconception and antenatal care for women with Type 2 diabetes from Black, Asian and other ethnic minority group who live in deprived areas?
- How do we manage mounting numbers of referrals of women with diabetes in pregnancy to the obstetric diabetes antenatal clinic?
- Should we have nationally agreed upon obstetric/diabetes medical notes?
- Do community midwives have a role to play in the care of women with gestational diabetes?
- Should the diabetes specialist nurse be based in the obstetric unit to support non-specialized staff in diabetes care and free the diabetes specialist midwife to fulfil her role delivering midwifery care?

BACKGROUND

A multidisciplinary team operating in a secondary or tertiary care setting is a commonly adopted model for the provision of pregnancy care to women with diabetes.[1] Our own clinic started in the 1960s and our practice has evolved over the years in response to changes in patient population, clinical evidence, and local resources. It mirrors practice elsewhere in the UK. Here we offer simple practical advice on how to provide a diabetes pregnancy service meeting the standards recommended in the latest UK CEMACH report.[2]

GUIDELINES FOR THE PROVISION OF CARE

Cutchie and coworkers published a review of 12 international guidelines for the care of women with diabetes in pregnancy.[3] Among women with known diabetes, the guidelines for preconception care are similar apart from folic acid doses varying between 0.4 and 5 mg daily. The guidelines for antenatal care rarely differentiate between patients with Type 1 or Type 2 diabetes, but there are significant differences among the different guidelines in glycemic targets during pregnancy, frequency of antenatal appointments, ultrasound scans, and gestational age at induction or cesarean section. However, recommendations for labor and postnatal management are similar.

For gestational diabetes mellitus (GDM), there is great variation within and between countries in the selection process for screening, screening methodology, and oral glucose tolerance testing (OGTT), including number of samples taken and the diagnostic criteria. For example, the selection for screening varies from none, to specified groups only, to all women. Screening methodology includes a 50-g non-fasting OGTT performed between 24 and 28 weeks; a random serum glucose at 28 weeks; and a 75-g OGTT. Diagnostic criteria vary with fasting: values from 5.3 to 7.0 mmol/L (95–126 mg/dL) and/or 2-hour glucose from 7.8 to 11.1 mmol/L (140–200 mg/dL) following a 75-g oral glucose load.[4,5]

In the management of GDM areas of disagreement involve fasting glucose targets (5.5–6.0 mmol/L [99–108 mg/dL]), postprandial targets (1 or 2 h; <7.0–<8.0 mmol/L [126–144 mg/dL]), timing of delivery (38 weeks to term), and timing of postnatal OGTT (4–26 weeks, but usually 6 weeks).[5]

There is therefore no international consensus on the management of women with diabetes in pregnancy, and especially for the diagnosis and management of GDM. These latter issues are addressed in chapter 6. The authors emphasize the advantages of a single international guideline based on consensus, best evidence, and best practice.

AIMS OF MULTIDISCIPLINARY JOINT METABOLIC ANTENATAL CARE

The overall aims are to allow the mother to have a good experience of pregnancy, excellent glycemic control, and normal delivery of a healthy baby

Prepregnancy care

The reader is referred to chapter 8. The barriers to achieving these aims are discussed in detail in the section below on Special needs.

Pregnancy care

The aims of pregnancy care for women with diabetes during pregnancy are:
- Referral to a combined (diabetes and obstetric care) antenatal clinic when pregnancy is suspected
- Maintenance of near-normal blood glucose levels throughout pregnancy if this can be achieved safely:
  - Premeal capillary glucose levels 3.5–5.9 mmol/L (63–106 mg/dL)[6]
  - 1-hour postprandial capillary glucose levels less than 7.8 mmol/L (140 mg/dL)[6]
- Cessation of any potentially teratogenic medication:
  - Patients are often prescribed statins and drugs affecting the renin angiotensin system prior to pregnancy

- Prescription of folic acid 5 mg daily during the first trimester
- Detection, monitoring, and appropriate management of any diabetes-related complications
- Accurate pregnancy dating
- Early identification of fetal abnormalities
- Assessment of fetal well-being
- Determination of the most appropriate time and mode of delivery
- In women at high risk of preterm delivery, inhospital administration of steroids with hourly glucose monitoring and, if necessary, with intravenous insulin therapy
- Provision of patient-centered care and support appropriate to the patient's educational, cultural, religious, and social background.
  Major factors limiting the standard of care include:
- Late referral due to inadequate patient education or compliance
- Severe hypoglycemia and hypoglycemia unawareness:
  - Major risk factors for pregnant women with Type 1 diabetes, particularly in the first trimester
  - Aggravation by nausea, vomiting, and/or autonomic neuropathy.

Postnatal care

The aims for postnatal care are to:
- Have a written plan of management for blood glucose control and neonatal care. Ideally this should be decided 1–4 weeks prior to delivery, with the understanding that plans often change depending on clinical circumstances
- Encourage skin-to-skin contact and breastfeeding within an hour of birth
- Enable all babies to remain with their mothers unless there are neonatal complications
- Encourage early feeding after delivery with monitoring of neonatal blood glucose if clinically indicated (see chapter 22)
- Maintain acceptable maternal blood glucose control to reduce the risk of hypoglycaemia:
  - Target 4–7 mmol/L (72–126 mg/dL) premeals as non-pregnant goal. Avoid prebreakfast values less than 5 mmol/L (<90 mg/dL) for 4–6 weeks
  - Close monitoring of blood glucose if breastfeeding
- Discuss and provide (e.g. for oral or injectable) contraception and arrange for contraception (e.g. intrauterine contraceptive device [IUCD] insertion) at 5–6 weeks postpartum
- Arrange a 6-week follow-up clinic visit

- Offer women with GDM:
  - A 6-week 75-g OGTT
  - Advice on weight management, diet, and exercise
  - An annual screening test for diabetes by their primary care physician
  - Glucose testing prior to discontinuation of contraception when future pregnancy is desired.

ORGANIZATION: MEMBERS OF THE MULTIDISCIPLINARY TEAM

The composition of the clinical team will vary according to local circumstances. Essential members of the team include an obstetrician and a diabetes physician supported by a diabetes specialist midwife, a diabetes specialist nurse, and a dedicated dietician. In US centers, other members may include a perinatologist and social worker. On the basis of clinical experience, we suggest that important characteristics of a multidisciplinary team should include that:
- It is comprised of motivated individuals with good interpersonal skills, and ideally possessing training in interview techniques and behavior change counseling
- The team members should meet regularly to discuss organization of the service, protocols, national standards, adverse events, audit, research and education.

The organization of clinics will vary according to local circumstances. In our practice, we have eight clinic rooms to enable individual (one-to-one) consultations, and team members utilize a "high-tech" colored peg system outside each room to indicate which staff are required to see patients that week. This is determined by the week of gestation and the previous visit assessment (Fig. 9.1). At the end of each clinic the investigations required at the next clinic visit are agreed upon, thus reducing phlebotomy and scanning waiting time.

The diabetes specialist midwife and diabetes specialist nurse provide telephone support, sometimes on a daily basis, to optimize glycemic control. The obstetricians and physicians have an on-call system providing continuous cover for emergency.

Roles of the multidisciplinary team members

Team members have some specific roles and some shared and/or exchangeable roles. Good communication between team members, including regular team meetings, and having clearly defined team goals facilitate task sharing. The role of each team member as developed

Date	Type of diabetes
Name	Date of diagnosis
Hospital number	Date GTT
	Results: fasting 2-h
DOB	Age

| Obstetric history | Parity |
| BMI prepregnancy | Gestation at first visit |

| Past medical history | Medication inc folic acid 5 mg |
| Social/family history/smoking | Allergies |

| Pre-con diabetes treatment | Diabetes complications |

Hypoglycemia (frequency/severity/awareness

| Pre-con care: Y/N – why? | Folic acid 5 mg od R'xd Y/N |

| Fundi: dates and findings | 1.   2.   3. |

| Glucagon prescribed Y/N | Ketostix prescribed Y/N |

| High risk: Y/N – why? | Date   Action |

Diabetes Management: For spontaneous labor. At induction of labor or C. section and postnatally

Refer to policy: "Intra- and Postpartum Management of Women with Type 1, Type 2 or Gestational Diabetes" and manage according to "Type of Diabetes" as listed above

Specific instructions:

Management of the neonate

Refer to policy: "Immediate care of the newborn immediately after birth," see section on thermoregulation and hypoglycemic control

Fig. 9.1 Diabetes in pregnancy proforma.

Name   Hospital number

Glucose targets; premeal: 3.5–5.9 mmol/L (63–106 mg/dL); 1–2 h postmeal: <7.8 mmol/L (140 mg/dL)

Date	Week	Special visit	Weight (kg)	HbA1c	Glucose: pre/post meal representative results				Insulin dose. Current/new Circle long – acting dose Write name above column				
					B'fast	Lunch	Eve meal	Before bed					
	4				/	/	/	/	/	/	/	/	/
	5	Booking			/	/	/	/	/	/	/	/	/
	6	Bloods Scan 7–8			/	/	/	/	/	/	/	/	/
	7	wk Folic acid			/	/	/	/	/	/	/	/	/
	8	Hb U&E			/	/	/	/	/	/	/	/	/
	9	LFT TFT			/	/	/	/	/	/	/	/	/
	10	HbA1c Fundi			/	/	/	/	/	/	/	/	/
	11	Glucagon Ketostix			/	/	/	/	/	/	/	/	/
	12				/	/	/	/	/	/	/	/	/
	13				/	/	/	/	/	/	/	/	/
	14				/	/	/	/	/	/	/	/	/
	15				/	/	/	/	/	/	/	/	/
	16	Screening tests			/	/	/	/	/	/	/	/	/
	17				/	/	/	/	/	/	/	/	/
	18				/	/	/	/	/	/	/	/	/
	19				/	/	/	/	/	/	/	/	/
	20	Anomoly scan			/	/	/	/	/	/	/	/	/
	21				/	/	/	/	/	/	/	/	/
	22				/	/	/	/	/	/	/	/	/
	23				/	/	/	/	/	/	/	/	/
	24	Fundi scan			/	/	/	/	/	/	/	/	/
	25				/	/	/	/	/	/	/	/	/
	26	Scan			/	/	/	/	/	/	/	/	/

Fig. 9.1 *Continued*

	27				/	/	/	/	/	/	/	/	/
	28	Anti-D scan			/	/	/	/	/	/	/	/	/
	29				/	/	/	/	/	/	/	/	/
	30	Scan			/	/	/	/	/	/	/	/	/
	31				/	/	/	/	/	/	/	/	/
	32	Scan			/	/	/	/	/	/	/	/	/
	33				/	/	/	/	/	/	/	/	/
	34	Fundi scan			/	/	/	/	/	/	/	/	/
	35				/	/	/	/	/	/	/	/	/
	36	Scan			/	/	/	/	/	/	/	/	/
	37				/	/	/	/	/	/	/	/	/
	38				/	/	/	/	/	/	/	/	/
	39				/	/	/	/	/	/	/	/	/
	40				/	/	/	/	/	/	/	/	/

Shading = obstetric review

Fig. 9.1 *Continued*

from our own clinical experience is summarized in Table 9.1.

STANDARDIZATION OF SCHEDULES AND DOCUMENTATION

National guidance is particularly useful when quality of care is variable and the standard is often suboptimal.[2] Here we describe our local practice which is broadly in line with the recommendations of the UK CEMACH guidelines.[2]

Preconception care tools

These will depend on the specific needs of the population served and local resources. The majority of our patients come from a multiethnic inner city population. With the help of our colleagues in primary care and the local hospital Diabetes Centre we have made, or are in the process of making, the following changes with the aim of improving preconception care:

- Recruitment of an Urdu-speaking diabetes specialist nurse to:
  - Supervise the management of all patients referred for preconception care
  - Develop links with the local ethnic communities and improve the acceptance and uptake of Western medical care
  - Coordinate preconception services between primary and secondary care
- Creation of an educational poster to be displayed in all diabetes clinics in primary and secondary care
- Production of an educational DVD to be sent to all women with diabetes with child-bearing potential. This was developed with the participation of women who use our service
- Production of an educational leaflet to be mailed annually to all women with diabetes with child-bearing potential
- Sending annual educational text messaging and e-mail reminders to all women with diabetes with child-bearing potential.

Table 9.1 Roles of multidisciplinary team members.

Team member	Roles
Team leader	• Chair monthly team meetings • Liaise with primary care physicians • Coordinate regional policies and procedures • Have responsibility for clinical governance, including auditing adverse outcomes
Obstetrician	• Counsel women on risks to mother and baby associated with diabetes • Educate all women about screening for anomalies, including spina bifida and Down syndrome (serum screening with or without nuchal thickness measurement), and diagnostic tests (amniocentesis) • Assess fetal well-being, including Doppler, fetal growth scans and antepartum testing • Decide on timing and mode of delivery and intrapartum management • Counsel parents and staff regarding adverse events • Take a lead role in audit and research with the diabetes physician
Diabetes physician	• Identify women of child-bearing age for preconception care • Give preconception advice including medication review • Optimize glycemic control before, during and after pregnancy • Manage and/or refer to appropriate subspecialists for treatment of complications such as retinopathy or nephropathy • Manage insulin: prescription, education and dose adjustment • Educate, including partner/friend/support person, about diagnosis and treatment of hypoglycemia, including use of glucagon • Offer emergency advice, e.g. on recognition of hypoglycemia and ketoacidosis
Diabetes specialist midwife (equivalent to certified diabetes educator in the US, who is frequently a registered nurse)	• Provide educational support during preconception, antenatal, intrapartum and postnatal stages • Explain potential risks to mother and baby • Offer advice on blood glucose monitoring, insulin use, hypoglycemia, hyperglycemia, ketoacidosis, and sickness • Optimize glycemic control • Liaise with partner/family and offer telephone support between clinics • Give advice to delivery suite staff on management of diabetes in labor • Give advice on the benefits of breastfeeding the neonate
Diabetes specialist nurse	• Provide educational support during preconception, antenatal and postnatal stages • Offer advice on blood glucose monitoring, insulin use, hypoglycemia, hyperglycemia, ketoacidosis, and sickness • Optimize glycemic control • Liaise with partner/family, including telephone support
Dietitian	• Give dietary advice in the preconception, antenatal, and postnatal phases • Give advice about a healthy balanced diet, carbohydrate counting, folic acid, weight management, and strategies for coping with illness • Optimize glycemic control • Promote and encourage breastfeeding
Primary care team	• Identify women with diabetes of child-bearing age for preconception care • Inform about contraception and prepregnancy management • Refer to specialist multidisciplinary team in a timely fashion
Ward staff	• Provide high-quality diabetes and obstetric care to inpatients • Optimize glycemic control, e.g. glucose/insulin infusion during labor

Provision of care for women with pregestational diabetes

Referral

In our centre we facilitate early clinic attendance once conception is confirmed by encouraging phone call referrals from patients, physicians, or diabetes specialist nurses. Our diabetes specialist midwives make immediate telephone contact with the patient. Advice given includes home blood glucose monitoring, blood glucose targets, the rationale for excellent glycemic control, folic acid 5 mg, stopping of potentially teratogenic medication, and providing contact numbers for future support. Women with a history of GDM or impaired glucose tolerance (IGT) during a previous pregnancy are also referred directly to our diabetes specialist midwife at booking (<12 weeks of gestation) and are given similar advice.

First visit following conception

This first clinic visit is offered within 1 week of referral and includes a review by all members of the multidisciplinary team and a dating ultrasound scan. At the dietary assessment we consider the appropriateness of a "carbohydrate-counting" approach to insulin dose adjustment. Women and their partners receive education on the management of hypoglycemia, including the use of glucagon, and the management of hyperglycemia, including the use of ketostix.

All women are provided with an individualized care plan from onset of pregnancy to 6 weeks postdelivery (Fig. 9.1). This document includes blood glucose targets, retinal and renal screening and follow-up, fetal surveillance including anomaly and serial growth scans, and plans for delivery and diabetes management after delivery. The care plan is part of the women's notes and is used by all team members.

At the first visit women are screened for the presence of all diabetes-related complications. Fundoscopy is advised in the first trimester and at least once in each trimester thereafter by digital imaging with mydriasis using tropicamide. Women with preproliferative or proliferative retinopathy are referred to an ophthalmologist. All women are screened for proteinuria at each visit. If persistent proteinuria (>1+) is confirmed and urine culture is negative, 24-hour urine protein, renal function, and blood pressure are obtained. Patients with nephrotic range proteinuria (≥3 g/day), progressive renal impairment, or uncontrolled hypertension are referred to a nephrologist for further evaluation and treatment.

Follow-up

Clinic visits are weekly from booking until glycemic control is satisfactory. For the remainder of the pregnancy, women are normally seen at least every 1–3 weeks until 36 weeks and then weekly until delivery.

All patients are offered screening for fetal abnormalities using a 20-week anomaly ultrasound scan, which includes a cardiac four-chamber view and outflow tract visualization in accordance with UK national recommendations.[2] Serial ultrasound scans for growth and liquor volume continue until delivery. If there is concern about a reduced fetal growth rate, additional tests such as Doppler umbilical artery profiles and cardiotocographs may be indicated, just as in the woman without diabetes.

Pregnancies in which the fetus is estimated to be macrosomic have a clear management plan that includes fetal surveillance and the timing of delivery.[7] If a preterm delivery (<36 weeks) is anticipated, then admission to the hospital for corticosteroid treatment is advised, covered by an intravenous sliding-scale insulin regime.

In the final weeks of pregnancy the timing and mode of delivery is discussed, along with the management of diabetes, and if necessary an anesthetic assessment is arranged. In uncomplicated pregnancies, we aim for a spontaneous vaginal delivery by no later than 40 weeks of gestation.[2,8] Postnatal management, including the plan to reduce or stop insulin depending on diabetes type, supervision of the neonate, and the initiation of breastfeeding and its effect on glycemic control are explained.

Delivery

Continuous cardiotocographs are performed on all women during labor with fetal scalp blood sampling performed if indicated. We administer intravenous dextrose and insulin during labor, delivered using glucose and insulin infusions to maintain maternal normoglycemia and reduce the risk of neonatal hypoglycemia (see chapter 20).[7] Delivery occurs in the presence of a pediatrician, with resuscitation facilities available if required. Glycemic targets, glucose management, and contraception are discussed prior to hospital discharge.

Postnatal care

All women are reviewed postnatally at around 6 weeks after delivery when they receive further advice on contraception and preconception care for future pregnancies. Contraception is prescribed or supplied at this visit if not already provided at hospital discharge. Patients are advised to not discontinue contraception when a future pregnancy is desired until maternal glucose concentrations are at a level that provides minimal risk of diabetes-related birth defects. Those with pre-existing diabetes are referred back to their prepregnancy care providers.

Provision of care for women with gestational diabetes.

Women are usually referred to the joint clinic at the time of diagnosis of GDM, usually at ~ 28 weeks of gestation. They are taught how to perform blood glucose monitoring and are reviewed within 1 week of diagnosis to assess their response to dietary advice from our dietitian. Women who have raised preprandial (>5.9 mmol/L [>106 mg/dL]) and/or 1-hour postprandial glucose levels (>7.7 mmol/L [>139 mg/dL]) after appropriate dietary advice are advised to start insulin (our team is not yet convinced about the safety of oral agents). Subsequent management is the same as for women with pre-existing diabetes (see above).

Women with GDM are offered a 75-g OGTT around 6 weeks postpartum and non-attenders are followed up. Their primary care physician is advised that women diagnosed with normal or impaired glucose tolerance should have annual diabetes screening by fasting glucose, and, ideally, a repeat OGTT 3-yearly. Subjects with postnatal Type 2 diabetes are referred either to their primary care physician or the local diabetes clinic, depending on clinical need and complexity. Advice is offered on weight management, diet, and exercise to all patients with GDM, along with the need for diabetes screening prior to future pregnancies.

SPECIAL NEEDS

Several barriers limit the provision of good quality diabetes care in pregnancy. These include external factors such as socioeconomic status, the healthcare system, the availability of and access to healthcare personnel, and the attitudes of healthcare professionals. Psychosocial factors include group pressure, prejudice, family demands, communication difficulties, and lack of support. Psychologic factors include cultural, religious, and health beliefs, poor motivation, low self-efficacy, difficulty setting priorities, the precontemplative stage of change, and emotional issues, including anxiety and depression.

Social deprivation

Social deprivation contributes to diabetes through dietary factors, higher levels of obesity and psychologic stress, and lower levels of physical activity, education, and employment. Those who develop diabetes in poor communities generally experience poorer access to diabetes care and that available is often of a quality lower than that required for reproductive-aged women. People from socially deprived communities have been shown to be less compliant with diabetes interventions and have lower levels of diabetes knowledge compared to more affluent individuals.[9]

Ethnicity

Type 2 diabetes and GDM are more common in ethnic minority groups compared to whites.[7] In the UK and Europe there are large numbers of high-risk women from South Asia and the Middle East. In the US, while there are also many South Asians, Latinas, particularly those of Mexican and Central American provenance, comprise a high-risk group for GDM. There is conflicting data regarding whether US-born African–Americans are at increased risk for GDM.

People from different ethnic groups may not speak or understand English and they may have different cultural and health beliefs. For example, Bangladeshi immigrants have been found to have very different healthcare beliefs about diabetes, and particularly about diet and exercise, compared to whites.

British South Asians report lower levels of physical activity than the general population, particularly among women and older people.[10] Social rules and cultural expectations, such as restrictions on women leaving the home to socialize and take part in other outdoor activities, could partly explain this.

Members of ethnic minorities tend to report more knowledge gaps about diabetes than the native population. Patients who do not speak English may also have poor literacy skills in their own language. The production of culturally appropriate patient information in the language understandable by the patient can be helpful. The provision of audio, video tapes, and CDs may be more appropriate for those with poor literacy skills.

PROBLEMS WITH PROVISION OF MATERNITY CARE AND CLINICAL GOVERNANCE

The 2007 UK Confidential Enquires into Maternal and Child Health (CEMACH) reported detailed alarmingly poor outcomes for women with either Type 1 or Type 2 diabetes when compared to women without diabetes.[2] Fewer than one in five of NHS Hospital Trusts had any kind of preconception service. Fewer than two in five women with established diabetes took folic acid or had some documentation of prepregnancy glycemic control and more than two-thirds of these women had a cesarean section. Rates for congenital malformations (10-fold), perinatal mortality (four- to seven-fold), and stillbirth (five-fold) were all higher in association with diabetes. The report has brought into sharp focus the urgent need to improve quality of care for women with diabetes.

THE WAY FORWARD

CEMACH has made several recommendations about best practice.[2] This guideline emphasizes the importance of prepregnancy counseling and of structured care delivered by a multidisciplinary team. The UK National Institute for Health and Clinical Excellence (NICE) guideline[6] highlighted the importance of preconception care and contraception, along with ambitious pregnancy glucose targets (see above).

Sufficient knowledge is now available to inform best practice. The universal implementation of this best practice could transform the outcomes for women with diabetes in pregnancy. Our challenge is how to deliver this quality of care to all women with diabetes.

EDITOR'S NOTE: A US PERSPECTIVE

In the US, many problems that impact on the care of women of reproductive age who have diabetes originate from the lack of availability of healthcare coverage. Approximately 16% of all Americans do not have health insurance. For those who do, insurance coverage is provided primarily by private insurers. The latter may, and in all but a few states do, refuse to provide insurance to patients who have pre-existing chronic conditions. Virtually all insurers refuse to pay for preconception care. The unwillingness of insurers to pay for contraception, the availability of federal funds to teach only abstinence in the public schools as the method of family planning, and the refusal of some pharmacists to provide "morning

after" contraception, undoubtedly contribute to the US's dubious distinction of having one of the highest rates of unplanned pregnancies in the industrialized world (nearly 50%).[11] It is therefore both disheartening and enlightening to learn that in the UK, a country that provides healthcare to all its citizens, many of the problems in caring for women with diabetes who are or may become pregnant remain to be solved. In reviewing the CEMACH data, it is clear that the mere availability of healthcare is not the sole determinant in reducing the risk for these women and their progeny. There is a universal need for us to learn how to improve compliance with elements of preconception and prenatal care for diabetic women that have been shown to be effective.

There are a few other cross-Atlantic differences in the care of women who have diabetes that bear comment. In the US, no distinction is made between the recommended dose of folic acid for reproductive-age women with and without diabetes. However, the American College of Obstetricians and Gynecologists (ACOG) recommends a daily dose of 0.4 mg for those who have not and 4 mg for those who have had a baby with an open-tube neural tube defect.[12]

Both preconception and prenatal care are less structured and utilize fewer personnel. Particularly in larger facilities and in university settings, reproductive care for women who have diabetes is provided by a team consisting of a perinatologist (subspecialist in materno–fetal medicine), a dietitian, a certified diabetes educator (the latter is usually a registered nurse with certification in advanced training in diabetes education), and a consulting endocrinologist. In other settings, the obstetrician provides prenatal care while a generalist or endocrinologist regulates medication doses (insulin and/or oral hypoglycemic agents).

First- and second-generation immigrants from Mexico and Central America comprise the largest growing ethnic groups in the American population. These ethnic groups have a higher incidence of obesity and diabetes than most other ethnic and racial groups in this country. The provision of healthcare to these immigrants, many of whom have no insurance, is a major unresolved public health concern.

REFERENCES

1 Dornhorst A, Hadden DR. *Diabetes and Pregnancy: An International Approach to Diagnosis and Management.* Chichester: John Wiley & Sons Ltd, 1996.

2 CEMACH. *Diabetes in Pregnancy: Are We Providing the Best Possible Care? Findings of a National Enquiry* 2007. www.cemach.org.uk.

3 Cutchie WA, Cheung NW, Simmons D. Comparison of international and New Zealand guidelines for the care of pregnant women with diabetes. *Diabet Med* 2006;**23**:460–8.

4 Agarwal MM, Dhatt GS, Punnose J, Koster G. Gestational diabetes: dilemma caused by multiple international diagnostic criteria. *Diabet Med* 2005;**22**:1731–6.

5 Hollander MH, Paarlberg KM, Huisjes AJ. Gestational diabetes: a review of the current literature and guidelines. *Obstet Gynecol Surv* 2007;**62**:125–36.

6 National Institute for Health and Clinical Excellence. *Diabetes in Pregnancy: Management of Diabetes and its Complications from Pre-conception to the Postnatal Period*, 2008. www.nice.org.uk/guidance/

7 Department of Health. *National Service Framework for Diabetes: Standards*, 2001. www.dh.gov.uk/en/Publicationsandstatistics/Publications/PublicationsPolicyAndGuidance/DH_4002951

8 Scottish Intercollegiate Guidelines Network. *Management of Diabetes: A National Clinical Guideline*, 2001. www.sign.ac.uk/pdf/sign55.pdf

9 Bachmann MO, Eachus J, Hopper CD, *et al.* Socio-economic inequalities in diabetes complications, control, attitudes and health service use: a cross-sectional study. *Diabet Med* 2003. **20**:921–9.

10 Hayes L, White M, Unwin N, *et al.* Patterns of physical activity and relationship with risk markers for cardiovascular disease and diabetes in Indian, Pakistani, Bangladeshi and European adults in a UK population. *J Public Health Med* 2002;**24**:170–8.

11 Finer LB, Henshaw SK. Disparities in rates of unintended pregnancy in the United States, 1994 and 2001. *Perspect Sex Reprod Health* 2006;**38**:90–6.

12 American College of Obstetricians and Gynecologists. *ACOG Practice Bulletin #60: Pregestational Diabetes Mellitus.* Washington, DC: ACOG, 2005.

10 Insulin regimes in pregnancy

David R. McCance[1] & Valerie A. Holmes[2]

[1]Regional Centre for Endocrinology and Diabetes, Royal Victoria Hospital, Belfast, Northern Ireland
[2]School of Nursing and Midwifery, Queen's University Belfast, Belfast, Northern Ireland

PRACTICE POINTS

- Optimal glycemic control is pivotal to the successful outcome of diabetic pregnancy.
- Most patients are now using a multiple dose insulin regime, although evidence for this is limited.
- The efficacy and safety of long-acting insulin analogs needs to be established.
- It is unclear how tight glycemic control must be to achieve a good outcome.
- Any strategy to intensify diabetes control must be balanced against the risk of hypoglycemia.

CASE HISTORY

A 21-year-old single woman with a 15-year history of Type 1 diabetes presented at 10 weeks of gestation in her first pregnancy. Her HbA1c at booking was 8.9%. Prior to pregnancy, her diabetes was controlled on a multiple-dose insulin regime (MDI) of insulin aspart and glargine and she performed only occasional self-monitoring. On examination there was evidence of background retinopathy and microalbuminuria; blood pressure was 140/80 mm/Hg. She was commenced on folic acid (5 mg/day), instructed regarding capillary glucose monitoring with targets, seen by the dietitian, and referred to ophthalmology. Follow-up was at 2-weekly intervals. Optimizing glycemic control initially was difficult due to glucose fluctuation and hypoglycemic unawareness. At 14 weeks she had a severe nocturnal hypoglycemic episode requiring intramuscular glucagon administered by her mother. By 14 weeks her HbA1c had fallen to 6.2%. During pregnancy she required laser photocoagulation for proliferative retinopathy and was commenced on methyldopa for rising blood pressure. Towards the end of pregnancy

A Practical Manual of Diabetes in Pregnancy, 1st Edition.
Edited by David R. McCance, Michael Maresh and David A. Sacks.
© 2010 Blackwell Publishing

hypoglycemic awareness improved and her insulin requirements had doubled compared with booking. At 36 weeks of gestation she developed pre-eclampsia and was delivered by emergency cesarean section of a normal live infant weighing 2890 g. By 6 hours after delivery she was tolerating food orally and insulin was prescribed approximating to that which she had taken prepregnancy. Prior to discharge her medication was reviewed and she was advised about the importance of contraception and future pregnancy planning.

- Why do insulin requirements change during pregnancy?
- What advice should be given regarding the frequency and targets for glucose monitoring?
- What is the recommended insulin regime for Type 1 diabetic pregnancy?
- Should insulin glargine be used either in women desiring to conceive or during pregnancy?
- What is the relevance of intensification of glycemic control to retinopathy?
- What are the risks of hypoglycemia?

BACKGROUND

Before the advent of insulin in 1922, pregnancy in a woman who had diabetes was uncommon and perinatal mortality rates ranged from 40% to 60%. While the discovery of insulin was revolutionary, White reported in 1928 that 25% of pregnancies in women with diabetes resulted in stillbirth.[1] Even as late as 1980, women were still being advised to avoid pregnancy because of the persisting poor obstetric history in 30–50% of women with diabetes.[2] In the intervening years, perinatal mortality rates have finally improved, most likely as a consequence of increasing sophistication of obstetric and neonatal care, widespread use of cesarean delivery and the advent of capillary home glucose monitoring. Despite these advances, perinatal mortality and congenital malforma-

99

tion rates remain three- to five-fold higher than in the general maternity population.

The relevance of hyperglycemia to maternal and perinatal outcomes is now clearly established. Poor control in early pregnancy contributes to an increased risk of spontaneous abortion and fetal malformations, and in late pregnancy to an increased risk of pre-eclampsia, hydramnios, macrosomia, operative delivery, and stillbirth. Unfortunately patients still present late in gestation with poor glycemic control. Optimizing insulin delivery remains demanding for both the patient and clinician.

This chapter will review the current approaches to optimizing insulin delivery in diabetic pregnancy. The primary focus will be on Type 1 diabetes and data from randomized trials, but the literature is limited. The key question is whether any treatment strategy is safe and superior to another in improving maternal/fetal outcome.

PHYSIOLOGY

An understanding of "normal" carbohydrate metabolism of pregnancy is necessary to the achievement of normoglycemia.[2] The pregnant woman with Type 1 diabetes requires sufficient insulin to compensate for increasing caloric needs, increasing adiposity, decreasing exercise, and increasing anti-insulin hormones (Table 10.1). There is also increased degradation of insulin in pregnancy and a reduced rate of glucose disposal. The normal pancreas can adapt to these factors by increasing the insulin secretory capacity. As the mechanism of disease in Type 1 diabetes involves destruction of beta (insulin-producing) islet cells, the need for insulin increases, and failure to increase insulin doses accordingly results in hyperglycemia.

PATHOPHYSIOLOGY

In vivo and *in vitro* studies have clearly shown that hyperglycemia is toxic to the embryo. Clinically, the picture is that of fasting and postprandial hyperglycemia. The presumption is that either sustained or intermittent hyperglycemia stimulates fetal insulin secretion with consequent increased fetal growth. Reports of macrosomia despite excellent metabolic control may possibly be explained by unrecognized glucose spikes, especially postprandially. Placental transfer of insulin complexed with IgGs has been associated with fetal macrosomia in mothers with normal glycemic control during gestation. However, in a prospective study of 42 women with gestational diabetes

Table 10.1 Metabolic alterations in Type 1 diabetic pregnancy.

Early pregnancy
- Loss of glucose and gluconeogenic substrates
- Blood glucose control is more unstable than usual
- Nocturnal hypoglycemia is common
- Insulin requirements can fall by 10–20% at end of the first trimester, possibly due to a fall in progesterone or change in human chorionic gonadotropin (hCG) or thyroid hormone and/or decreased nutrient intake due to pregnancy-related nausea

Mid pregnancy
- Change to a lipid-based energy economy
- Insulin requirements begin to increase
- Progressive increase in insulin resistance at the level of the skeletal muscle and fat cells

Late pregnancy
- Increased production of anti-insulin hormones
- Anti-insulin hormones include human placental lactogen, prolactin, estrogen, maternal production of cortisol
- Insulin requirements increase to twice or more the prepregnancy total daily dosage
- Insulin requirements may plateau or even decrease towards term

mellitus (GDM) who failed diet control, there was no difference in anti-insulin antibody levels, gestational age at birth or birthweight between women randomized to either insulin lispro (n = 19) or regular insulin (n = 23). The area under the glucose curve during a test meal was significantly lower in the lispro group.[3]

Glucose levels during pregnancy and in relation to adverse outcome

Much interest has centered on fetal macrosomia defined as birthweight greater than 4000 g or at or above the 90th centile for gestational age (large for gestational age). Two US studies reported on diabetic patients using the White classification, which categorizes patients by age of onset, diabetes duration, and presence of vascular complications rather than mechanisms of disease; most of these patients were likely to have had Type 1 diabetes. In the first study, Landon *et al*[4] showed that among 75 women with White Class B through D, those with a mean capillary blood glucose greater than 6 *versus* less than 6 mmol/L (108 mg/dL) during the second and third trimester had significantly increased rates of fetal macrosomia (28% *vs*

17%, respectively; p < 0.05) and neonatal respiratory distress (21.1% *vs* 2.3%; p < 0.01). In the other study, Jovanovic *et al*[5] reported that 52 insulin-dependent women with diabetes (White class B through F), who maintained "normal" blood glucose levels from 12 weeks of gestation (fasting 3.0–3.6 mmol/L [54–65 mg/dl], mean glucose 4.4–4.8 mmol/L [79–87 mg/dL], and postprandial <7.7 mmol/L [139 mg/dL]) had infants with a mean birthweight of 2910 g and none was above the 75th centile or developed respiratory distress. More recently, Nielsen *et al*[6] described a dose-dependent association between HbA1c levels greater than 7% in the first trimester and risk of adverse outcome among 573 Danish women with Type 1 diabetes.

PREPRANDIAL *VERSUS* POSTPRANDIAL CAPILLARY GLUCOSE MONITORING

Traditional approaches have measured capillary glucose before meals. Prolonged postprandial hyperglycemia, however, is the primary manifestation of hypoinsulinemia and its relevance to outcome has come under increasing scrutiny. Several studies have compared pre- and post-prandial glucose measurements with neonatal macrosomia, but the results are conflicting. Among three studies which controlled for confounders, two reported that postprandial, but not fasting, glucose was predictive of birthweight percentile[7] and macrosomia.[8] In contrast, the third study found that fasting, but not postprandial, glucose was significantly associated with relative birthweight.[9]

Two randomized trials compared fasting and preprandial (target 3.3–5.9 mmol/L [60–106 mg/dL]) with postprandial glucose monitoring (target < 7.8 mmol/L [<140 mg/dlL]). De Veciana *et al*[10] randomized 66 insulin-requiring Latina women with gestational diabetes mellitus at less than 30 weeks of gestation and found that the postprandial group had a lower mean HbA1c predelivery (8.1% *vs* 6.5%; p < 0.001), lower rates of cesarean section due to cephalopelvic disproportion (12% *vs* 36%; p ≤ 0.04), and large for gestational age offspring less frequently (12% *vs* 42%; p = 0.01) than the preprandial group. Manderson *et al*[11] randomized 61 Type 1 diabetic women at 16 weeks and reported a significantly reduced incidence of pre-eclampsia (55% *vs* 30%; p < 0.001), greater success in achieving glycemic control targets (55% *vs* 30%; p < 0.001) and smaller neonatal triceps skinfold thickness (4.5 ± 0.9 *vs* 5.1 ± 1.3; p = 0.05) in

those whose insulin dose was based on postprandial glucose measurements.

GLUCOSE AND HbA1c VALUES IN NORMAL PREGNANCY

In pregnant women without diabetes Parretti *et al*[12] reported a mean capillary glucose of 3.11 mmol/L (56.0 mg/dL) between 28 and 38 weeks of gestation, with the mean peak postprandial response occurring at 1 hour and never exceeding 5.84 mmol/L (105 mg/dL). There was a significant association between fetal abdominal circumference and 1-hour postprandial glucose (p < 0.0003).

Neilsen *et al* showed that healthy pregnant women have significantly lower HbA1c concentrations than non-pregnant women.[13] In addition, the upper limit of normal of HbA1c decreased from 6.3% in early pregnancy to 5.6% by late pregnancy, which is of clinical importance when defining a reference range for HbA1c during pregnancy.[13]

RECOMMENDATIONS FOR GLUCOSE MONITORING AND TARGETS

Current guidelines are outlined in Table 10.2. Glucose targets vary somewhat depending on the expert body recommendation.[14,15] Women should be supported and encouraged to monitor their blood glucose regularly. The evidence suggests that additional benefit is to be gained from a combination of pre- and post-prandial monitoring. The 1-hour postprandial time point is

Table 10.2 Recommended targets for capillary whole blood glucose during pregnancy.

American Diabetes Association (ADA)[14]*

• Preprandial glucose	≤5.8 mmol/L (105 mg/dL)
• 1 h Postprandial glucose	≤7.8 mmol/L (140 mg/dL)
	or
• 2 h Postprandial glucose	≤6.7 mmol/L (120 mg/dL)

National Institute for Health and Clinical Excellence (NICE) (2008)[15]**

• Fasting	3.5–5.9 mmol/L (63–106 mg/dL)
• 1-h postprandial	<7.8 mmol/L (140 mg/dL)

* ADA does not distinguish between different type of diabetes
** NICE states that targets should be individualized; monitoring is advised fasting and 1-h postprandially (and for insulin treated, at bedtime)

optimal as it corresponds most closely to the postprandial glucose peak and has been related to fetal outcome. In Type 1 diabetes, blood glucose should be measured eight times daily (before and after each meal, at bedtime and in the middle of the night). In Type 2 diabetes/GDM, the frequency of monitoring is to some extent dictated by the treatment strategy, but more frequent measurements identify more frequent hyperglycemia, leading to a higher insulin usage and a lower incidence of macrosomia. Although interpretation of HbA1c results is made difficult by methodologic variation and the fall in HbA1c during normal pregnancy, it provides an important index of periconceptional hyperglycemia. While the UK National Institute for Health and Clinical Evidence (NICE) guidelines do not recommend serial HbA1c measurements during pregnancy, the authors believe that knowledge of periodic HbA1c readings, with reference to a non-pregnant reference range, may be reassuring to the patient, and if raised, provides the clinician with an additional pointer to the problematic pregnancy.

INTENSIVE INSULIN REGIMES

In most countries intensive insulin regimes usually comprise an MDI of short-acting insulin before meals and intermediate-acting insulin at bedtime (often given with a pen device). Some advocate the need to give the basal isophane insulin more than once daily,[5] and there may be justification for this approach with the increasing use of insulin analogs, and if the gap between meals is greater than 3 hours. In the US, a greater proportion of subjects who have Type 1 diabetes use continuous subcutaneous insulin infusion (CSII) outside of pregnancy and this method is then continued in the maternity setting (see below). Some patients, particularly those with Type 2 diabetes, use a twice-daily fixed mixture insulin regime prepregnancy, but are often changed to an MDI regime for the duration of pregnancy.

The advantage of MDI over traditional regimes is that blood glucose levels can be tightly controlled by frequent self-regulated adjustment of dose, necessary because of the dynamic insulin requirements of pregnancy. To some extent this has evolved with changes of diabetes care. The Diabetes Control and Complications Trial (DCCT) (1990s) was pivotal in leading to the acceptance that MDI regimes prevented long-term consequences of diabetes, but data supporting such regimes in pregnancy are limited. *Post hoc* analysis of the DCCT trial of women who subsequently became pregnant on the different

regimes did demonstrate better outcome for multiple injections than more conventional regimes.[16]

Nachum *et al*[17] reported a randomized trial comparing outcomes in women with diabetes who received insulin four times daily (138 GDM and 58 pregestational) with twice daily (136 GDM, 60 pregestational). Glycemic control was better with the four times daily regime: in GDM women mean blood glucose concentrations decreased by 0.19 mmol/L (3.5 mg/dL) (95% CI 0.13–0.25) and HbA1c by 0.3% (95% CI 0.2–0.4%); in women with pregestational diabetes; corresponding values for mean blood glucose were 0.44 mmol/L (8.0 mg/dL) (95% CI 0.28–0.60) and HbA1c 0.5% (0.2–0.8%). In women with GDM, the four times daily regime resulted in lower rates of neonatal hyperbilirubinemia (RR 0.51, 95% CI 0.29–0.91) and hypoglycemia (RR 0.12, 95% CI 0.02–0.97). The relative risk of neonatal hypoglycemia in women with pregestational diabetes was 0.17 (95% CI 0.04–0.74).

Insulin treatment in gestational diabetes mellitus and Type 2 diabetes

Prospective studies of insulin treatment for GDM have generally shown a reduction in the likelihood of macrosomia.[14] In a small study of women with GDM randomized to receive only porcine regular insulin before each meal or a morning dose of Neutral Protamine Hagedorn (NPH) insulin, those receiving premeal short-acting insulin had infants with lower birthweight (3.079 ± 0.722 vs 3.943 ± 0.492 kg) and a lower rate of macrosomia.[18] As the mechanisms of disease are similar for both GDM and Type 2 disease (i.e. increased insulin resistance resulting in beta cell exhaustion), the management of insulin-requiring GDM and Type 2 diabetes is identical.

Comment on insulin regimes

Most patients are now using an MDI regime although data supporting such regimes in pregnancy are limited. Patients must be encouraged to check their blood glucose regularly and record the results in a form that permits recognition of glycemic patterns and which allows gradual prospective insulin adjustments (Table 10.3).

INSULIN ANALOGS

There has been increasing interest in the role of insulin analogs outside of pregnancy. Their main advantages are fewer episodes of hypoglycemia, a reduction in postprandial glucose excursions, and an improvement in overall glycemic control and patient satisfaction. A Cochrane review, however, concluded that evidence for their benefit over regular and NPH insulin was minimal. Although physiologically attractive in pregnancy, data here are even more limited and have largely been provided by clinical experience. Relevant issues include potential teratogenicity, mitogenicity, and interaction with the insulin-like growth factor (IGF-1) receptor.

Table 10.3 Insulin-adjustment examples.

- If 1-h postprandial glucose is >7.8 mmol/L(140 mg/dL) add 2 U of regular insulin to dose impacting that meal the following day
- If 1-h postprandial glucose is <3.3 mmol/L (59 mg/dL), decrease dose of regular insulin impacting that meal by 2 U following day or increase interval between insulin injection and meal
- If fasting glucose is >5.5 mmol/L (99 mg/dL), add 2 U to 2200-h intermediate-acting insulin, but check 0300-h blood glucose level before 2200-h insulin dose is increased. A 0300-h plasma glucose <3 mmol/L (54 mg/dL) would point to unrecognized nocturnal hypoglycemia as an explanation for the elevated fasting glucose. In this case, decrease the 2200-h intermediate-acting insulin by 2 U while carefully monitoring the fasting glucose level
- If fasting glucose is <3.3 mmol/L (59 mg/dL), decrease 2200-h long-acting insulin by 2 U
- If glucose is elevated during late afternoon, increase morning dose of intermediate-acting insulin following morning (if taking intermediate-acting insulin) or increase noon dose of short-acting insulin (if on prandial insulin)
- If glucose is low mid-morning and mid-afternoon, reduce morning dose of short-acting insulin (frequently to resolve both problems)

Three short-acting human insulin analogs and two long-acting human analogs are currently commercially available (Table 10.4).

Randomized trials

Several small randomized trials of insulin lispro in pregnancy have been published. Among women with GDM[3,19] or Type 1 diabetes treated from week 15,[20] those for whom insulin lispro analogs were added to basal NPH insulin had fewer hypoglycemic episodes[3] and lower 1-hour postprandial glucose levels,[19,20] but no difference in overall blood glucose levels or HbA1c[3,20] compared with subjects receiving regular human insulin. Birthweight, macrosomia, cesarean delivery, neonatal hypoglycemia, and anti-insulin antibody levels[3] were similar between the two groups.[3,20] Cypryk et al[21] reported pregnancy outcome among 25 women with Type 1 diabetes treated with lispro compared with 46 controls (who were maintained on the same type of insulin as prepregnancy); maternal and fetal outcomes in the two groups were similar.

Two studies have been reported using insulin aspart.[22,23] Pettitt et al[22] randomized 27 women with GDM to aspart or regular human insulin before meals, and found safety and effectiveness were comparable in the two groups. In the largest randomized controlled trial to date,[23] 157 pregnant women with Type 1 diabetes were randomized to insulin aspart and 165 to regular human insulin. There were fewer episodes of nocturnal hypoglycemia (RR 0.48, 95% CI 0.20–1.14; $p = 0.10$) and severe hypoglycemia (RR 0.72, 95% CI 0.36–1.46; $p = 0.36$) in the aspart group, although neither of these achieved statistical significance. Prandial increments were significantly lower in the aspart group in the first and third trimester. No differences were observed in 24-hour mean glucose profiles or HbA1c. Perinatal outcomes were similar between the

Table 10.4 Pharmacokinetic properties of regular human insulin and rapid-acting analogs.

Type of insulin	Onset of action	Peak plasma values	Duration of action
Regular human insulin	30–60 min	1–3 h	5–7 h
NPH insulin	60–90 min	8–12 h	18–24 h
Insulin lispro	15–60 min	0.5–1 h	2–4 h
Insulin aspart	10–20 min	1–3 h	3–5 h
Insulin glulisine	10–20 min	1–2 h	3–5 h
Glargine	4–5 h	No peak	>24 h
Detemir	4–6 h	No peak	20 h

two groups. It was concluded that aspart was at least as safe as human insulin regarding perinatal outcome.[23]

Safety issues

The mitogenic potential of insulin lispro and insulin aspart correlates with their relative affinity for the IGF-1 receptor. Both analogs, with insulin receptor affinity less than that of human insulin, also have mitogenic potencies less than those of human insulin. In one retrospective report of 10 pregnant women treated with insulin lispro either before or early in pregnancy, three progressed from no retinopathy to proliferative retinopathy; however, this was not confirmed in two larger studies and other pregnancy factors may have been relevant.[2] Four case series of women with Type 1 diabetes exposed to insulin lispro in pregnancy (n = 696) and a systematic review found that insulin lispro improved glycemic control with no adverse maternal or fetal effects.[2,15]

Detemir has a lower insulin receptor affinity than does human insulin, and an even lower IGF-1 receptor affinity and mitogenic potential. Glargine has an IGF-1 receptor affinity and mitogenic potency approximately seven-fold greater than human regular insulin. The clinical implications of these findings remain to be determined.[24]

Few clinical data exist on the use of long-acting insulin analogs, but a retrospective multicentre study involving 127 pregnancies found no difference in outcomes between subjects receiving isophane insulin and those receiving glargine.[25] A multicenter randomized controlled trial comparing basal isophane *versus* detemir (with prandial aspart) is currently in progress (Novo Nordisk).

Insulin aspart is licensed for the treatment of diabetes in pregnancy. In the US, the Food and Drugs Administration (FDA) has approved a pregnancy category B rating for insulin aspart (www.medscape.com/viewarticle/551560). (The FDA classifies drugs for use in pregnancy by an alphabetically ordered classification system, primarily on the basis of reported human and/or animal teratogenicity. All insulins are classified as B or C. Currently this classification system is undergoing revision.) Data on the role and safety of long-acting analogs in pregnancy are needed. Issues of teratogenicity are less relevant to GDM, but careful discussion of the risks and benefits is required when women present using long-acting analogs either before or in early pregnancy.

CONTINUOUS SUBCUTANEOUS INSULIN INFUSION

An alternative method of insulin administration is continuous subcutaneous insulin infusion (CSII). Modern pumps are small and light weight, battery operated, and hold enough short- or ultra-short-acting insulin for several days. Different basal rates can be preset and boluses given as required. Potentially, CSII reduces the risk of hypoglycemia, decreases the risk of fasting hyperglycemia (the dawn phenomenon), and improves patient compliance as the woman does not have to constantly inject insulin. Despite widespread use of CSII in the US, Germany, France and Italy, it is used infrequently in other countries, including the UK. The reasons are likely to include conservatism, complexity, cost, and concern regarding reports of diabetic ketoacidosis (DKA). A recent meta-analysis of randomized controlled trials assessing glycemic control with CSII compared with MDI did not identify an increased risk of DKA with CSII.[26] The authors suggested that previous reports of DKA may have been explained by the short duration of trials and poor reporting, though improvement in pump technology is also likely to be relevant.

Although insulin infusion pumps have been used for treatment for over two decades, experience with these devices in pregnancy is limited; most are observational, often uncontrolled, and numbers of subjects are generally small. In addition, few trials have been published in the last 10–15 years. Six randomized controlled trials of CSII *versus* MDI found no difference in glycemic control, or obstetric or neonatal outcomes (Table 10.5).[27–33] Other cohort observational studies have reported no or only minor benefits with CSII over conventional therapy.[2,15] Most of the women in these trials had pump treatment started in the second or third trimesters.

It seems that pump therapy is not necessary in order to achieve and maintain optimal control for the majority of patients. There is a need for randomized controlled trials comparing CSII with MDI using insulin analog therapy. Selective use of pumps for those who are motivated and with difficult to control diabetes is an alternative to its widespread use. All studies should include an estimation of quality of life.

CONTINUOUS GLUCOSE MONITORING SYSTEMS

Several studies have shown that in pregnancies complicated by diabetes, complications such as fetal macro-

Table 10.5 Randomized controlled trials of continuous subcutaneous insulin infusion (CSII) versus multiple dose injection (MDI) regimes in diabetic pregnancy.[27-32] (Adapted from Mukhopadhyay et al[33].)

Author	Randomization	Study detail	Start of treatment	Comment
Coustan et al (1986)[27]	Truly randomized	11 CSII (Autosyringe: AS-SC, AS 6-C; AS 6-C[U-100]; Lilly CPI-9100) vs 11 MDI (2–4 daily injections of intermediate/ isophane/actrapid)	Preconception/ first trimester	No difference in mean glucose, symptomatic hypoglycemia or HbA1c
Carta et al (1986)[28]	Unclear	14 CSII (Microjet MC20) vs 15 MDI (3–4 regular daily doses)	Preconception/ first and second trimester	No significant differences in mean insulin requirements at different stages of gestation; "perinatal outcome satisfactory in both groups"; control of fetal growth better with MDI than CSII
Burkart et al (1988)[29]	Quasi randomized	48 CSII (open loop, not clear) vs 41 MDI (conventional, not clear)	First trimester	No difference in the rate of pregnancy complications or in fetal outcome
Nosari et al (1993)[30]	Truly randomized	16 CSII (Microjet MC20 /DahediBV) vs 16 MDI (3–4 regular daily doses)	Not clear	No difference in maternal and neonatal mortality, fetal anomaly, hypoglycemia, mean 24-h blood glucose, mean HbA1c, gestational age at delivery, birthweight
Laatikainen et al (1987)[31]	Unclear	13 CSII (Autosyringe AS 6-C) vs 18 MDI (1–3 daily injections of intermediate/short acting)	First trimester	No difference in mean HbA1c. While not significant, worsening retinopathy more evident in CSII group
Botta et al (1986)[32]	Quasi randomized	5 CSII (CPI 9100 Lilly) vs 5 MDI (2–3 daily injections of intermediate/short acting/retard)	Not clear	No difference in insulin requirements, maternal body weight gain, gestational age at delivery, mode of delivery, birthweight or maternal and fetal complications

somia still occur at a considerably higher frequency than in a healthy population, even with good glycemic control.[34] This suggests that HbA1c may not sufficiently reflect the complexities of glycemic control or that current criteria for strict glycemic control are not "safe". Kerssen et al[35] reported that the frequency of hyperglycemia is underestimated in pregnant women who seem to be well-controlled using home self-monitoring records and HbA1c.

Continuous glucose monitoring systems (CGMS) provide a dynamic picture of interstitial glucose levels, converting these to an electrical signal which produces a recording of average glucose level every 5 minutes. Studies using CGMS have reported hyperglycemic episodes undetected by self-monitoring of blood glucose,[36,37] which may be relevant to fetal outcome. The studies showed that examination of 72-hour glucose profiles can help identify patterns of glucose control, allow a better targeting of insulin treatment, assist in patient education, and improve dietary adherence.[37] Devices with built-in alarms triggered at preset glucose levels are now available. CGMS, however, have also shown just how variable results can be from day to day in pregnant women with Type 1 diabetes.

It seems unlikely that this technology will be widely available given the cost of each sensor but its selected use in problematic patients may supplement home blood glucose monitoring data.

HYPOGLYCEMIA

Efforts to intensify glycemic control must be balanced against the risk of maternal hypoglycemia, particularly in the first trimester when pregnancy-associated nausea and vomiting may occur. Up to 70% of women who have Type-1 diabetes report hypoglycemic episodes in pregnancy with one-third being severe.[38] Many pregnant women lose the ability to detect "warning signs" of impending hypoglycemia as a result of decreased autonomic response to low glucose. Hypoglycemia in intensively controlled pregnant women with Type 1 diabetes may be attributed to defective counter-regulation (i.e. decreased secretion of glucagon, epinephrine), placental or pituitary growth hormone, and/or decreased sensitivity to epinephrine in response to maternal hypoglycemia. Hypoglycemia unawareness may lead to serious consequences, including seizures, comas, accidents, and death. Risk factors for defective maternal glucose counter-regulation and hypoglycemia unawareness include a history of hypoglycemia preceding pregnancy, prolonged duration of diabetes, intensive glycemic control, and pregnancy itself.[38]

Clinical studies which have examined the relationship between adverse fetal outcome and exposure to maternal hypoglycemia in pregnant women with Type 1 diabetes may seem reassuring but cannot dispel all concerns. The association of hypoglycemia with subsequent blood glucose fluctuations into the hyperglycemia range has been offered as an explanation for the continuing occurrence of macrosomia despite excellent HbA1c levels through pregnancy. Animal studies in rodents indicate that hypoglycemia occurring early in gestation may be teratogenic.[38] Also, severe hypoglycemia can rapidly deteriorate into a life-threatening situation with profound psychologic sequelae for the patient and her family. Moreover, it is an entirely iatrogenic complication.

HOW TIGHT MUST GLYCEMIC CONTROL BE TO ACHIEVE A GOOD OUTCOME?

Some 30 years after the initial evidence suggesting that pregnancy outcome was improved by lowering maternal glucose concentrations, the question of how strict control should be remains unanswered. The Cochrane review of tight *versus* less tight glycemic control included two trials, both of which were associated with more frequent hypoglycemia, and both of which had methodologic flaws. More recently, Sacks *et al*[39] reported a feasibility study of 22 subjects with Type 1 diabetes randomized either to "rigid" (fasting and premeal targets 3.3–5.0 mmol/L [60–90 mg/dL] and 1-hour postprandial 6.7–7.8 mmol/L [120–140 mg/dL]) or "less rigid" (5.3–6.4 mmol/L [95–115 mg/dL] and 8.6–9.7 mmol/L [155–175 mg/dL], respectively) groups. Mean maternal glucose levels were significantly greater in the first and second trimesters among the "less rigid" group. Both subjective and objective hypoglycemia episodes were more frequent in the "rigid" group. There were no differences between groups in cesarean deliveries, birthweights, and neonatal glucose concentrations.

SUMMARY AND FUTURE DIRECTIONS

Despite modern technology, optimizing glycemic control remains demanding for both the patient and clinician. Increasing evidence suggests that capillary home glucose monitoring should include a combination of both pre- and 1-hour post-prandial measurements. Most patients are now using an MDI insulin regime, although there is little evidence to support the use of one particular regime over another. Data on the safety of long-acting analogs are needed. There are no convincing data that CSII is superior to MDI for the majority of women, but trials comparing these two approaches using insulin analogs are now indicated. It is unclear how tight glycemic control must be to achieve good outcome and any strategy to intensify diabetes control must constantly be balanced against the risk of maternal hypoglycemia. It seems likely that capillary glucose monitoring reveals only a minor fraction of glucose variability and this may be relevant to adverse fetal outcome. While the selective use of CGMS may facilitate management in problematic patients, the possibility of closing the glucose sensing and/or CSII/insulin administration loop is the tantalizing ideal.

REFERENCES

1 White P. Diabetes in pregnancy. In: Joslin EP (ed). *The Treatment of Diabetes Mellitus*, 4th edn. Philadelphia: Lea and Febiger, 1982:861–72.

2 Jovanovic L, Kitzmiller JL. Insulin therapy in pregnancy. In: Hod M, Jovanovic L, Di Renzo GC, de Leiva A, Langer O (eds). *Textbook of Diabetes and Pregnancy*, 2nd edn. London: Informa Healthcare, 2008:205.

3 Jovanovic L, Llic S, Pettitt DJ, *et al.* Metabolic and immunologic effects of insulin lispro in gestational diabetes. *Diabetes Care* 1999;**22**:1422–7.

4 Landon MB, Gabbe SG, Piana R, *et al.* Neonatal morbidity in pregnancy complicated by diabetes mellitus: predictive value of maternal glycemic profiles. *Am J Obstet Gynecol* 1987;**156**:1089–95.

5 Jovanovic L, Druzin M, Peterson CM. Effect of euglycaemia on the outcome of pregnancy in insulin-dependent diabetic women as compared with normal control subjects. *Am J Med* 1981;**71**:921–7.

6 Nielsen GL, Moller M, Sorensen HT. HbA1c in early diabetic pregnancy and pregnancy outcomes: A Danish population-based cohort study of 573 pregnancies in women with type 1 diabetes. *Diabetes Care* 2006;**29**:2612–6.

7 Jovanovic-Peterson L, Peterson CM, Reed GF, *et al.* Maternal postprandial glucose levels and infant birthweight: the Diabetes in Early Pregnancy Study. *Am J Obstet Gynecol* 1991;**164**:103–11.

8 Combs CA, Gunderson E, Kitzmiller JL, *et al.* Relationship of fetal macrosomia to maternal postprandial glucose control during pregnancy. *Diabetes Care* 1992;**25**:1251–7.

9 Persson B, Hanson U. Fetal size at birth in relation to quality of blood glucose control in pregnancies complicated by pregestational diabetes mellitus. *Br J Obstet Gynaecol* 1996;**103**:427–33.

10 De Veciana M, Major CA, Morgan MA, *et al.* Postprandial versus preprandial blood glucose monitoring in women with gestational diabetes mellitus requiring insulin therapy. *N Engl J Med* 1995;**333**:1237–41.

11 Manderson JG, Patterson CC, Hadden DR, *et al.* Preprandial versus postprandial blood glucose monitoring in type 1 diabetic pregnancy: a randomized controlled clinical trial. *Am J Obstet Gynecol* 2003;**189**:507–12.

12 Parretti E, Mecacci F, Papini M, *et al.* Third-trimester maternal glucose levels from diurnal profiles in nondiabetic pregnancies: correlation with sonographic parameters of fetal growth. *Diabetes Care* 2001;**24**:1319–23.

13 Nielsen LR, Ekbom P, Glumer C, *et al.* HbA1c levels are significantly lower in early and late pregnancy. *Diabetes Care* 2004;**27**:1200–1.

14 American Diabetes Association. Executive Summary: Standards of Medical Care in Diabetes- 2008. *Diabetes Care* 2008;**31** (Suppl 1):S5–S54.

15 National Institute for Health and Clinical Excellence. *Diabetes in Pregnancy. Management of Diabetes and its Complications from Pre-conception to the Post Natal Period. 2008.* NICE clinical guideline 63, July 2008. www.nice.org.uk/CG063

16 The Diabetes Control and Complications Trial Research Group. Pregnancy outcomes in the Diabetes Control and Complications Trial. *Am J Obstet Gynecol* 1996;**174**:1343–53.

17 Nachum Z, Ben Shlomo I, Weiner E, *et al.* Twice daily versus four times daily insulin dose regimens for diabetes in pregnancy: randomized controlled trial. *BMJ* 1999;**319**:1223–7.

18 Poyhonen-Alho M, Teramo K, Kaaja R. Treatment of gestational diabetes with short or long acting insulin and neonatal outcome: a pilot study. *Acta Obstet Gynecol Scand* 2002;**81**:258–9.

19 Mecacci F, Carignani L, Cioni R, *et al.* Maternal metabolic control and perinatal outcome in women with gestational diabetes mellitus treated with regular or lispro insulin: comparison with non-diabetic pregnant women. *Eur J Obstet Gynecol Reprod Biol* 2003;**111**:19–24.

20 Persson B, Swahn ML, Hjertberg R, *et al.* Insulin lispro therapy in pregnancies complicated by type 1 diabetes mellitus. *Diabetes Res Clin Pract* 2002;**58**:115–21.

21 Cypryk K, Sobczak M, Pertynska-Marczewska M, *et al.* Pregnancy complications and perinatal outcome in diabetic women treated with Humalog (insulin lispro) or regular human insulin during pregnancy. *Med Sci Monit* 2004;**10**:129–32.

22 Pettitt DJ, Ospina P, Howard C, *et al.* Efficacy, safety and lack of immunogenicity of insulin aspart compared with regular human insulin for women with gestational diabetes mellitus. *Diabet Med* 2007;**24**:1129–35.

23 Mathiesen E, Kinsley B, McCance DR, *et al.* Maternal hyperglycemia and glycemic control in pregnancy. A randomized trial comparing insulin aspart with human insulin in 322 subjects with type 1 diabetes. *Diabetes Care* 2007;**30**:771–6.

24 Kustzhals P, Schaffer L, Sorensen A, *et al.* Correlations of receptor binding and metabolic and mitogenic potencies of insulin analogs designed for clinical use. *Diabetes* 2000;**49**:999–1005.

25 Gallen IW, Jaap AJ, Roldan JM, Chirayath HH. Survey of insulin glargine use in 115 pregnant women with Type 1 diabetes. *Diabetic Med* 2008;**25**:165–9.

26 Pickup J, Mattock M, Kerry S. Glycemic control with continuous subcutaneous insulin infusion compared with intensive insulin injections in patients with type 1 diabetes: meta-analysis of randomized controlled trials. *BMJ* 2002;**324**:1–6.

27 Coustan DR, Reece EA, Sherwin RS, *et al.* A randomized clinical trial of the insulin pump vs intensive conventional therapy in diabetic pregnancies. *JAMA* 1986;**255**:631–6.

28 Carta Q, Meriggi E, Trossarelli GF, *et al.* Continuous subcutaneous insulin infusion versus intensive conventional insulin therapy in type 1 and type 2 diabetic pregnancy. *Diabet Metab* 1986;**12**:121–9.

29 Burkart W, Hanker JP and Schneider HP. Complications and fetal outcome in diabetic pregnancy. Intensified conventional versus insulin pump therapy. *Gynecol Obstet Invest* 1988;**26**:104–12.

30 Nosari I, Maglio ML, Lepore G, *et al.* Is continuous subcutaneous insulin infusion more effective than intensive conventional insulin therapy in the treatment of pregnant diabetic women? *Diabetes Nutr Metab Clin Exp* 1993;**6**: 33–7.

31 Laatikainen L, Teramon K, Hieta-Heikurainen H, *et al.* A controlled study of the influence of continuous subcutaneous insulin infusion treatment on diabetic retinopathy during pregnancy. *Acta Med Scand* 1987;**221**:367–76.

32 Botta RM, Sinagra D, Angelico MC, *et al.* Comparison of intensified traditional insulin therapy and micropump therapy in pregnant women with type 1 diabetes mellitus. *Minerva Med* 1986;**77**:657–61.

33 Mukhopadhyay A, Farrell T, Fraser RB, *et al.* Continuous subcutaneous insulin infusion vs intensive conventional insulin therapy in pregnant diabetic women: a systematic review and meta analysis of randomised controlled trials. *Am J Obstet Gynecol* 2007;**197**:447–56.

34 Evers IM, Valk HW, Mol BWJ, *et al.* Macrosomia despite good glycemic control in type 1 diabetic pregnancy: results of a nationwide study in the Netherlands. *Diabetologia* 2002;**45**:1484–9.

35 Kerssen A, De Valk HW, Visser GH. Do HbA1c levels and the self monitoring of blood glucose adequately reflect glycemic control during pregnancy in women with type 1 diabetes mellitus? *Diabetologia* 2006;**49**:25–8.

36 Kerssen A, Evers IM, de Valk HW, Visser GH. Poor glucose control in women with type 1 diabetes mellitus and "safe" haemoglobin values in the first trimester of pregnancy. *J Matern Fetal Neonatal Med* 2003;**13**:309–13.

37 Yogev Y, Chen R, Ben-Haroush A, *et al.* Continuous glucose monitoring for the evaluation of gravid women with type 1 diabetes mellitus. *Obstet Gynecol* 2003;**101**:633–8.

38 ter Braak EW, Evers IM, Erkelens, Visser GH. Maternal hypoglycemia during pregnancy in type 1 diabetes: maternal and fetal consequences. *Diabetes Metab Res Rev* 2002;**18**: 96–105.

39 Sacks DA, Feig DS, Liu ILA, Wolde-Tsadik G. Managing type 1 diabetes in pregnancy: how near normal is necessary? *J Perinatol* 2006;**26**:458–62.

11 Oral hypoglycemic agents in pregnancy

Mount Sinai Hospital, Toronto, Ontario, Canada

PRACTICE POINTS

- Metformin crosses the placenta while glyburide does not.
- Metformin and glyburide are unlikely to be teratogenic.
- Pregnant women with Type 2 diabetes on oral hypoglycemic agents (OHAs) are usually switched to insulin therapy during pregnancy.
- Metformin increases the rate of ovulation in women with polycystic ovary syndrome (PCOS). While there is some evidence that continuation of metformin up to the first trimester, or throughout pregnancy, may reduce the risk of spontaneous abortions and gestational diabetes in women with PCOS, more data are needed from randomized controlled trials before the drug is used for this indication.
- Insulin remains the mainstay of treatment for women with gestational diabetes; however, for those women who cannot afford insulin, or do not wish to take insulin, metformin or glyburide may be offered as an alternative, with appropriate explanation of the risks and benefits.
- Acarbose has been used in only very small studies in pregnancy to date, and tolerability is likely to be an issue.
- PPAR-gamma agonists cross the placenta and should be avoided in pregnancy until more safety data are available.

CASE HISTORY 1

A 32-year-old woman G2P0Sab1 with Type 2 diabetes and PCOS presents to clinic at 9 weeks of gestation. This is not a planned pregnancy. She is taking metformin 1 g twice daily and glyburide 10 mg twice daily. HbA1c is 9%.

What do you advise her?

A Practical Manual of Diabetes in Pregnancy, 1st Edition.
Edited by David R. McCance, Michael Maresh and David A. Sacks.
© 2010 Blackwell Publishing

CASE HISTORY 2

A 30-year-old woman G1P0 is diagnosed with gestational diabetes at 28 weeks of gestation. She is started on a diabetic diet but her blood sugars remain above target. She is extremely afraid of needles and asks if she can take pills.

What do you advise her?

BACKGROUND

The standard treatment for gestational diabetes mellitus (GDM) and Type 2 diabetes in pregnancy has been diet therapy, with the addition of insulin when blood sugar targets are not achieved. In the 1970s and early 1980s oral hypoglycemic agents gained usage in pregnancy, particularly in South Africa. However, this trend failed to gain popularity as experts in the field cautioned against their use because of fear of teratogenicity, and reports of prolonged neonatal hypoglycemia. In spite of these concerns, a growing body of literature has been accumulating on the use of oral agents in pregnancy. In this chapter we examine the evidence for the safety and efficacy of oral hypoglycemic agents in women with GDM, PCOS, and Type 2 diabetes in pregnancy.

SULFONYLUREAS AND MEGLITINIDES

Sulfonylureas and meglitinides are "insulin secretagogues" (Table 11.1). They both bind to receptors (although not at identical sites) on the pancreatic beta cell, causing insulin secretion. Examples of sulfonylureas include the first-generation sulfonylureas, tolbutamide, chlopropramide, and tolazamide, and the second-generation sulfonylureas, such as glyburide (glibenclamide), glipizide, and glimeperide. The meglitinides include nateglinide and repaglinide.

Table 11.1 Properties of oral hypoglycemic agents (OHAs).

Type of OHA	Examples	Mechanism of action
Sulfonylureas	First generation: tolbutamide, chloropropamide and tolazamide Second generation: glyburide or glibenclamide, glipizide and glimeperide	Insulin secretagogue: bind to the sulfonylurea receptor on the beta cell of the pancreatic islets, leading to closure of the ATP-sensitive potassium channel, leading to insulin secretion
Meglinitides	Nateglinide and repaglinide	Insulin secretagogue: bind to a receptor close to the sulfonylurea binding site on the beta cell, causing closure of the ATP-sensitive potassium channel, leading to insulin secretion
Biguanides	Metformin	Reduce hepatic glucose output, increase peripheral glucose uptake in skeletal muscle and adipocytes, and reduce intestinal glucose absorption
Glucosidase Inhibitors	Acarbose and voglibose	Slow carbohydrate absorption and reduce postprandial glucose by inhibiting the alpha-glucosidase enzymes present on the brush border of the small intestine
Peroxisome proliferator-activated receptor-gamma (PPAR-gamma) agonists	Rosiglitazone, pioglitazone, and troglitazone	Insulin sensitizers: bind to the nuclear transcription factor peroxisome proliferator-activated receptor-gamma (PPAR-gamma) which modulates gene expression in adipose tissue, skeletal muscle, and the liver, leading to changes in several metabolic pathways which involve glucose transport, lipoprotein lipase, and insulin signaling

Placental transfer

In light of earlier reports of neonatal hypoglycemia in infants of mothers taking sulfonylureas, researchers investigated whether sulfonylureas crossed the placenta by using the human placental cotyledon perfusion model. In this model, a human placental cotyledon is obtained from a healthy mother at the time of delivery. The drugs in question are perfused on the maternal side, and transfer of the drug is measured on the fetal side. Studies found that, although the first-generation sulfonylureas crossed the placenta in moderate amounts (tolbutamide 21.5% and chlorpropramide 11%), the second-generation sulfonylureas crossed less (glipizide 6.6%), with glyburide crossing the least (3.9%).[1] A similar finding was noted in a study using glyburide in women with GDM. Glyburide was measurable in the serum of these women at the time of delivery; however, no glyburide was detected in cord blood.[2] There are no studies to date looking at the placental transfer of the meglitinides.

Clinical experience: cohort studies and randomized trials

Congenital anomalies
Women with Type 2 diabetes
The majority of studies looking at the rate of congenital anomalies in women using sulfonylureas in the first tri-

mester have not shown an increased rate of congenital anomalies.[3–6] Only two studies found an increased rate (n = 20 and n = 43, respectively); however, glycemic control was either not ideal[7] or not described.[8] A meta-analysis of 471 women exposed to oral agents (sulfonlyureas and/or biguanides) in the first trimester compared with 1344 women not exposed, found no significant difference in the rates of major malformations.[9] In the largest retrospective cohort study to date (n = 342), congenital anomalies were associated with poor glycemic control rather than the specific oral hypoglycemic agent (OHA) used (glyburide/glibenclamide or metformin).[3] In summary, sulfonylureas are unlikely to be teratogenic.

There are limited data on congenital anomalies with meglitinide use, but two recent case reports of three women exposed to repaglinide during the first trimester of pregnancy did not report any congenital malformations.[10,11]

Perinatal mortality
Women with Type 2 diabetes
In early cohort studies of women with Type 2 diabetes in pregnancy, treatment with either sulfonylureas alone, or in combination with metformin, resulted in reduced rates of perinatal mortality when compared with those who were "untreated". However, perinatal mortality rates were higher than those in women who were con-

Table 11.2 Glyburide failure rates* in women with gestational diabetes.

Study	Number treated with glyburide	Glyburide failures (%)	Study design
Langer et al (2000)[2]	201	4	Randomized controlled trial
Kremer & Duff (2004)[18]	73	19	Observational
Conway et al (2004)[14]	75	16	Observational
Chmait et al (2004)[15]	69	18.8	Observational
Jacobson et al (2005)[19]	316	17	Cohort
Bertini et al (2005)[13]	24	20	Randomized controlled trial
Kahn et al (2006)[16]	95	19	Observational
Rochon et al (2006)[17]	101	21	Observational
Total	954	16–21	

*"Glyburide failures" are those patients who were switched to insulin; the majority for inadequate glycemic control, the minority because of hypoglycemia

verted to insulin. This was attributed to better glycemic control in those treated with insulin.[4,5,12] In a more recent retrospective cohort study by the same group in South Africa, the use of OHAs *throughout* pregnancy (glyburide [glibenclamide] alone, or in combination with metformin) was associated with an increased rate of perinatal mortality.[3] However, there were no perinatal deaths in infants of women taking metformin exclusively. The perinatal mortality rate was significantly higher in the group that used OHAs throughout compared with those who switched to insulin at the beginning of the pregnancy, or those who were treated with insulin alone. This could not be explained by differences in glycemic control, maternal age, body mass index (BMI), parity, booking gestational age or comorbidities between groups. The reason for this increased rate of perinatal mortality is unclear but until more definitive data are available, the use of insulin is preferred in women with Type 2 diabetes. Other studies, some of higher quality (randomized controlled trials) in women with gestational diabetes, have not found this association (see below).[2]

Other morbidity

Women with gestational diabetes mellitus

In 2000, Langer and colleagues conducted a landmark randomized controlled trial involving 404 women with GDM.[2] Those women who failed to meet targets on diet were randomized at 11–33 weeks of gestation to receive either insulin or glyburide therapy (starting at 2.5 mg in the morning and titrated to 20 mg/day when necessary). They found no significant differences in glycemic control or neonatal outcomes between the two groups, including large birthweight for gestational age (LGA), macrosomia, birthweight, neonatal hypoglycemia and pulmonary complications, admission to the neonatal intensive care

unit (NICU), congenital anomalies or perinatal mortality. Eight patients (4%) in the glyburide group needed insulin. While this study was groundbreaking, one of the main criticisms was that it was underpowered to assess neonatal outcomes. Since publication of this trial there has been only one other very small randomized trial (<30 women per arm), where women with GDM were randomized to glyburide, insulin or acarbose.[13] No difference was found in glycemic control or birthweight, although there were significantly more infants with neonatal hypoglycemia in the glyburide group.

Several observational studies have been published looking at how often GDM women treated with glyburide need to be switched to insulin (i.e. "glyburide failure").[14–17] In these studies glyburide "failure rates" ranged from 16% to 21% (Table 11.2), the majority being because of poor glycemic control and a minority because of hypoglycemia. Predictors of "failure" included a glucose challenge test result greater than or equal to 11.1 mmol/L (≥200 mg/dL), diagnosis before 25 weeks, increased maternal age, multiparity, and pretreatment fasting capillary blood glucose values of greater than 6.1 mmol/L (>110 mg/dL). Target values in these studies were fasting values of 5.0–5.3 mmol/L (90–95 mg/dL), 1-hour values of 7.2–7.8 mmol/L (130–140 mg/dL), and 2-hour values of 6.4–6.7 mmol/L (115–120 mg/dL).

There are no data on the use of glipizide or the meglitinides in women with gestational diabetes or Type 2 diabetes.

Use of sulfonylureas during pregnancy: summary and existing concerns

Glyburide (glibenclamide) does not appear to be teratogenic, nor does it cross the placenta to an appreciable extent. In women with Type 2 diabetes there is some concern regarding increased perinatal mortality with continued use of glyburide throughout pregnancy, and until further studies are available, women should be switched to insulin during pregnancy. In women with GDM, glyburide is associated with good glycemic control in the majority, with failure rates of approximately 16–21% (Table 11.1). Most studies found no differences in neonatal outcomes between women on glyburide and those using insulin. However, because there is only one randomized controlled trial of moderate size that was not powered to assess neonatal outcomes, some concerns remain.

METFORMIN

Metformin is a biguanide which acts by reducing hepatic glucose output, increasing peripheral glucose uptake in skeletal muscle and adipocytes, and reducing intestinal glucose absorption (Table 11.1). This leads to improved insulin sensitivity. It does not cause insulin secretion and hence does not cause hypoglycemia or weight gain. It is contraindicated in patients with renal dysfunction or abnormal creatinine clearance from any cause.

Placental transfer

Metformin freely crosses the placenta. This was demonstrated in a placental transfer study which showed that metformin transferred readily from the maternal to the fetal side of placentas from women with GDM.[20] Two studies throughout pregnancy found that levels were 50–100% as high as maternal blood concentrations, and in some infants the level was even higher.[21,22]

Clinical experience: cohort studies and randomized trials

Ovulation induction, pregnancy, and live birth rates
Women with polycystic ovary syndrome
Metformin has been shown to decrease insulin resistance in women with PCOS, which has resulted in improved rates of ovulation.[21] Evidence, however, is conflicting regarding the benefits of metformin to increase pregnancy and live birth rates compared with clomiphene.[23,24]

Congenital anomalies
Women with Type 2 diabetes
The majority of studies during pregnancy using metformin alone or with sulfonlyureas have not found an increased rate of congenital malformations in offspring.[3–5,9,25]

Women with polycystic ovary syndrome
While hyperglycemia is a major confounding factor in those studies that have looked at congenital anomalies in women with Type 2 diabetes exposed to OHAs in the first trimester, this problem does not arise in women with PCOS whose blood sugar levels are normal. Studies in over 500 women with PCOS using metformin, either in the first trimester or throughout pregnancy, showed no increased rate of congenital malformations.[26–33]

Other morbidity and mortality
Women with Type 2 diabetes
In early cohort studies, perinatal mortality rates in women taking metformin (and/or sulfonylureas) were elevated, most likely due to poor glycemic control.[4,5,12] Perinatal mortality rates decreased when glycemic control improved after 1977.[25] In a later study, metformin use was associated with an increase in pre-eclampsia and perinatal mortality compared with those women on insulin.[34] In this latter study, however, patients taking metformin were more obese than women on insulin, suggesting this may have accounted for the increased rates. A more recent retrospective cohort study from South Africa (discussed above), found that while perinatal mortality was increased in women taking glyburide (glibenclamide) alone or in combination with metformin, no increase in perinatal mortality was seen in patients treated solely with metformin.[3]

Women with gestational diabetes mellitus
The metformin in gestational diabetes (MiG) trial was a large randomized controlled trial in which 751 women with GDM at 20–33 weeks of gestation and with inadequate glycemic control on diet therapy were randomized to receive either metformin (starting at 500 mg once or twice daily and titrated to a maximum of 2500 mg as necessary) or insulin.[35] The rate of the primary composite outcome of neonatal morbidity, which included neonatal hypoglycemia, respiratory distress, need for phototherapy, birth trauma, 5-minute Apgar score less than 7 and prematurity, was not significantly different in women assigned to metformin (32.0%) and those assigned to

insulin (32.2%) (RR 0.99, 95% CI 0.80–1.23). Severe neonatal hypoglycemia (<1.6 mmol/L [<28.8 mg/dL]) was decreased in the metformin group (3.3% *vs* 8.1%; p = 0.008), but preterm birth was more common in the metformin group (12.1% *vs* 7.6%; p = 0.04). There was no significant difference in glycemic control between the groups, although 46.3% of women in the metformin group required supplemental insulin to maintain good glycemic control. Follow-up of these infants is planned (the MiG TOFU study) to look at the long-term effects of metformin.

Women with polycystic ovary syndrome

Several observational and cohort studies have now been published looking at maternal and fetal outcomes in women with PCOS given metformin throughout pregnancy. These have shown no adverse pregnancy outcomes, and possibly some potential benefits, such as decreased rates of spontaneous abortion[31,36] and gestational diabetes.[28,30] In a prospective study of 90 women with PCOS who conceived on metformin 1.5–2 g/day there were no differences in pre-eclampsia rates, gestational diabetes rates, perinatal mortality, or birthweight compared with 252 healthy controls.[28] In a recent prospective cohort study, 200 non-diabetic patients with PCOS who took 1–2 g of metformin/day throughout pregnancy were compared to 80 women with PCOS who conceived on metformin but stopped the drug at the time of conception.[37] Rates of early pregnancy loss were significantly lower in the metformin group who continued to take the drug throughout pregnancy. Finally, a retrospective study of infants of mothers who took metformin in pregnancy found normal height, weight, motor and social development at 6 months of age.[38] Prospective randomized controlled trials are needed to confirm these findings.

Use of metformin in pregnancy: summary and existing concerns

Metformin freely crosses the placenta. It does not appear to be teratogenic. Metformin increases the rate of ovulation in women with PCOS; however, the use of clomiphene may be more efficacious for induction of a successful pregnancy. In one large randomized controlled trial, metformin was as efficacious as insulin *vis à vis* a composite neonatal outcome of neonatal hypoglycemia, respiratory distress, need for phototherapy, birth trauma, 5-minute Apgar score less than 7, and prematurity in women with gestational diabetes, without adverse

effects. We await long-term studies of neonates exposed to metformin throughout pregnancy. Randomized trials are needed to inform us regarding the ability of metformin to decrease spontaneous abortions and gestational diabetes in women with PCOS, and its role in pregnant women with Type 2 diabetes.

ALPHA-GLUCOSIDASE INHIBITORS

The alpha-glucosidase inhibitors, which include acarbose and voglibose, slow carbohydrate absorption and reduce postprandial glucose by inhibiting the alpha-glucosidase enzymes present on the brush border of the small intestine. These drugs are not absorbed into the bloodstream in any significant amount. Only acarbose has been studied in pregnancy. In one case series, six women with GDM not controlled on diet alone were given acarbose three times a day before meals. In all six patients, the fasting and postprandial glucose values normalized and the infants were healthy.[39] Acarbose, however, was associated with intestinal discomfort that persisted throughout the pregnancy. Finally, acarbose was used in a small randomized controlled trial where women with GDM who were not successfully controlled on diet therapy were randomized to receive insulin (n = 27), glyburide (n = 24) or acarbose (n = 19).[13] No differences were observed in the maternal glucose levels achieved, rate of LGA or birthweight among patients in each of the three groups. There was no mention of the tolerability of acarbose in this study. Larger randomized controlled trials are needed to elucidate further the benefits of acarbose in pregnancy. Tolerability is likely to be an issue.

PPAR-GAMMA AGONISTS

The peroxisome proliferator-activated receptor (PPAR)-gamma agonists, also known as thiazolidinediones, include rosiglitazone, pioglitazone, and troglitazone (the latter has been taken off the market because of hepatic toxicity). They bind to the nuclear transcription factor PPAR-gamma, which modulates gene expression in adipose tissue, skeletal muscle, and the liver, leading to changes in several metabolic pathways which involve glucose transport, lipoprotein lipase, and insulin signaling. They are known as "insulin sensitizers" as they enhance insulin action in these tissues. They are used in patients with Type 2 diabetes and do not cause hypoglycemia. They have been associated with weight gain, fluid retention, and an increase in heart failure due to water retention. Rosiglitazone has recently been shown possibly to increase cardiac events in a retrospective meta-analysis[40] and in a nested case–control study of older patients.[41] Further studies are needed to clarify this.

Placental transfer

In a study of 31 women between 8 and 12 weeks of gestation, two doses of rosiglitazone 4 mg were given prior to surgical termination of pregnancy.[42] Rosiglitazone was detected in fetal tissue, especially after 10 weeks of gestation, suggesting it does cross the placenta.

Clinical experience

There is little experience with PPAR-gamma agonists in pregnancy. No teratogenic effects have been noted in studies of rats and rabbits.[43] Two cases of exposure to rosiglitazone in the first trimester, and a third case exposed in the second trimester, have been described, but with no congenital anomalies or neonatal complications reported.[44,45] Rosiglitazone has been used in two randomized trials of women with PCOS for ovulation induction (n = 25 in each trial) (one comparing rosiglitazone and clomiphene *vs* metformin plus clomiphene, and the other comparing rosiglitazone plus placebo *vs* rosiglitazone plus clomiphene).[46,47] In the first trial, rosiglitazone improved ovulatory rates; in the second, the addition of clomiphene to rosiglitazone was superior. No congenital anomalies were described in the 14 pregnancies, although there were three early fetal losses.

Summary

PPAR-gamma agonists cross the placenta and to date there are few data on the safety of these drugs in pregnancy. Therefore, these drugs should not be used in pregnancy, and should only be used for ovulation induction if potential benefits outweigh the potential risks to the fetus.

BREASTFEEDING

Women with Type 2 diabetes are often on OHAs prior to pregnancy, and after delivery, the question of when these drugs can safely be restarted frequently arises. The main issue is whether these drugs will be secreted into breast milk, posing a risk to infants.

Sulfonylureas

The first-generation sulfonylureas, tolbutamide and chlorpropamide, cross into breast milk. To date only one study has looked at the transfer of glyburide and glipizide into breast milk.[48] In this study of women with Type 2 diabetes, eight women received a single oral dose of 5 or 10 mg of glyburide, while five women were given 5 mg of glyburide or glipizide daily from the first day postpartum. Neither glyburide nor glipizide was detected in the breast milk of any of the women.

Metformin

In three studies which looked at the transfer of metformin into breast milk, all three found that metformin crosses into breast milk, albeit in very small quantities.[49–51] The mean estimated infant dose as a percentage of the mother's weight-adjusted dose was 0.65%, far below the arbitrary cut-off level of 10%. In addition, blood glucose levels taken from three infants of nursing mothers were normal.[50] At 6 months of age, the weight, height, and motor–social development of infants of mothers taking metformin while breastfeeding did not differ from those for formula-fed infants.[52]

Other drugs

There are no data on PPAR-gamma agonists or alpha-glucosidase inhibitors and breastfeeding.

Summary

Glyburide, glipizide and metformin appear compatible with breastfeeding, but their use is still not universally recommended in all practice guidelines.[53]

CASE HISTORY 1

In this 32-year-old woman with Type 2 diabetes and PCOS metformin and glyburide are unlikely to be teratogenic; however, with an elevated HbA1c there is an increased risk of congenital malformations. This should be assessed with an anatomy ultrasound and fetal echocardiogram at 18–20 weeks of gestation. For better glycemic control, metformin and glyburide should be discontinued and insulin should be initiated. While there is some evidence that continuation of metformin up to the first trimester, or throughout pregnancy, may reduce the risk of spontaneous abortions in women with PCOS, more data are needed from randomized controlled trials before using metformin for this indication.

CASE HISTORY 2

Both glyburide and metformin have been used in randomized controlled trials of women with gestational diabetes, and both were as efficacious as insulin in achieving glycemic control. Metformin crosses the placenta, while glyburide does not, making it an attractive drug to use in pregnancy. However, only one randomized controlled trial has been done using glyburide and it was underpowered to look at differences in neonatal outcomes. Metformin has the advantage of lowering insulin resistance, which is elevated in gestational diabetes. The MiG trial, which looked at the use of metformin in women with GDM, was powered to look at neonatal outcomes and did not show a difference in the primary neonatal composite outcome. Both glyburide and metformin can be offered to this patient, with appropriate discussion of the risks and benefits.

REFERENCES

1 Elliot BD, Langer O, Schenker S, et al. Comparative placental transfer of oral hypoglycemic agents in humans: a model of human placental drug transfer. Am J Obstet Gynecol 1994;171:653–60.
2 Langer O, Conway DL, Berkus MD, et al. A comparison of glyburide and insulin in women with gestational diabetes mellitus. N Engl J Med 2000;343:1134–8.
3 Ekpebegh CO, Coetzee EJ, van der Merwe L, Levitt NS. A 10-year retrospective analysis of pregnancy outcome in pregestational type 2 diabetes: comparison of insulin and oral glucose-lowering agents. Diabet Med 2007;24:253–8.
4 Coetzee EJ, Jackson WPU. Pregnancy in established non-insulin-dependent diabetics. S Afr Med J 1980;58:795–9.
5 Coetzee EJ, Jackson WPU. Oral hypoglycemics in the first trimester and fetal outcome. S Afr Med J 1984;65:635–7.
6 Towner D, Kjos SL, Leung B, et al. Congenital malformations in pregnancies complicated by type 2 diabetes. Diabetes Care 1995;18:1446–51.
7 Picquadio K, Hollingsworth DR, Murphy H. Effects of in utero exposure to oral hypoglycaemic drugs. Lancet 1991;338:866–9.
8 Botta RM. Congenital malformations in infants of 517 pregestational diabetic mothers. Annali Dell'Istituto Superiore di Sanita 1997;33:307–11.
9 Gutzin SJ, Kozer E, Magee LA, Feig DS, Koren G. The safety of oral hypoglycemic agents in the first trimester of pregnancy: a meta-analysis. Can J Clin Pharmacol 2003;10:179–83.
10 Napoli A, Ciampa F, Colatrella A, Fallucca F. Use of repaglinide during the first weeks of pregnancy in two type 2 diabetic women. Diabetes Care 2006;29:2326–7.
11 Mollar-Puchades MA, Martin-Cortes A, Perez-Calvo A, Diaz-Garcia C. Use of repaglinide on a pregnant woman during embryogenesis. Diabet Obesity Metab 2007;9:146–7.
12 Coetzee EJ, Jackson WPU. The management of non-insulin-dependent diabetes during pregnancy. Diabet Res Clin Pract 1986;1:281–7.
13 Bertini AM, Silva JC, Taborda W, et al. Perinatal outcomes and the use of oral hypoglycemic agents. J Perinat Med 2005;33:519–23.
14 Conway DL, Gonzales O, Skiver D. Use of glyburide for the treatment of gestational diabetes: the San Antonio experience. J Matern Fetal Neonatal Med 2004;15:51–5.
15 Chmait R, Dinise T, Moore T. Prospective observational study to establish predictors of glyburide success in women with gestational diabetes mellitus. J Perinatol 2004;24:617–22.
16 Kahn BF, Davies JK, Lynch AM, Reynolds RM, Barbour LA. Predictors of glyburide failure in the treatment of gestational diabetes. Obstet Gyncol 2006;107:1303–9.
17 Rochon M, Rand L, Roth L, Gaddipati S. Glyburide for the management of gestational diabetes: risk factors predictive of failure and associated pregnancy outcomes. Am J Obstet Gynecol 2006;195:1090–4.
18 Kremer CJ, Duff P. Glyburide for the treatment of gestational diabetes. Am J Obstet Gynecol 2004;190:1438–9.
19 Jacobson GF, Ramos GA, Ching JY, Kirby RS, Ferrara A, Field. Comparison of glyburide and insulin for the management of gestational diabetes in a large managed care organization. Am J Obstet Gynecol 2005;193:118–24.
20 Nanovskaya TN, Nekhayeva IA, Patrikeeva SL, Hankins GD, Ahmed MS. Transfer of metformin across the dually perfused human placental lobule. Am J Obstet Gynecol 2006;195:1081–5.
21 Charles B, Norris R, Xiao X, Hague W. Population pharmacokinetics of metformin in late pregnancy. Ther Drug Monit 2006;28:67–72.
22 Vanky E, Zahlsen K, Spigset O, Magnus Carlsen S. Placental passage of metformin in women with polycystic ovary syndrome. Fertil Steril 2005;83:1575–8.
23 Lord JM, Flight IHK, Norman RJ. Metformin in polycystic ovary syndrome: systematic review and meta-analysis. BMJ 2003;327:951–3.
24 Legro RS, Barnhart HX, Schlaff WD, et al. Clomiphene, metformin, or both for infertility in the polycystic ovary syndrome. N Engl J Med 2007;356:551–66.
25 Coetzee EJ, Jackson WP. Metformin in management of pregnant insulin-dependent diabetics. Diabetologia 1979;16:241–5.
26 Turner MJ, Walsh J, Byrne KM, et al. Outcome of clinical pregnancies after ovulation induction using metformin. J Obstet Gynecol 2006;26:233–5.

27 Thatcher SS, Jackson EM. Pregnancy outcome in infertile patients with polycytic ovary syndrome who were treated with metformin. *Fertil Steril* 2006;**85**:1002–9.

28 Glueck CJ, Goldenberg N, Wang P, *et al*. Metformin during pregnancy reduces insulin, insulin resistance, insulin secretion, weight, testosterone, and development of gestational diabetes: prospective longitudinal study of women with polycystic ovary syndrome from pre-conception through pregnancy. *Hum Reprod* 2004;**19**:510–21.

29 Glueck CJ, Bornovali S, Pranikoff J, *et al*. Metformin, pre-eclampsia, and pregnancy outcomes in women with polycystic ovary syndrome. *Diabet Med* 2004;**21**:829–36.

30 Glueck CJ, Wang P, Kobayashi S, *et al*. Metformin therapy throughout pregnancy reduces the development of gestational diabetes in women with polycystic ovary syndrome. *Fertil Steril* 2002;**77**:520–5.

31 Jakubowicz DJ, Iuorno MJ, Jakubowicz S, *et al*. Effects of metformin on early pregnancy loss in the polycystic ovary syndrome. *J Clin Endocrinol Metab* 2002;**87**:524–9.

32 Vanky E, Salvesen KA, Heimstad R, Fougner KJ, Romundstad P, Carlsen SM. Metformin reduces pregnancy complications without affecting androgen levels in pregnant polycystic ovary syndrome women: results of a randomized study. *Hum Reprod* 2004;**19**:1734–40.

33 Kovo M, Weissman A, Gur D, *et al*. Neonatal outcome in polycystic ovarian syndrome patients treated with metformin during pregnancy. *J Matern Fetal Neonatal Med* 2006;**19**:415–19.

34 Hellmuth E, Damm P, Molsted-Pederson I. Congenital malformations in offspring of diabetic women treated with oral hypoglycaemic agents during embryogenesis. *Diabet Med* 1994;**11**:471–4.

35 Rowan JA, Hague WM, Gao W, Battin MR, Moore MP for the MiG trial Investigators. Metformin versus insulin for the treatment of gestational diabetes. *N Engl J Med* 2008;**358**:2003–15.

36 Glueck CJ, Wang P, Goldenberg N, Sieve-Smith L. Pregnancy outcomes among women with polycystic ovary syndrome treated with metformin. *Hum Reprod* 2002;**17**:2858–64.

37 Khattab S, Abdel Mohsen I, Abourl Foutouh I, *et al*. Metformin reduces abortion in pregnant women with polycstic ovary syndrome. *Gynecol Endocrinol* 2006;**22**:680–4.

38 Glueck CJ, Godenberg N, Pranikoff J, *et al*. Height, weight and motor-social development during the first 18 months of life in 126 infants born to 109 mothers with polycystic ovary syndrome who conceived on and continued metformin through pregnancy. *Hum Reprod* 2004;**19**:1323–30.

39 Zarate A, Ochoa R, Hernandez M, Basurto L. Effectiveness of acarbose in the control of glucose tolerance worsening in pregnancy. *Ginecol Obstet Mex* 2000;**68**:42–5.

40 Nissen SE, Wolski K. Effect of rosiglitazone on the risk of myocardial infarction and death from cardiovascular causes. *N Engl J Med* 2007;**356**:2457–71.

41 Lipscombe L, Gomes T, Levesque LE, Hux JE, Juurlink DN, Alter D. Thiazolidinediones and cardiovascular outcomes in older patients with diabetes. *JAMA* 2007;**298**:2634–43.

42 Yik-Si Chan L, Hok-keung Yeung J, Kin Lau T. Placental transfer of rosiglitazone in the first trimester of human pregnancy. *Fertil Steril* 2005;**83**:955–80.

43 Briggs GG, Freeman RK, Yaffe SJ. *Drugs in Pregnancy and Lactation*, 7th edn. Philadelphia: Lippincott Williams & Wilkins, 2005:1316 & 1438.

44 Brooks Vaughan T, Bell DSH. Stockpiling of ovarian follicles and the response to rosiglitazone. *Diabetes Care* 2005;**28**:2333–4.

45 Kalyoncu NI, Yaris F, Ulku C, *et al*. A case of rosiglitazone exposure in the second trimester of pregnancy. *Reprod Toxicol* 2005;**19**:563–4.

46 Rouzi AA, Ardawi MSM. A randomized controlled trial of the efficacy of rosiglitazone and clomiphene citrate versus metformin and clomiphene citrate in women with clomiphene citrate-resistant polycystic ovary syndrome. *Fertil Steril* 2006;**85**:428–35.

47 Ghazeeri G, Kutteh WH, Bryer-Ash M, Haas D, Ke RW. Effect of rosiglitazone on spontaneous and clomiphene citrate-induced ovulation in women with polycystic ovary syndrome. *Fertil Steril* 2003;**79**:562–6.

48 Feig DS, Briggs GG, Kraemer JM, *et al*. Transfer of glyburide and glipizide into breast milk. *Diabetes Care* 2005;**28**:1851–5.

49 Hale TW, Kristensen JH, Hackett LP, *et al*. Transfer of metformin into human milk. *Diabetologia* 2002;**45**:1509–14.

50 Briggs GG, Ambrose PJ, Nageotte MP, *et al*. Excretion of metformin into breast milk and the effect on nursing infants. *Obstet Gynecol* 2005;**105**:1437–41.

51 Gardiner SJ, Kirkpatrick CM, Begg EJ, *et al*. Transfer of metformin into human milk. *Clin Pharmacol Ther* 2003;**73**:71–7.

52 Glueck CJ, Salehi M, Sieve L, Wang P. Growth, motor, and social development in breast- and formula-fed infants of metformin treated women with polycystic ovary syndrome. *J Pediatr* 2006;**148**:628–32.

53 National Institute for Health and Clinical Excellence. *Diabetes in Pregnancy: Management of Diabetes and its Complications from Pre-conception to the Postnatal Period.* NICE Clinical Guideline 63, March 2008 (reissued July 2008). www.nice.org.uk/CG063

12 Fetal surveillance in diabetes in pregnancy

Joanna Girling & Archana Dixit

West Middlesex University Hospital NHS Trust, Isleworth, Middlesex, UK

PRACTICE POINTS

- Pregnancy in women with diabetes is associated with increased perinatal morbidity and mortality.
- Fetal compromise in women with diabetes with vasculopathy or pre-eclampsia is related to placental vascular disease.
- The mechanism of fetal compromise in fetuses with normal or accelerated growth is not well understood and is likely to be mutifactorial.
- No currently available fetal surveillance technique has been proven to predict fetuses at risk or to prevent poor outcome in diabetic pregnancies.
- Surveillance methods are of proven value only in pregnancies with vascular complications of diabetes, pre-eclampsia or fetal growth restriction.
- Serial growth scans in the second half of pregnancy are recommended to detect accelerated fetal growth and/or polyhydramnios or growth restriction.

CASE HISTORY

A 26-year-old nullipara with Type 1 diabetes booked at 8 weeks of gestation. She had chronic hypertension treated with ramipril prior to conception. Her diabetic retinopathy had been treated by laser therapy 2 years ago. She did not have proteinuria. Ramipril was stopped on confirmation of pregnancy and she was commenced on low-dose aspirin. Blood pressure did not require treatment until 24 weeks of gestation when she was started on methyldopa.

Glycemic control was chaotic in the first trimester, but good glycemic control was achieved by 20–24 weeks with increasing doses of insulin and improved attention to diet. There was no deterioration of the diabetic retinopathy.

A Practical Manual of Diabetes in Pregnancy, 1st Edition.
Edited by David R. McCance, Michael Maresh and David A. Sacks.
© 2010 Blackwell Publishing

In view of the increased risk of pre-eclampsia, uterine artery Doppler examination was arranged for 24 weeks, which showed bilateral notches. Serial growth scans were commenced from 28 weeks of gestation, which showed fetal growth just below the 50th centile, normal liquor volume, and normal umbilical Doppler flow.

At 32 weeks of gestation, she was admitted with pre-eclampsia (significant proteinuria and rise in blood pressure). Ultrasound scan revealed a slowing of growth velocity to the 5th centile, reduced liquor volume, and normal umbilical Dopplers. She remained an inpatient with twice daily cardiotocographs (CTGs), weekly scans for liquor volume and umbilical Doppler measurements, and fortnightly scans for fetal growth, which showed low liquor volume, normal umbilical Dopplers, and maintenance of growth along the 5th centile. Glycemic control remained excellent.

She was delivered at 35 weeks of gestation for worsening pre-eclampsia (further increments in anti-hypertensive therapy were required) and a suboptimal CTG, by cesarean section of a healthy male baby weighing 1.9 kg. Following 5 days on the special care baby unit he was discharged with his mother after 7 days.

- Is this pattern of fetal growth typical in diabetes? Why is the pattern like this?
- What is another common pattern of fetal growth in women with diabetes?
- What is the optimal fetal surveillance in women with diabetes?
- Should all women with diabetes be offered CTGs in pregnancy?
- What is the significance of the normal umbilical Doppler measurements in this woman? Should they be measured in all women with diabetes?
- Is assessment of fetal lung maturation justified before delivery? If so, what are the options for doing this?

• Why is fetal death more common in women with diabetes?

BACKGROUND

Historically, pregnancy in women with diabetes is associated with high perinatal morbidity and mortality. The fetal and neonatal complications include increased risk of congenital malformations, miscarriage, preterm delivery, stillbirth, accelerated fetal growth with its attendant risk of traumatic vaginal delivery and shoulder dystocia, cardiomyopathy, respiratory distress syndrome, and neonatal metabolic derangements, especially hypoglycemia. Fetuses of women with vascular complications of long-standing diabetes, notably diabetic nephropathy with or without accompanying hypertension, are also at risk of intrauterine growth restriction (IUGR) as a result of placental insufficiency. Many of the late fetal and neonatal complications in diabetic pregnancies can be explained by the Pedersen hypothesis.[1] This states that maternal hyperglycemia resulting in fetal hyperglycemia causes marked fetal hyperinsulinemia via fetal pancreatic beta cell overstimulation. This in turn causes accelerated fetal growth, excess subcutaneous fat, and increased hepatic glycogen storage, features often referred to as macrosomia and all of which can contribute to traumatic delivery and neonatal metabolic derangements. This theory has driven the clinical management of diabetes in pregnancy, with the belief that better glycemic control in the mother can reduce perinatal morbidity and mortality. This chapter focuses on the surveillance required in the third trimester in order to minimize perinatal mortality and morbidity in structurally normal fetuses.

The 2002–2003 UK Confidential Enquiry into Maternal and Child Health (CEMACH)[2] showed that babies of women with Type 1 or Type 2 diabetes are five times more likely to be stillborn and three times more likely to die in their first month of life compared with those of mothers without diabetes. The perinatal mortality rate was 31.8 per 1000 births, compared to the national rate of 8.5 per 1000 births. Approximately 80% of these losses were stillbirths, 80% of these babies being structurally normal. Perinatal mortality in European countries and other UK regional studies is comparable, and ranges from 27.8 to 48 per 1000 births.

The goal of obstetric surveillance is to identify fetuses at risk, in order to intervene in a timely and appropriate fashion and reduce perinatal morbidity and mortality. However, the CEMACH enquiry[3] during 2002–2003 found that fetal surveillance was poor in 20% of 37 pregnancies with antenatal evidence of fetal growth restriction and in 45% of 129 pregnancies with antenatal evidence of accelerated growth; the enquiry did not explain what the deficiencies were nor make recommendations regarding optimal surveillance.

PATHOPHYSIOLOGY OF FETAL COMPROMISE IN DIABETES IN PREGNANCY

Before choosing a test to assess fetal well-being, it is important to understand the pathophysiology of fetal compromise in diabetes in pregnancy. When fetal death occurs, it is usually in the final weeks of pregnancy in the context of poor glycemic control, polyhydramnios, and/or accelerated fetal growth.[4,5] In contrast, diabetic women with vasculopathy and/or pre-eclampsia may develop IUGR and fetal demise as early as the second trimester, probably related to placental vascular disease.

The pathophysiology of fetal compromise in diabetic pregnancy where the fetus is normally grown or large for dates is likely to be multifactorial. It is probable that the majority of unexplained stillbirths result from chronic fetal hypoxia and/or fetal acidemia secondary to maternal/fetal hyperglycemia and fetal hyperinsulinemia.

Evidence of fetal hypoxia is seen in the form of raised fetal erythropoietin (EPO) levels in infants with intrauterine growth acceleration.[6] Extramedullary hematopoiesis is found more often in stillborn infants of mothers with diabetes.[7] Thickening of the basement membrane of chorionic villi has been described in placentae of pregnancies in women with diabetes,[8] which potentially could reduce oxygen transfer.

Maternal hemoglobin A1c (HbA1c) concentrations in the third trimester correlate with fetal umbilical venous EPO at delivery[9] suggesting that antepartum control of maternal hyperglycemia is a significant factor associated with fetal hypoxia. A recent systematic review of four studies of adverse pregnancy outcome in women who have Types 1 and 2 diabetes found increased perinatal mortality associated with poor glycemic control (pooled OR 3.23, 95% CI 1.87–4.92),[10] although the studies reviewed had methodologic limitations. Marked oscillations in maternal glycemic control may explain accelerated fetal growth and fetal compromise seen in some pregnancies with apparently excellent diabetic control.[11] Maternal hypoglycemia does not seem to impact the fetus significantly; however, there are few studies addressing this issue.

Hyperglycemia and hyperinsulinemia in fetal lambs increase oxygen consumption with a simultaneous decrease in oxygen content.[12] Hyperglycemia increases fetal glycosylated hemoglobin, which shifts the fetal oxygen dissociation curve, thus reducing red cell oxygen delivery at tissue level.[13] In late pregnancy, the switch from HbF to HbA production is delayed in women with diabetes, and this may further reduce tissue oxygen availability. Fetal amniotic fluid insulin levels correlate significantly with fetal plasma EPO levels independently of maternal glycemia, suggesting that insulin exerts an effect on fetal oxygenation beyond that of maternal and fetal glycemia.[9] Fetal hyperinsulinemia may also result in hypokalemia in the fetus (possibly predisposing to fatal cardiac arrhythmia). There is a significant association between fetal plasma insulin levels and the degree of fetal acidemia,[14] and significant acidemia has been observed even in the absence of hypoxia.[15] Glucose oxidation and oxygen consumption are increased by hyperinsulinism, this effect being independent of that caused by hyperglycemia. The reduced capacity of the fetus for oxidative metabolism and low pyruvate dehydrogenase activity result in hyperlactinemia. Diabetic ketoacidosis is dangerous for both the mother and the fetus, the risks to the latter probably being related to acidosis (see chapter 19).

ACCELERATED FETAL GROWTH

Various definitions of accelerated fetal growth are in use, such as birthweight over 4000 g, over the 90th centile, or two standard deviations above the mean weight for gestation corrected for sex. The last mentioned is preferred, but even this does not characterize the selective organomegaly seen in the infant of the woman with diabetes. The CEMACH report[2] found that 21% of singleton babies of women with diabetes weighed over 4000 g compared with 11% in the general population, and over 1% of babies of women with diabetes weighed under 1000 g compared with 0.5% in the general population.

A strong relationship between fetal weight and umbilical plasma insulin,[16] and a direct relationship with amniotic fluid EPO levels, have been observed, suggesting that the larger the fetus is, the greater the risk of fetal hypoxia. Growth acceleration may start as early as 18 weeks of gestation.[17] However, the growth potential of fetuses seems to be determined by prevailing maternal glycemia before then and excessive growth can continue despite optimum glycemic control subsequently.[18] Nonetheless, optimal glycemic control during pregnancy is associated with a reduced incidence of accelerated fetal growth[19] and therefore with improved perinatal outcome.

Accelerated fetal growth is associated with a significant increase in the risk of fetal death in the presence but not the absence of maternal diabetes. Seeds et al reported an OR of 3.4 (95% CI 1.1–9.6; p < 0.01) for intrauterine death at or beyond 24 weeks of gestation for a birthweight over the 95th centile and an OR of 3.2 (CI 1.3–7.4; p < 0.01) for a birthweight between the 90th and 95th centiles compared with birthweights between the 25th and 75th centiles.[20]

One of the major challenges relates to the best way to minimize the likelihood of shoulder dystocia, brachial plexus injury, and other major birth trauma in babies with scan-detected accelerated growth. The UK CEMACH[2] report into pregnancies in women with pregestational diabetes found an incidence of Erb palsy of 4.5 per 1000 births, 10-fold greater than for the general population, but 25% of babies with Erb palsy born to women with diabetes were delivered by cesarean section. It also confirmed that shoulder dystocia is more common in larger babies, ranging from 1% in babies less than 2500 g to 43% in babies over 4500 g. In addition, it has been reported that babies of women with diabetes have a three- to seven-fold greater risk for shoulder dystocia at each given weight category compared with non-diabetic women.[21] This can be explained by anthropometric differences between babies of diabetic and non-diabetic mothers.[22] While both detection of accelerated fetal growth (see below) and prediction of shoulder dystocia, which relates to more than fetal size alone, are poor, studies using ultrasound weight prediction followed by cesarean for those cases where birthweight is predicted to be more than 4250 g have shown a reduction in shoulder dystocia, but at the expense of an increase in cesarean section rate (see also chapter 20). In addition, many babies estimated by scan to be large have actual birthweights less than 4250 g:[23] 443 cesarean sections with a scan-estimated fetal weight (EFW) threshold of 4500 g would need to be performed to prevent one permanent brachial plexus injury, or 489 with an EFW threshold of 4000 g.[24]

FETAL SURVEILLANCE METHODS

Surveillance includes monitoring of fetal growth and assessment of fetal well-being. Given the multifactorial nature of the etiology and the timing of fetal demise in pregnancies *with diabetes*, it is difficult to know which forms of monitoring, if any, are appropriate. It is generally considered that standard clinical assessment needs to be supplemented by other methods of surveillance, although two recent reviews of fetal monitoring in diabetic pregnancy[7,25] show that no currently available technique has been proven to predict the fetuses at risk or *to* prevent poor outcome. This is not surprising as the methods assessed were not designed to predict the pathologic processes likely to precede fetal demise. Accordingly, some clinicians reserve surveillance only for those pregnancies with additional issues, such as vasculopathy, hypertension or growth restriction, that have more predictable fetal complications and better-established modes of surveillance.

The tools available for fetal surveillance include:
- Antenatal CTG
- Ultrasound assessment of fetal growth
- Ultrasound assessment of amniotic fluid volume
- Biophysical profile
- Umbilical artery Doppler velocimetry
- Amniocentesis – assessment of fetal lung maturity, fetal insulin, EPO
- Magnetic resonance imaging (MRI) spectroscopy.

Antenatal cardiotocography

Antenatal CTG records fetal heart rate and displays it in relation to spontaneous uterine activity, a technique sometimes referred to as a non-stress test (NST). Antenatal contraction stress tests, in which the fetal heart rate is observed during uterine activity induced by, for example, an infusion of oxytocin, are rarely used.

Outside of diabetes, antenatal CTG is used to detect antenatal fetal compromise in high-risk pregnancies. A Cochrane Systematic Review however revealed only four published studies including a total of 1588 high-risk pregnancies, only one of which pertained to diabetes.[26] These failed to show a significant effect of antenatal CTGs on perinatal morbidity or mortality. There are no randomized controlled trials assessing the value of antenatal CTG for fetal surveillance in diabetes in pregnancy. Non-randomized studies indicate that the tool is a poor predictor of fetal compromise in diabetes with fetal demise reported hours after a normal trace.[27] This is not surprising considering the probable pathogenesis of fetal demise in diabetes in pregnancy.

Barrett *et al* reviewed seven studies of antepartum CTGs for fetal surveillance and found that within 7 days of a normal CTG there was a stillbirth rate of 1.4% in pregnancies with diabetes, similar to the figure for pregnancies complicated by IUGR (2%); there were no stillbirths in pregnancies with other risk factors, such as being postdates or pre-eclampsia.[28] Attempts to correlate CTG patterns with maternal glycemic status have been unsuccessful.[29,30] Tincello *et al*[29] found that 10.7% of computerized CTG recordings in pregnancies complicated by Type 1 diabetes had no episodes of high variation (defined as long-term variation exceeding a gestation-dependent threshold, with the presence of high variation considered to be a sensitive indicator of fetal well-being in normal pregnancy), compared with the expected value of 0.8% in uncomplicated singleton pregnancies, a difference of 9.5% (95% CI 4.5–15.3). The authors concluded that along with other differences in short-term variation, basal heart rate, frequency of fetal movements, and heart rate accelerations, these changes may represent a delay in fetal maturation. They did not identify any relationship between these changes and adverse fetal outcome, and therefore computerized CTG must be used with caution in women with diabetes.

In conclusion, available evidence does not support the routine use of antenatal CTG in pregnancies with diabetes outside the usual indications, including reduced fetal movements, fetal growth restriction or antepartum hemorrhage.

Ultrasound estimation of fetal growth

There is no clear consensus that monitoring fetal size by ultrasound in pregnancies with diabetes without risk factors for IUGR is beneficial[31] or necessary. The UK National Institute for Health and Clinical Excellence (NICE) guidelines[32] state that three growth scans, including estimation of amniotic fluid index, should be carried out at 28, 32, and 36 weeks of gestation, but no guidance is offered as to how the information obtained should subsequently be used.

Conventional ultrasound biometry is based on predicting IUGR, and is less accurate for detecting large babies, including those babies whose mothers have diabetes:[33] it overlooks 10–20% of babies with accelerated growth.[31] This is an important deficiency as diabetes influences the abdominal circumference (AC) but not bony measurements via its effect on insulin-sensitive tissues such as the liver (glycogen storage) and abdominal wall adipose tissue (Fig. 12.1). Accordingly, ultrasound measurements made to detect accelerated fetal growth are unreliable and therefore cannot be expected to predict trauma at delivery for these babies;[22] as such they are of debatable value.

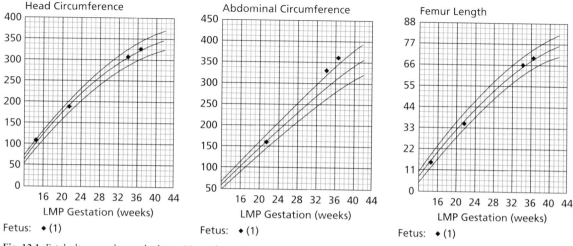

Fig. 12.1 Fetal ultrasound growth charts. Normal growth of head and femur with accelerated growth of abdominal circumference.

A systematic review[31] of 63 studies including a total of 19 117 women concluded that there was no difference in accuracy between ultrasonographic EFW and AC in the prediction of birthweight over 4000 g. These studies were in women without diabetes and therefore cannot be extrapolated directly to pregnancies in women with diabetes, but it is likely that accuracy would be even lower in the latter. In two studies of pregnant women with diabetes, the sensitivity of ultrasound for predicting fetal weight over 4000 g was relatively poor, ranging from 33% to 83%, and specificity from 77% to 98%.[34] The correlation between ultrasound determination of fetal size or fetal growth and fetal hyperinsulinemia (measured using amniotic fluid insulin levels) is also poor, and therefore ultrasound is not likely to be able to predict those babies at risk of the consequences of fetal hyperinsulinemia, such as intrauterine death and neonatal hypoglycemia.[35] In addition, growth continues to accelerate late into the third trimester, thereby further reducing the accuracy and usefulness of scanning as delivery approaches.[36]

Three-dimensional (3D) ultrasound volumetric assessments of fetal weight within 7 days of delivery has been shown to be superior to conventional two-dimensional (2D) biometry in a cross-sectional study in women without diabetes.[37] Fetal liver volume may also be assessed using 3D ultrasound. In a cross-sectional study, fetal liver volume was significantly greater in fetuses of 32 women with diabetes compared with matched controls, even after normalization for EFW. Fetal liver volume also correlated significantly with glycosylated hemoglobin.[38]

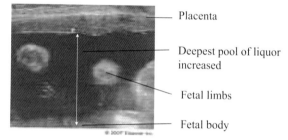

Fig. 12.2 Polyhydramnios on ultrasound scan.

More research is needed in this area before incorporation into routine clinical practice can be recommended.

In conclusion, serial growth scans in pregnancy with diabetes can be helpful for identifying growth restriction. Normal growth on ultrasound examinations does not reliably exclude accelerated growth or risks for shoulder dystocia. If the ultrasound suggests accelerated fetal growth, it is not known what risks this may pose to the fetus either antenatally or at delivery, and therefore the information is of debatable value. Accelerated growth may indicate poor glycemic control and so may be useful for intensifying insulin therapy and dietary advice.

Ultrasound assessment of amniotic fluid volume

Between 27 and 42 weeks, amniotic fluid volume (AFV) measurements are greater in pregnancies with diabetes than other pregnancies (Fig. 12.2).[39] This probably reflects fetal polyuria secondary to hyperglycemia-induced osmotic diuresis. There is a significant positive correlation between elevated AFV and both birthweight centiles and AC in both pregnancies with and without diabetes.[39,40] This relationship is linear in diabetic patients with poor glycemic control.[41] In pregnancies without diabetes, there is a four-fold increase in perinatal mortality when the AFV is increased, partly related to structural anomaly, prematurity, and malpresentation; however, there have been no prospective studies looking at the value of AFV measurements in predicting fetal outcome in structurally normal, term pregnancies with diabetes.

In conclusion, in structurally normal fetuses, raised AFV may trigger a further search for anomalies associated with swallowing difficulties. This finding may predict the possible need for nasogastric aspiration prior to first feeding, but it does not seem to be helpful in predicting antenatal fetal compromise. It may be a useful trigger for intensifying glycemic control.

Biophysical profile

The biophysical profile (BPP) involves ultrasound assessment of fetal breathing, fetal tone, fetal body movements, and AFV, and analysis of a CTG. Each of the five parameters scores either 0 (absent or low) or 2 (normal or present), giving a possible maximum of 10. It was originally validated for growth-restricted pregnancies in the absence of a major congenital anomaly. In maternal diabetes a number of problems in interpretation can be predicted. First, pregnancy with diabetes is commonly associated with an increased AFV. Second, increased fetal breathing can occur in pregnancies with diabetes[42] and with higher maternal blood glucose values. Where fetal acidemia is secondary to uteroplacental insufficiency, fetal breathing is reduced, whereas in fetal acidemia secondary to maternal hyperglycemia, fetal breathing movements are either normal or increased.[43] Salvesen et al[43] found that BPP was a poor predictor of fetal acidemia (as determined by cordocentesis performed after the BPP) in pregnancy with diabetes. Dicker et al performed almost 1000 BPPs in 98 pregnant women with diabetes, and found that while 3% were abnormal, that this was not helpful in determining Apgar scores or abnormal intrapartum CTG recordings.[44] BPP in pregnancies with diabetes has a higher false-negative rate than in pregnancies without diabetes.[25]

In conclusion the use of the BPP in pregnancy with diabetes in which fetal growth is normal or accelerated is not routinely advised.

Umbilical artery Doppler velocimetry

Doppler assessment of the umbilical arteries (UAs) is a commonly used method in the evaluation of the fetus in high-risk pregnancies (Fig. 12.3). A Cochrane Systematic Review found a trend to reduction in perinatal deaths (OR 0.71, 95% CI 0.50–1.01) with the use of Doppler ultrasound in high-risk pregnancies, especially those complicated by hypertension or presumed impaired fetal growth.[45]

In diabetes, however, the fetal hemodynamic and metabolic response to maternal hyperglycemia is complex and dependent on the duration of insult. The fetus increases its oxidative metabolism, becoming more hypoxemic. Perfusion of the brain and kidneys increases even in the absence of any changes in the feto-placental perfusion. In maternal diabetes, UA Doppler velocimetry therefore remains unchanged despite fetal hypoxemia (unless there is also vasculopathy or placental insufficiency and fetal growth restriction) and the presence of normal Doppler indices does not exclude fetal compromise.

There is conflicting evidence regarding the value of UA Doppler in the assessment of fetal well-being in pregnancy with diabetes. Three studies,[46–48] involving a total of 249 patients, found that UA Doppler is not helpful in predicting adverse outcome in diabetic pregnancy in the absence of growth restriction or pre-eclampsia. One study[49] including 207 pregnancies with diabetes suggested that UA Doppler ultrasound (systolic-to-diastolic ratio >3) within 1 week of delivery was associated with a raised relative risk of adverse outcome (RR 2.6, 95% CI 1.9–3.5) compared with a BPP of 6 or less (RR 1.7, 9.5% CI 0.9–2.9) and non-reactive CTG (RR 1.7, 95% CI 1.2–2.5). However, the main endpoints relate to growth restriction, prematurity, and pre-eclampsia; pregnancies complicated by accelerated growth were excluded, and there was no correlation between outcome and diabetic control.

In conclusion, there is no evidence that UA Doppler velocimetry is of routine value in pregnancy with diabetes. It should only be used in pregnancy with diabetes when this is complicated by growth restriction or pre-eclampsia. This recommendation was echoed in the recent UK NICE guideline on pregnancy with diabetes.[27]

Amniocentesis

Sampling of the amniotic fluid in pregnancy with diabetes may be useful to assess fetal lung maturity (FLM)

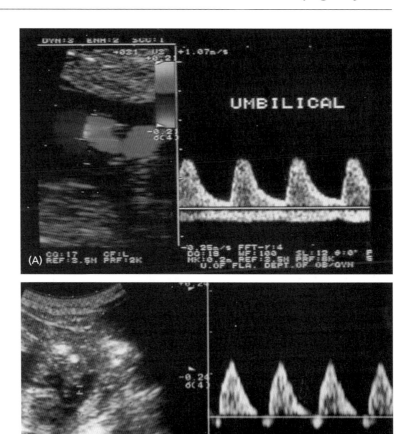

Fig. 12.3 (A) Normal umbilical artery Dopplers showing forward flow in both systole and diastole. (B) Abnormal umbilical artery Dopplers showing reversed end-diastolic flow.

prior to planned preterm delivery. In an attempt to identify the "at-risk" fetus, it also facilitates the measurement of amniotic fluid insulin and more recently amniotic fluid EPO, although these measurements are still confined to research. The risks of amniocentesis at this gestation are small, but include provoking a non-reassuring fetal heart rate, preterm labour, and introduction of infection.

Assessment of fetal lung maturity

Historically, the determination of FLM in pregnancy with diabetes has helped guide obstetricians when to deliver near-term fetuses, aiming to both minimize the risk of respiratory distress syndrome (RDS) and to avoid late stillbirth. Various amniotic fluid analyses are used to assess FLM, such as the lecithin-to-sphingomyelin (L:S) ratio, presence of phosphatidylglycerol (PG), surfactant-to-albumin ratio, lamellar body counts (LBCs), foam stability index (FSI), and optical density.[50] All have good correlation with the absence of RDS. LBC is the test of choice, followed by other tests if a transitional result is obtained;[50] the choice of test may be determined by local availability.

Poorly controlled maternal diabetes is associated with delayed FLM[51] of uncertain etiology, while women with good glycemic control show no delay in lung maturation and risks are similar to those of women without diabetes.[52] Kjos et al[53] found a low (<1%) but similar rate of RDS in neonates delivered at term (beyond 37 completed weeks) in whom no assessment of FLM was performed compared with a group of historic controls, and concluded that the test should be abandoned. However, delivery of these infants by elective cesarean section was associated with increased RDS when compared with vaginal delivery, as is found in pregnancy without diabetes.

In conclusion, FLM testing is not required beyond 37 weeks of gestation when maternal diabetes is well-controlled and the gestation is known accurately through early ultrasound estimation. There may still be a place for FLM testing if diabetic control is poor, if early ultrasound confirmation of estimated delivery date is uncertain and elective preterm delivery is considered, or on the rare occasion that administration of steroids between 34 and 36 weeks is contemplated. However, usually the indications for delivery will be sufficiently strong to override concerns about FLM.

Amniotic fluid insulin

High fetal insulin levels in the third trimester have been implicated in accelerated fetal growth, as well as fetal acidemia.[14] Conceptually, identification of the hyperinsulinemic fetus before delivery might allow the intensification of maternal insulin therapy, leading to a reduction in the incidence and severity of diabetic fetopathy.[54] However, published data are limited. While studies in women with Type 1 and diet-treated gestational diabetes mellitus (GDM) showed that high amniotic fluid insulin concentrations correlated with accelerated fetal growth, and increased rates of symptomatic neonatal hypoglycemia,[54] it is unclear whether this might have been predicted by the usual assessment of glycemic control or other clinical determinants.

A retrospective study of 121 pregnancies in German and Middle Eastern women with diabetes attempted to establish whether ultrasound can reduce the need for amniocentesis. They found that only 21% (10 of 47) of fetuses with an AC over the 75th centile in the third trimester had hyperinsulinism (amniotic fluid insulin levels >16 µU/mL, a level reported to be associated with considerable neonatal and long-term morbidity). Therefore ultrasound alone cannot determine which fetuses have hyperinsulinism, and if accurate determination of amniotic fluid insulin were thought to be required, 80% of amniocenteses would be done unnecessarily. The negative predictive value of AC under the 75th centile was 100% (74 of 74; p < 0.0001). Although this suggests that ultrasound might help to identify babies at low risk of hyperinsulinism, there is insufficient evidence to support this conclusion in other populations.[55]

In conclusion, there are not enough data yet to warrant measuring antenatal levels of amniotic fluid insulin in routine clinical practice, nor for using ultrasound to identify "high-risk" pregnancies.

Amniotic fluid erythropoietin

Tissue hypoxia is the major stimulus for EPO synthesis and high amniotic fluid EPO levels are a surrogate marker for chronic fetal hypoxia. EPO neither crosses the placenta nor is stored. Fetal plasma and amniotic fluid levels are therefore indicative of fetal EPO synthesis and elimination. Amniotic fluid EPO levels correlate well with cord plasma levels in both normal and abnormal pregnancies. Repeated amniotic fluid EPO measurements reveal exponential increases during fetal hypoxia in pregnancies with diabetes and other high-risk pregnancies.[56]

Teramo et al[56] found that in Type 1 diabetes, neonatal hypoglycemia, hypertropic cardiomyopathy, and admission to the neonatal intensive care unit occurred significantly more often in cases with amniotic fluid EPO levels over 63.0 mU/mL.

It is possible that weekly measurements of amniotic fluid EPO from 37 weeks, with delivery if levels are rising towards a threshold, could be the way forward in the management of these complex high-risk pregnancies with diabetes.

In conclusion, while this appears attractive in potentially identifying the "at risk" fetus, it remains a research tool and its use requires confirmation in randomized controlled trials.

MRI spectroscopy

Given the limitations of the above procedures, ongoing research is examining the role of MRI spectroscopy as a non-invasive method to assess FLM by measuring a variety of compounds, including choline and lecithin.[57] The technique is also being assessed as a tool to identify the fetus at risk of intrauterine death by analysis of spectra for fetal metabolic products, such as lactate, in the amniotic fluid.[58]

FETAL SURVEILLANCE IN PREGESTATIONAL DIABETES (TYPE 1 OR TYPE 2) COMPARED WITH GESTATIONAL DIABETES MELLITUS

Although much data assessing fetal risk and antepartum surveillance pertain to Type 1 diabetes, evolving evidence suggests that outcomes in Type 2 diabetes are similarly poor.[2] In fact, the risk of accelerated fetal growth and perinatal morbidity/mortality may be greater in Type 2 diabetes given the frequent occurrence of other risk factors for poor obstetric outcome, such as advanced maternal age, raised maternal body mass index (BMI), non-Caucasian ethnicity, and social deprivation.

The issue of fetal surveillance is even more controversial in GDM than pre-existing diabetes. There are few data in the literature to support or refute antenatal fetal surveillance in GDM. The optimal method, timing, and frequency of fetal surveillance in GDM remains unclear and will only be resolved by prospective, randomized controlled trials. It would seem reasonable, however, that women with poorly controlled GDM, whose babies have accelerated growth and who require insulin or have other risk factors such as hypertension or adverse obstetric history, should have fetal surveillance similar to women with pre-existing diabetes.[59] Ultrasound measurement of abdominal circumference may also serve to guide the clinician as to the need for insulin therapy in conjunction with the results from home blood glucose monitoring.[59]

PRACTICAL APPROACHES TO FETAL SURVEILLANCE (Table 12.1)

Given the lack of an ideal fetal monitoring test, the limitations of the available tests and lack of rigorous scientific trials, including randomized controlled trials, all protocols used for fetal surveillance are empiric, rather than evidence-based, and all have limitations.

Serial ultrasound growth scans measuring AC and liquor volume in the second half of pregnancy help to detect IUGR and accelerated growth. The former should be monitored in the same manner as any other pregnancy complicated by fetal growth restriction. In the latter, the appropriate tests for fetal monitoring are still unknown. When diabetic control is excellent, growth scans are normal, and there is no vascular disease or other diabetic complications, it is reasonable not to offer other routine tests of fetal well-being.

In poorly controlled diabetes and where the fetus has accelerated growth and/or polyhydramnios, some form of fetal surveillance should be offered, although at present it is not known which is the best test, and the optimal frequency of testing also remains unknown. Twice-weekly CTGs with a BPP when the CTG was non-reassuring have been suggested;[60] however, fetal deaths have been reported following a normal CTG.[27] Weekly UA Dopplers may be better at recognizing fetal well-being,[32,49] although this is unclear and cannot be routinely recommended.

The financial impact on health resources, the maternal anxiety generated, and the lack of evidence regarding the efficacy of the tests must all be considered when local

Table 12.1 Summary of usefulness of available tests for fetal well-being in clinical practice in the context of a pregnancy with diabetes.

Fetal surveillance test	Recommendation
Serial growth scans	Recommended routinely
Antenatal CTGs	Recommended in specific cases *viz* IUGR, reduced FM, etc
Fetal movement count	Not recommended routinely
Estimation of liquor volume	Not recommended as a test of fetal well-being but is of other clinical significance
Biophysical profile	Not recommended
Umbilical artery Doppler velocimetry	Recommended in specific cases *viz* coexisting pre-eclampsia or IUGR
Assessment of fetal lung maturity	Not routinely recommended
Amniotic fluid insulin*	Not recommended in routine clinical practice
Amniotic fluid erythropoietin*	Not recommended in routine clinical practice
MRI spectroscopy*	Not recommended in routine clinical practice

* Potentially useful test, but more research needed before being incorporated into routine clinical practice
CTG, cardiotocograph; IUGR; intrauterine growth restriction; FM, fetal movements; MRI, magnetic resonance imaging

protocols are developed. The National Service Framework for Diabetes (England) Standards[61] includes serial ultrasound scans for fetal growth during the third trimester and consideration of CTG monitoring from 36 weeks. The UK NICE guideline[32] recommends that ultrasound monitoring of fetal growth and AFV should be offered every 4 weeks from 28 to 36 weeks and that routine monitoring of fetal well-being is only needed for pregnancies complicated by IUGR. On the basis of the current information, this seems reasonable.

RESEARCH DIRECTIONS

- Understanding the mechanism of fetal demise in pregnancy with diabetes.
- The use of 3D ultrasound for the identification of accelerated fetal growth.
- The most appropriate management strategy following detection of accelerated fetal growth antenatally.
- Randomized controlled trials to determine the optimal surveillance tests and the frequency of testing.

- Randomized controlled trials of amniotic fluid EPO to detect the "at-risk" fetus.
- Non-invasive methods to assess FLM and fetal compromise.

REFERENCES

1 Pedersen J. *Diabetes and Pregnancy. Blood Sugar of Newborn Infants.* PhD thesis. Copenhagen: Danish Science Press, 1952.

2 Confidential Enquiry into Maternal and Child Health. *Pregnancy in Women with Type 1 and Type 2 Diabetes in 2002–03, England, Wales and Northern Ireland.* London: CEMACH, 2005.

3 Confidential Enquiry into Maternal and Child Health. *Diabetes in Pregnancy: Are We Providing the Best Care? England, Wales and Northern Ireland.* London: CEMACH, 2007.

4 Seeds JW, Peng CC. Does augmented growth impose an increased risk of fetal death? *Am J Obstet Gynecol* 2000;**183**:316–23.

5 Mondestin MAJ, Ananth CV, Smulian JC, *et al.* Birth weight and fetal death in the United States: The effect of maternal diabetes during pregnancy. *Am J Obstet Gynecol* 2002;**187**: 922–6.

6 Jazayeri A, O'Brien WF, Tsibris JC, *et al.* Are maternal diabetes and pre-eclampsia independent stimulators of erythropoietin production? *Am J Perinatol* 1998;**15**:577–80.

7 Landon MB, Vickers S. Fetal surveillance in pregnancy complicated by diabetes mellitus: is it necessary? *J Matern Fetal Neonat Med* 2002;**12**:413–6.

8 Bjork O, Persson B. Villous structure in different parts of the cotyledon in placentas of insulin dependent diabetic women. *Acta Obstet Gynecol Scand* 1984;**63**:37–43.

9 Widness JA, Teramo KA, Clemons GK, *et al.* Direct relationship of antepartum glucose control and fetal erythropoietin in human Type 1 (insulin dependent) diabetic pregnancy. *Diabetologia* 1990;**33**:378–83.

10 Inkster ME, Fahey TP, Donnan PT, *et al.* Poor glycated haemoglobin control and adverse pregnancy outcomes in type 1 and type 2 diabetes mellitus: Systematic review of observational studies. *BMC Pregnancy Childbirth* 2006;**6**: 30.

11 Kyne-Grzebalski D, Wood L, Marshall SM, *et al.* Episodic hyperglycaemia in pregnant women with well-controlled Type 1 diabetes mellitus: a major potential factor underlying macrosomia. *Diabet Med* 1999;**16**:621–2.

12 Phillips AF, Widness JA, Garcia JF, *et al.* Erythropoeitin elevation in the chronically hyperglycaemic fetal lamb. *Proc Soc Exp Biol Med* 1982;**170**:42–7.

13 Salvesen DR, Brudenell JM, Nicolaides KH. Fetal polycythaemia and thrombocytopenia in pregnancies complicated by maternal diabetes. *Am J Obstet Gynecol* 1992; **166**:1287–92.

14 Salvesen DR, Brudenell JM, Proudler A, *et al.* Fetal pancreatic beta-cell function in pregnancies complicated by maternal diabetes mellitus. *Am J Obstet Gynecol* 1993; **168**:1363–9.

15 Bradley RJ, Brudenell JM, Nicolaides KH. Fetal acidosis and hyperlactinemia diagnosed by cordocentesis in pregnancies complicated by maternal diabetes mellitus. *Diabet Med* 1991;**8**:464–8.

16 Schwartz R, Gruppuso PA, Petzold K, *et al.* Hyperinsulinaemia and macrosomia in the fetus of the diabetic mother. *Diabetes Care* 1994;**17**:640–8.

17 Wong SF, Chan FY, Oats JJN, *et al.* Fetal growth spurt and pregestational diabetic pregnancy. *Diabetes Care* 2002;**25**: 1681–4.

18 Raychaudhuri K, Maresh MJA. Glycemic control throughout pregnancy and fetal growth in insulin-dependent diabetes. *Obstet Gynecol* 2000;**95**:190–4.

19 Page RCL, Kirk Ba, Fay T, *et al.* Is macrosomia associated with poor glycaemic control in diabetic pregnancy? *Diabetic Med* 1996;**13**:170–4.

20 Seeds JW, Peng CC. Does augmented growth impose an increased risk of fetal death? *Am J Obstet Gynecol* 2000;**183**: 316–23.

21 Langer O, Berkus MD, Huff RW, *et al.* Shoulder dystocia: Should the fetus weighing >4000 grams be delivered by caesarean section? *Am J Obstet Gynecol* 1991;**165**:831–7.

22 MacFarland MB, Trylovich CG, Langer O. Anthropometric differences in macrosomic infants of diabetic and non diabetic mothers. *J Matern Fetal Neonatal Med* 1998;**7**: 292–5.

23 Conway DL, Langer O. Elective delivery of infants with macrosomia in diabetic women: Reduced shoulder dystocia versus increased caesarean deliveries. *Am J Obstet Gynecol* 1998;**178**:922–5.

24 Rouse DJ, Owen J. Prophylactic caesarean delivery for fetal macrosomia diagnosed by means of ultrasonography – A Faustian bargain? *Am J Obstet Gynecol* 1999;**181**: 332–8.

25 Siddiqui F, James D. Fetal monitoring in type 1 diabetic pregnancies. *Early Hum Dev* 2003;**72**:1–13.

26 Pattison N, McCowan L. Cardiotocography for antepartum fetal assessment. *Cochrane Database Syst Rev* 2002, Issue 2: CD001068.

27 Shaxted EJ, Jenkins HM. Fetal death immediately following a normal antenatal fetal heart rate pattern. *Br J Obstet Gynaecol* 1981;**88**:747–8.

28 Barrett JM, Salyer SL, Boehm FH. The non-stress test: an evaluation of 1,000 patients. *Am J Obstet Gynecol* 1981;**141**: 153–7.

29 Tincello D, White S, Walkinshaw S. Computerised analysis of fetal heart rate recordings in maternal type 1 diabetes. *Br J Obstet Gynaecol* 2001;**108**:853–7.

30 Serra-Serra V, Camara R, Sarrion P, *et al.* Effects of prandial glycemic changes on objective fetal heart rate parameters. *Acta Obstet Gynecol Scand* 2000;**79**:953–7.

31 Coomarasamy A, Connock M, Thornton J, *et al*. Accuracy of ultrasound biometry in the prediction of macrosomia: a systematic quantitative review. *BJOG* 2005;**112**:1461–6.

32 National Institute of Health and Clinical excellence. *Diabetes in Pregnancy: Management of Diabetes and its Complications from Pre-conception to the Postnatal Period. NICE Guideline*. London: NICE, 2007. www.nice.org.uk

33 Benacerraf BR. Sonographically estimated fetal weights: accuracy and limitations. *Am J Obstet Gynecol* 1988;**159**: 118–21.

34 O'Reilly-Green C, Divon M. Sonographic and clinical methods in the diagnosis of macrosomia. *Clin Obstet Gynecol* 2000;**43**:309–20.

35 Farrell T, Owen P, Kernaghan D, *et al*. Can ultrasound fetal biometry predict fetal hyperinsulinaemia at delivery in pregnancies complicated by maternal diabetes? *Eur J Obstet Gynecol Reprod Biol* 2007;**131**:146–50.

36 Wong SF, Lee-Tannock A, Amaraddio D, *et al*. Fetal growth patterns in fetuses of women with pregestational diabetes mellitus. *Ultrasound Obstet Gynecol* 2006;**28**:934–8.

37 Schild RL, Fimmers R, Hansmann M. Fetal weight estimation by three-dimensional ultrasound. *Ultrasound Obstet Gynecol* 2000;**16**:445–52.

38 Boito SM, Struijk PC, Ursem NTC, *et al*. Assessment of fetal liver volume and umbilical venous volume flow in pregnancies complicated by insulin-dependent diabetes mellitus. *BJOG* 2003;**110**:1007–13.

39 Kofinas A, Kofinas G. Differences in amniotic fluid patterns and fetal biometric parameters in third trimester pregnancies with and without diabetes. *J Matern Fetal Neonatal Med* 2006;**19**:633–8.

40 Hackmon R, Bornstein E, Ferber A, *et al*. Combined analysis with amniotic fluid index and estimated fetal weight for prediction of severe macrosomia at birth. *Am J Obstet Gynecol* 2007;**196**:333.e1–4.

41 Vink JY, Poggi SH, Ghidini A, *et al*. Amniotic fluid index and birth weight: Is there a relationship with poor glycaemic control? *Am J Obstet Gynecol* 2006;**195**:848–50.

42 Boddy K, Dawes G. Fetal breathing. *Br Med Bull* 1975; **31**:3–7.

43 Salvesen DR, Freeman J, Brudenell JM, *et al*. Prediction of fetal acidemia in pregnancies complicated by maternal diabetes mellitus by biophysical profile scoring and fetal heart rate monitoring. *Br J Obstet Gynaecol* 1993;**100**:227–33.

44 Dicker D, Feldberg D, Yeshaya A, *et al*. Fetal surveillance in insulin dependent diabetic pregnancy: predictive value of the biophysical profile. *Am J Obstet Gynecol* 1988;**159**: 800–4.

45 Neilson JP, Alfirevic Z. Doppler ultrasound for fetal assessment in high-risk pregnancies. *Cochrane Database Syst Rev* 2002, Issue 2: CD000073.

46 Kofinas AD, Penry M, Swain M. Uteroplacental Doppler flow velocity waveform analysis correlates poorly with gly-

caemic control in diabetic pregnant women. *Am J Perinatol* 1991;**8**:273–7.

47 Johnstone FD, Steel JM, Haddad NG, *et al*. Doppler umbilical artery flow velocimetry waveforms in diabetic pregnancy. *Br J Obstet Gynaecol* 1992;**99**:135–40.

48 Reece EA, Hagay Z, Assimakopoulos E, *et al*. Diabetes mellitus in pregnancy and the assessment of umbilical artery waveforms using pulsed Doppler ultrasonography. *J Ultrasound Med* 1994;**13**:73–80.

49 Bracero LA, Figueroa R, Byrne DW, *et al*. Comparison of umbilical artery Doppler velocimetry, nonstress testing and biophysical profile in pregnancies complicated by diabetes. *J Ultrasound Med* 1996;**15**:301–8.

50 Ventolini G, Neiger R, Hood D, *et al*. Update on assessment of fetal lungaturity. *J Obstet Gynaecol* 2005;**25**:535–38.

51 DeRoche ME, Ingardia CJ, Guerette PJ, *et al*. The use of lamellar body counts to predict fetal lung maturity in pregnancies complicated by diabetes mellitus. *Am J Obstet Gynecol* 2002;**187**:908–12.

52 Piazze JJ, Anceschi MM, Maranghi L, *et al*. Fetal lung maturity in pregnancies complicated by insulin dependent and gestational diabetes: a matched cohort study. *Eur J Obstet Gynaecol Reprod Biol* 1999;**83**:145–50.

53 Kjos SL, Berkowitz KM, Kung B. Prospective delivery of reliably dated term infants of diabetic mothers without determination of fetal lung maturity: comparison to historical control. *J Mat Fetal Neonat Med* 2002;**12**:433–7.

54 Fraser RB, Bruce C. Amniotic fluid insulin levels identify the fetus at risk of neonatal hypoglycaemia. *Diabet Med* 1999;**16**:568–72.

55 Schafer-Graf UM, Kjos SL, Buhling KJ, *et al*. Amniotic fluid insulin levels and fetal abdominal circumference at the time of amniocentesis in pregnancies with diabetes. *Diabet Med* 2003;**20**:349–54.

56 Teramo K, Kari MA, Eronen M, *et al*. High amniotic fluid erythropoietin levels are associated with an increased frequency of fetal and neonatal morbidity in type 1 diabetic pregnancies. *Diabetologia* 2004;**47**:1695–703.

57 Clifton MS, Joe BN, Zektzer AS, *et al*. Feasibility of magnetic resonance spectroscopy for evaluating fetal lung maturity. *J Paediatr Surg* 2006;**41**:768–73.

58 Robinson JN, Cleary JG, Arias FM, *et al*. Detection of fetal lactate with two-dimensional-localized proton magnetic resonance spectroscopy. *Obstet Gynecol* 2004;**104**:1208–10.

59 American College of Obstetricians and Gynecologists. ACOG Practice Bulletin No. 39. Gestational diabetes. *Obstet Gynecol* 2001;**98**:525–38.

60 Landon MB, Langer O, Gabbe SC, *et al*. Fetal surveillance in pregnancies complicated by insulin-dependent diabetes mellitus. *Am J Obstet Gynecol* 1992;**167**:617–21.

61 Department of Health. *National Service Framework for Diabetes (England) Standards*. London: The Stationery Office, 2001.

13 Diet and exercise in diabetes in pregnancy

Anita Banerjee & Anne Dornhorst

Queen Charlotte's & Chelsea Hospital, Imperial College NHS HealthCare Trust, London, UK

PRACTICE POINTS

- Diet and exercise are important lifestyle determinants for health. During pregnancy minor modification to the diet is required to cover the energy costs. Exercise patterns also need to be modified to accommodate the physiologic and anatomic changes that occur with increasing gestation.
- Pregnant women with Type 1 diabetes need to balance their dietary intake with their changes in insulin therapy required to achieve glycemic control. The increased risk of hypoglycemia in the first half of pregnancy necessitates careful meal planning and regular low glycemic snacks between meals. Proactive adjustments to dietary intake and insulin dose help to prevent exercise-related hypoglycemia.
- For obese women with Type 2 diabetes or gestational diabetes, dietetic advice should be aimed at minimizing excess weight gain. Simple adjustments to dietary intake that include low glycemic carbohydrates can help to reduce postprandial hyperglycemia.
- All women should be encouraged to be physically active in pregnancy, this can usually be achieved by including short walks in their daily regime.

CASE HISTORY 1

Angela is a 28-year-old dental nurse who was diagnosed with Type 1 diabetes when 8 years old and is currently 15 weeks' pregnant in her first pregnancy. Angela attended preconception counseling and had taken folic acid 400 μg/day prior to and during the first 12 weeks of this pregnancy. Although she has no diabetic complications, there is a previous history of anorexia and bulimia for 3 years in her early 20s. More recently Angela has managed to maintain her BMI at 22 kg/m^2 by jogging 30–40 minutes daily and sensible eating.

A Practical Manual of Diabetes in Pregnancy, 1st Edition.
Edited by David R. McCance, Michael Maresh and David A. Sacks.
© 2010 Blackwell Publishing

When Angela was reviewed at 15 weeks she was maintaining her fasting blood glucoses between 4.5 and 5.0 mmol/L (81–90 mg/dL). However, her awareness of hypoglycemia had deteriorated and she was experiencing frequent hypoglycemic episodes that were followed by extremely high blood glucose values. As a consequence, she was performing glucose monitoring eight times a day, including a reading before bed. Angela had not so far gained any weight during her pregnancy and was continuing to jog after work.

CASE HISTORY 2

Senita is a 34-year-old Asian mother of two who attended the antenatal diabetic obstetric clinic following the diagnosis of gestational diabetes mellitus (GDM) at 17 weeks. Senita had an oral glucose tolerance test at 16 weeks of gestation as she had had GDM in her previous two pregnancies, both diagnosed at 28 weeks and managed with diet alone. Senita's body mass index (BMI) was 31 kg/m^2 at her 12-week booking visit and when reviewed at 17 weeks, she had already gained 6 kg from her prepregnancy weight. Lifestyle assessment revealed she took no regular exercise and her diet was predominately vegetarian, high in saturated fat and refined carbohydrates.

- What are the basic physiologic energy needs in pregnancy?
- What is the weight gain in normal pregnancy and in pregnancy in women with diabetes?
- What advice should be given regarding diet in normal pregnancy and pregnancy in women with diabetes?
- What advice should be given regarding exercise in normal pregnancy and pregnancy in women with diabetes?
- What advice should be given after pregnancy?

Table 13.1 Components of maternal weight gain in a term pregnancy.[1]

Tissue	Fetus	Uterus	Placenta	Amniotic fluid	Breast Tissue	Circulatory fluid/blood	Adipose tissue	Total weight gain
Weight gain (kg)	3.5	0.9	0.66	0.8	0.4	3.25	1.7*	11.2

* The average total adipose weight gain is >4 kg in the first half of pregnancy; however, by late pregnancy there is a loss in maternal adipose mass.

BACKGROUND

Pregnancy is associated with physiologic changes that optimize the transfer of maternal nutrients to the fetus. Maternal and fetal adaptation occurs throughout pregnancy to ensure the energy requirements of the feto-placental unit and subsequent lactation are met from a combination of maternal energy intake, maternal adipose stores, and energy conservation through decreased physical activity.

The average total weight gain in pregnancy for a fit non-obese woman is between 10 and 12.5 kg.[1] This extra weight relates to the feto-placental unit and the increase in maternal tissues (Table 13.1).

Weight gain accelerates in pregnancy with 25% in the first 20 weeks, 25% between 20 and 30 weeks of gestation, and the remaining 50% in the last 10 weeks of pregnancy.

CHANGES IN GLUCOSE METABOLISM RELEVANT TO DIET AND EXERCISE

Normal pregnancy

Glucose is the major fetal fuel substrate and maternal metabolic changes occur throughout pregnancy to optimize its uninterrupted supply to the fetus. Maternal postprandial glucose concentrations rise to facilitate materno-fetal transfer after meals. Paradoxically, in normal pregnancy fasting glucose concentrations decrease at about 10 weeks and remain at this level until birth. A rise in hepatic glucose output, however, ensures a continual glucose supply between meals.

Placental hormones promote maternal insulin resistance and maternal lipolysis; the latter further increases insulin resistance. This rise in maternal insulin resistance effectively diverts glucose away from maternal insulin-sensitive tissues to the fetus. As a consequence, maternal energy requirement becomes increasingly reliant on fat metabolism as the pregnancy progresses (see chapter 2 for more detail).

Pregnancy with diabetes

The pregnancy-related rise in maternal insulin resistance also occurs in women with diabetes. For women with Type 1 diabetes this is apparent by their two- to three-fold increase in insulin requirements by late pregnancy. For women with Type 2 diabetes, who can be managed with diet and oral agents alone prior to pregnancy, the further increase in insulin resistance that occurs inevitably necessitates the need for insulin therapy, with many women requiring a disproportionate increase in insulin demand and high doses of insulin by the third trimester. Similarly, many women with gestational diabetes mellitus (GDM) who start their pregnancy with normal glucose tolerance but with increasing insulin resistance, require therapy (either with oral hypoglycemic drugs or insulin) by the third trimester to maintain adequate glycemic control.[2]

IS THERE A HEALTHY WEIGHT GAIN FOR PREGNANCY?

Normal pregnancy

There is no international consensus on what is the ideal weight gain for pregnancy. Current guidelines are outdated as they are based on antenatal populations that were less obese than today's and at a time when there was greater concern for preventing low birthweight infants.[3] Despite this, there is general agreement that pregnancy weight gain should reflect prepregnancy BMI. For normal weight women, a 10–12.5-kg pregnancy weight gain is considered optimal as it is associated with fewer pregnancy-related complications. By contrast, for underweight women (BMI < 19.8 kg/m²), a pregnancy weight gain of 12.5–18 kg is recommended.

The risk of hypertension, GDM, infections, and need for cesarean birth all increase when weight gain exceeds 10–12.5 kg, especially when women start their pregnancies overweight or obese. For obese (>30 kg/m²) and morbidly obese (>40 kg/m²) women, little or no weight

gain during pregnancy reduces the risk of large for gestational age (LGA) infants and cesarean births, while only
minimally increasing the risk of small for gestational age
(SGA) infants.[4,5] Normal and underweight women who
gain less than 7–10 kg are at increased risk of giving birth
to an SGA infant.

To date no national obstetric body has been prepared
to endorse no weight gain. This is despite the data for
obese or morbidly obese pregnant women (BMI > 35 kg/
m[2]) that the benefits gained in reducing the risk of GDM,
hypertension, and an operative birth are likely to outweigh any adverse risks. Many clinicians currently recommend that pregnancy should be weight neutral for
obese women, with no excess weight remaining after the
birth. However, there remains a concern about the negative relationship in women who have diabetes between
maternal ketonemia and intellectual and motor performance of their children aged 2–5 years.[6]

Pregnancy with diabetes

The pregnancy weight gain targets for women with Type
1 and Type 2 diabetes, and GDM should be the same
as for woman without diabetes. However, this may be
difficult to achieve for women on insulin due to their
greater dependency on frequent snacks to avoid hypoglycemia. Dietary advice around appropriate food choices
taken as snacks and for the management of hypoglycemia
is required to prevent unnecessary weight gain as
insulin management is intensified. Approximately 20 g
of oral carbohydrate is required to manage a typical
hypoglycemic episode; suitable food choices for the
immediate management for hypoglycemia are listed in
Table 13.2.

Table 13.2 Immediate management for hypoglycemia.

Food	Calories	Carbohydrate (g)
4 Jelly babies (Trebor, Nestle)	80	19
5 Liquorice allsorts (Bassett & Co Ltd, Beacon)	107	23
6 Wine gums (Bassett & Co Ltd, Maynards)	126	28
7 Dextrosol tablet	94	23
100 ml Lucozade Energy	73	26
250 ml Ribena Original (prediluted)	128	30
½ 330-ml can of Fanta Orange	48	16

Minimizing unnecessary weight gain in obese women
with Type 2 diabetes or GDM can improve maternal
glycemic control and improve pregnancy outcomes.
Current UK guidelines recommend women with a prepregnancy BMI of greater than 27 kg/m[2] to restrict their
calorie intake to around 25 kcal/kg/day in the second
trimester.[7] In comparison, the US Institute of Medicine
guidelines (not specific to diabetes) recommend that
women with a prepregnancy BMI of 26–29 kg/m[2] gain a
total weight of 7–11.5 kg during pregnancy.[3] They further
recommend a target weight gain of less than 6 kg for
women with a pregnancy BMI > 29 kg/m[2]. However, they
have subsequently reviewed these guidelines and concluded there is a need for further research, particularly in
view of the rising trends in obesity.[8]

For women with GDM, the introduction of metformin
rather than insulin for glycemic management if dietary
measures fail could potentially help to limit weight gain,
due to less defensive snacking as there is a reduced risk
of hypoglycemia associated with metformin compared to
insulin. However, there are still concerns around the
introduction of metformin in the first trimester as it does
cross the placenta and could theoretically be teratoge-
netic in humans.

FACTORS THAT LIMIT MATERNAL EXERCISE

Normal pregnancy

Sensible moderate exercise is to be encouraged in pregnancy; contact sports, high impact sports, and sport
undertaken alone or in remote places, together with those
commonly referred to as "extreme sports", are not recommended. Scuba diving should be avoided throughout
pregnancy as the fetus is not protected from problems
arising from decompression; both the risks of malformation and gas embolism have been associated with decompression disease.

Exercising in the supine position in late pregnancy can
potentially cause aorto-caval compression and should be
avoided. It is important to ensure adequate hydration
during exercise, especially in hot weather.

In fit and active women, a number of cardiovascular
and respiratory changes occur as pregnancy progresses
that directly affect and limit exercise tolerance (Table
13.3). As pregnancy advances there are also physical limitations due to the increasing size of the gravid uterus.
Exercise tolerance is further compromised by the third
trimester as the uterus splints the diaphragm (Table 13.3).

Table 13.3 Cardiovascular and respiratory changes in normal pregnancy.[9-11]

	Prepregnancy	First trimester	Second trimester	Third trimester
Heart rate (beats/min)	70	70	80	90–105
Cardiac output (L/min)	5	7	7	7.5
Tidal volume (mL)	500	650	–	700–740
Minute ventilation (L/min)	6	7.8	–	8.4–9
Extra energy cost (kcal/day)	–	20	85	310

Normal physiologic changes by late gestation result in a sensation of breathlessness and respiratory discomfort that may limit exercise. A combination of the increased resting and effort minute ventilation and tachycardia can be associated with a perception of anxiety and apprehension that by late pregnancy can limit exercise tolerance.[12]

With increasing gestation, joint laxity, pubic symphysis dysfunction, and backache can also limit a woman's ability to exercise. These muscular skeletal problems become more problematic with increasing parity and obesity.

Pregnancy with diabetes

All women with diabetes experience cardiovascular and muscular skeletal changes in pregnancy similar to those of women without diabetes. The problems encountered with exercise, however, are different for women with Type 1 diabetes than for women with Type 2 diabetes or GDM, and therefore need to be considered separately.

Exercise creates challenges throughout pregnancy for women with Type 1 diabetes, the most common and potentially most serious being hypoglycemia. The risk for exercise-induced hypoglycemia is increased in pregnancy due to decreased hypoglycemic awareness and the attenuated adrenergic response to a fall in blood glucose. Quite modest exercise, such as encountered traveling to work, doing the housework, and shopping, needs to be proactively and individually factored into daily insulin and dietary management. More strenuous exercise, such as aerobics, swimming, and jogging, that may outside pregnancy be well tolerated, will require ongoing individual review and assessment throughout pregnancy, and may need to be curtailed altogether if hypoglycemia persists.

Many women with Type 2 diabetes and GDM enter pregnancy with poor exercise tolerance, having done little or no regular exercise beforehand. Limitations in increasing physical activity in overweight gravid women with Type 2 diabetes and GDM include their increased risk for muscular skeletal problems and other comorbidities.

For all women with Type 2 diabetes or GDM, any increase in exercise, especially postprandial, is potentially beneficial to the pregnancy as it helps to limit postprandial hyperglycemia, weight gain, and insulin requirements. A physical activity program combined with dietary modification and intensive glycemic management has been shown to reduce perinatal complications in women with GDM.[13] Exercise programs based on 20 minutes of arm movements three times a week and/or weekly resistance exercises three times a week have been found to lower fasting blood glucose, 1-hour postprandial blood glucose, and hemoglobin A1c (HbA1c) in women with GDM, as well as reducing the need for insulin when compared with diet alone.[14,15] Exercise does, however, need to be sustained throughout pregnancy.[16]

All advice around physical activity needs to be tailored around that which is safely achievable. Small increases in physical activity can be incorporated in daily living by encouraging women to walk 20 minutes twice a day. Simple modifications around exercise, such as walking to the shops or taking the children to and from school, can, if taken after a meal, lower postprandial glucose values, allowing some women with GDM to require no or less insulin. In addition, encouraging women with GDM to continue their exercise postpartum along with a calorie-restricted diet upon cessation of breastfeeding, will lessen their likelihood of progression to Type 2 diabetes, as shown in the Diabetes Prevention Program.[17] Pregnancy provides a real opportunity for previously unfit women with Type 2 diabetes or GDM with poor lifestyle habits to receive motivational advice reinforced over several weeks around exercise. As with Type 1 diabetes, all exercise advice needs to be given around avoiding hypoglycemia for women on insulin.

DIETARY ADVICE

Normal pregnancy

The aim of all diets in pregnancy is to ensure that adequate maternal and fetal nutrition can be provided by a well-balanced diet. The extra daily calorie requirement for each trimester is modest, being approximately 100 kcal in the first trimester and rising to 200–300 kcal in the third; however, this is independent of any reduction in physical activity that might occur.

The proportion of the three main macronutrients, carbohydrate, protein and fat, should be similar to that of a healthy non-pregnant diet, with approximately 50% of total energy being provided by carbohydrate and less than 35% by fat. The type of dietary carbohydrate and fat is critically important, with fiber as non-starch polysaccharide, low glycemic index carbohydrates, and monosaturated and polyunsaturated fats being healthier than high glycemic index unrefined carbohydrates, and saturated and *trans*-fatty acid fats. Current UK recommendations are still based on the original 1991 Department of Health published dietary reference values (DRVs) for a range of nutrients (Table 13.4).

Throughout pregnancy, diet needs to provide sufficient mineral and vitamins for growth and development. Even today in our overfed Western society many diets are deficient in iron, calcium, vitamin D, folic acid, and vitamin B12, all essential for a healthy pregnancy outcome. The number of women choosing to be vegetarians is increasing in the UK, and many of these diets, especially if they are vegan diets, will require supplementation in pregnancy.

Table 13.4 UK dietary recommendations for adults based on the 1991 Department of Health published dietary reference values for a range of nutrients.[18]

	Food total energy (%)
Total dietary carbohydrate	**50**
Non-milk extrinsic sugars	<11
Intrinsic and milk sugars, and starch	39
Fiber as non-starch polysaccharide (g/day)	18*
Total dietary fat	**<35**
Saturated fatty acids	<11
Polyunsaturated fatty acids	6.5
Monounsaturated fatty acids	13
Trans-fatty acids	<2

While iron studies are routinely carried out in pregnancy and iron supplements prescribed when indicated, evaluation of vitamin D status is not. Current UK guidance from the National Institute for Health and Clinical Excellence (NICE) emphasizes the importance to maintain adequate vitamin D during pregnancy and breastfeeding, and those women may choose to take up to 10 µg of vitamin D a day during these periods, particularly if they have specific risk factors for vitamin D deficiency.

A number of dietary foods carry a risk of listeria, salmonella, and toxoplasmosis, and advice on avoiding these foods should be given (Table 13.5). Controversy remains whether complete avoidance of alcohol should be advised.

Pregnancy with diabetes

There are few evidenced-based dietary guidelines available for women with Type 1 or Type 2 diabetes, or GDM in pregnancy, and even fewer for obese women with diabetes. In addition to the general principles of a healthy diet for pregnancy as outlined above, diets for women with diabetes should aim to limit blood glucose values post meals and to provide sufficient slow-release carbohydrate to prevent hypoglycemia between meals. Encouraging foods that contain carbohydrates with a low glycemic index (GI) helps to achieve this (Table 13.6). Dietary modification that limits postprandial glycemia reduces the risk of macrosomia and other diabetic-related perinatal complications.[19,20]

The diets for women with Type 1 diabetes need to optimize glycemic control, while minimizing the risk of hypoglycemia and ketosis. For those women who adjust their bolus insulin according to the grams of dietary carbohydrate, the ratio of quick-acting insulin to grams of carbohydrate will rise throughout pregnancy and women should be prepared to adjust their insulin accordingly.

Table 13.5 Foods that increase the risk of listeria, salmonella, and toxoplasmosis.

- Soft and blue-veined cheese
- Pâté
- Raw or partially cooked eggs
- Unwashed raw fruit and vegetables
- Raw or undercooked meat
- Unpasteurized dairy products

Table 13.6 Examples of low glycemic foods and snacks.

Fruit	Banana, apple
Cereal	Bran cereals, porridge oats
Bread	Wholegrain, pumpernickel, rye, mixed grains
Legumes	Lentils, kidney beans, chick peas
Pasta/rice	Spaghetti, whole wheat, basmati rice
Nuts	Almonds, hazelnuts
Dairy	Low fat milk, cottage cheese, soft cheese, yoghurt

Both hypoglycemia and ketoacidosis contribute to the majority of avoidable diabetic-related maternal deaths. To minimize these risks carbohydrate needs to be incorporated into each meal and snack. Women with Type 1 diabetes must be encouraged not to restrict their dietary carbohydrates as this increases the risk of not only hypoglycemia but also ketosis in late pregnancy. Women with Type 1 diabetes are at increased risk of diabetic ketoacidosis at lower glucose concentrations in late pregnancy than in the non-pregnant state, due to increasing lipolysis, increasing dependency on fatty acids as an energy substrate, and increasing breakdown of fatty acids to ketones.

The background risk of celiac disease is increased in Type 1 diabetes and women with celiac disease must be encouraged and given support to be fully compliant with their gluten-free diet, as untreated celiac disease is associated with fetal growth restriction. Pernicious anemia due to vitamin B12 deficiency is another autoimmune disorder with higher background prevalence in Type 1 diabetes. In normal pregnancy, B12 tissue levels are normal while serum levels are low, making assessment of B12 deficiency unreliable. Women with pernicious anemia require regular injections of intramuscular B12 during pregnancy.

Dietary management for women with Type 2 diabetes and GDM is pivotal. Pregnancy often presents the obese diabetic woman with their first opportunity to see a trained dietitian. Simple basic dietary advice at this time, when reinforced throughout the pregnancy, can improve glycemic control and limit unnecessary weight gain. Many women will be performing regular daily self-glucose monitoring for the first time, and this will provide an important learning experience of how common foods affect their blood glucose levels.

All prescribed diets should be realistic, affordable, and culturally appropriate. Dietary habits and food choices vary among ethnic populations and this makes it impractical to have very detailed guidelines. Approximately half of all women with Type 2 diabetes in the 2002–2003

CEMACH audit on all pregestational diabetic pregnancies in England, Wales, and Northern Ireland were from ethnic minority communities with high levels of social deprivation.[21] Awareness around cultural foods and festivities, such as Ramadan and Eid, helps to promote acceptance of and compliance with the dietary advice given. The high preponderance of women with Type 2 diabetes or GDM from the Indian subcontinent and other cultures whose clothing allows little direct sunlight exposure, makes this group extremely at risk of vitamin D deficiency, and many will require 10 µg of vitamin D supplementation in pregnancy and throughout lactation. Low-fat dairy products, such as low-fat milk and yoghurts, are rich in calcium and vitamin D and should be recommended. Many of these women are also vegetarian and their diets may be low in B12; a useful vegetarian source for this vitamin is yeast extract that is widely available and easy to take.

For women with Type 2 diabetes or GDM, low GI diets provide other potential benefits over and above just reducing postprandial hyperglycemia. Studies on non-diabetic pregnant African women consuming traditional low GI–high fiber diets and pregnant Western women taking low GI diets demonstrate that the rise in insulin resistance and insulin levels is attenuated and maternal weight gain and birthweight are reduced with a low GI diet.[22–24] Typically, many Western meals, especially breakfast when it includes common brand-named cereals, fruit juice, toast, and preserves, have a very high GI content. The high postprandial breakfast blood glucose values commonly observed in diabetes in pregnancy has led some US authorities to advocate limiting dietary carbohydrate for breakfast to less than 30% of the total energy taken; however, informed food choices for breakfast (Table 13.6) can limit high glucose levels following breakfast.

There is considerable debate on what degree of caloric restriction, if any, is appropriate for the obese pregnant women with Type 2 diabetes or GDM. There are a number of small interventional studies in late pregnancy that restrict total energy intake by approximately a third, or between 20 and 25 kcal/kg/day, that are associated with reduced rates of macrosomia and reduced maternal weight gain.[25–28] Reducing energy intake to below 1200 kcal/day is associated with increased ketonemia and is therefore not recommended due to concerns raised in the 1960s about possible adverse fetal neurologic and psychologic development associated with ketonemia; however, these concerns have still to be fully substantiated.

ADVICE AFTER PREGNANCY

Women without diabetes

All women who have gained weight in pregnancy should be encouraged to return to their prepregnancy weight through healthy eating and physical activity over the following year. Lactation will help women to lose excess weight gained in pregnancy as mothers who fully breast-feed their babies produce approximately 800 ml/day of milk, which equates to 2.1 MJ or 500 kcal/day. Other women will meet this energy demand through a combination of eating more and reducing their physical activity. Women who are breastfeeding should keep themselves well hydrated with six to eight glasses of fluid a day and to take 10 μg/day of vitamin D from other foods or supplements. Women above 120% of their ideal body weight should be encouraged to lose weight by lifestyle intervention prior to any subsequent pregnancy.[29,30]

Women with diabetes

There are no contraindications to breastfeeding for women with diabetes. However, women with Type 1 diabetes need to receive specific advice about maintaining safe glycemic control while breastfeeding.

Almost immediately following birth the insulin requirements of a mother with Type 1 diabetes fall to those prior to pregnancy. Once she has successfully established breastfeeding her insulin requirements are likely to drop further. For those women who adjust their bolus insulin according to the grams of dietary carbohydrate, the ratio of quick-acting insulin to grams of carbohydrate will fall. It is important that all new mothers with Type 1 diabetes understand that hypoglycemia can be associated with breastfeeding. They should therefore also understand the importance of checking their blood glucose levels prior to feeding. Ideally, breastfeeding should occur after taking an adequate carbohydrate-containing meal or snack. Mothers should be advised to breastfeed sitting in a chair, not lying on a bed, and to always have an appropriate drink or snack within arm's reach that they can take if they feel their blood glucose level is falling.

It is important that women who have Type 2 diabetes or GDM understand the health advantages of continuing to follow the long-term dietary (minus the additional calories added for pregnancy and lactation) and exercise advice they received in pregnancy. As for women without diabetes, those who are overweight or obese should be encouraged to loose weight prior to any subsequent pregnancy. Those women with GDM should be informed that maintaining a healthy lifestyle and losing weight if overweight, will lessen their short-term risk of progression to Type 2 diabetes. They also need to know that they should be screened annually by their general practitioner for Type 2 diabetes and be screened again early in any subsequent pregnancy for GDM.

SUMMARY

A healthy lifestyle consisting of moderate physical activity and a well-balanced diet should be encouraged for all women during pregnancy. For women with Type 1 diabetes quite modest exercise can contribute to their added risk of hypoglycemic episodes, especially in early pregnancy. Individual advice around appropriate carbohydrate intake and adjustment of the bolus insulin prior to exercise needs to be given. For women with Type 2 diabetes or GDM, many of whom will have been previously unfit, realistic and appropriate exercise for pregnancy should be advocated. Encouraging 20 minutes of walking once or twice a day after meals is easily achievable and can lower postprandial blood glucose values. For women with GDM, combining exercise with a dietary program improves glycemic control and reduces the need for insulin treatment.

A healthy diet in pregnancy needs to ensure that appropriate weight gain targets are set; these should be based on the woman's prepregnancy weight. For women with Type 1 diabetes, adequate amounts of carbohydrate need to be provided in each meal and snack throughout the day to lessen the risk of hypoglycemia and ketosis. For women with Type 2 diabetes or GDM, education on food choices that constitute a well-balanced diet will help minimize excess pregnancy weight gain, improve glycemic control, and reduce the risk of a macrosomic infant. In addition, for women with GDM, continuing with a well-balanced diet and regular physical activity after pregnancy can delay or even avoid the progression to Type 2 diabetes.

CASE HISTORY 1

Dietary and exercise advice should be given in an informative manner, to help Angela understand how the pregnancy is going to affect her diabetes and how her diabetes may affect the pregnancy. Since Angela attended preconception counseling, she has already indicated she is open to advice on how to optimize her pregnancy. It is important to build on this positive start by explaining, while empathizing with her, why after 20 years of Type 1 diabetes it is so difficult to achieve the glycemic targets set for her in pregnancy. She needs to be given practical support to safely achieve the best glycemic control.

Angela needs to be given reassurance that hypoglycemia and poor hypoglycemic awareness are extremely common, especially in the first half of pregnancy, and both often improve as the pregnancy progresses. Advice around the rapid correction of hypoglycemia will prevent rebound hyperglycemia following these episodes (see Table 13.2). Advice on how to anticipate the likely effect of exercise on her blood glucose is needed. By taking slow-release carbohydrate prior to exercise and reducing her short-acting insulin for the meal before the exercise should lessen her risk of exercise-induced hypoglycemia. If this does not work, it may be necessary to suggest a less strenuous form of exercise. However, it is likely, due to the physiologic and anatomic changes occurring in the second trimester (see Table 13.3), that she will soon begin to reduce her exercise pattern herself.

Following a dietary review assessing energy content and ensuring that sufficient meals and snacks are being taken throughout the day, Angela should be given a healthy weight gain target during pregnancy of 10–12.5 kg based on her prepregnancy BMI. She should understand that this is the optimal weight gain for her baby. Meanwhile she can be reassured that with breastfeeding and a healthy lifestyle postpartum that she will likely return to her prepregnancy weight within the following year.

CASE HISTORY 2

Senita will need advice and support to change her diet in a way that she can continue with after the pregnancy. She will need encouragement to try new foods to replace previously unhealthy ones. Increasing the amounts of pulses in her diet, such as beans, chick peas, and lentils, will provide a good vegetarian source of protein, energy, and fiber. She will need to replace many of her high refined carbohydrate foods with ones that have a lower GI, such as basmati rice and cereal products made from whole grain or oats (see Table 13.6). Senita will be able to reduce her dietary fat content by being encouraged to grill rather than fry her food and ensuring all cooking oils are either mono- or poly-unsaturated.

As Senita is Asian it is likely that she will be vitamin D deficient. In addition to taking 10 μg of oral vitamin D, she should be encouraged to eat dairy products, such as low-fat milk and yoghurt, as well as green vegetables,

almonds, and sesame seeds, which are also a good source of calcium.

Senita should be encouraged to increase her daily walking, especially after breakfast and lunch, explaining this is likely to delay or lessen the likelihood of her requiring insulin in this pregnancy. As she has young children at home, incorporating 20 minutes of walking twice a day into her daily routine should be possible by taking the children to school or the local park. Reinforcing the benefits of simple regular walking should be a part of every antenatal clinic consultation with her.

Senita should be given a realistic pregnancy weight gain target that should not exceed 10 kg for the entire pregnancy. Given she has already gained 6 kg, this means limiting the rest of the pregnancy to only a 4-kg weight gain, effectively making her current pregnancy weight neutral. Dietary advice on how to limit further excess weight gain will require a degree of calorie restriction with an energy content of 25 kcal/kg. By adopting more healthy food choices, as outlined above, will in itself reduce her energy intake, making a diet based on 25 kcal/kg highly achievable.

Senita will need ongoing advice throughout the pregnancy and if she requires insulin treatment, her diet will need to be further modified to incorporate low GI snacks to avoid hypoglycemia.

Senita will need to be encouraged to continue with her healthier lifestyle after the pregnancy. She needs to be informed that continuing with these lifestyle changes will lessen the risk of her developing Type 2 diabetes over the next few years, and that she will need testing annually for diabetes by her general practitioner. If she is hoping to extend her family in the future, she should be informed of the benefits of weight loss prior to undertaking another pregnancy and of the need for early screening for GDM.

REFERENCES

1 Hytten FE. *Maternal Physiological Adjustments*. Washington, DC: National Academy of Sciences, 1970.

2 Langer O, Anyaegbunam A, Brustman L, Guidetti D, Levy J, Mazze R. Pregestational diabetes: insulin requirements throughout pregnancy. *Am J Obstet Gynecol* 1988;**159**: 616–21.

3 Institute of Medicine, Food and Nutrition Board, Committee on Nutritional Status During Pregnancy and Lactation, Subcommittee on Dietary Intake and Nutrient Supplements During Pregnancy, Subcommittee on Nutritional Status and Weight Gain During Pregnancy, National Academy of Sciences. *Nutrition During Pregnancy. Part I – Weight Gain.*

Part II – Nutrient Supplements. Washington, DC: National Academy Press, 1999.

4 Kiel DW, Dodson EA, Artal R, Boehmer TK, Leet TL. Gestational weight gain and pregnancy outcomes in obese women: how much is enough? *Obstet Gynecol* 2007;**110**: 752–8.

5 Nohr EA, Vaeth M, Baker JL, Sorensen TI, Olsen J, Rasmussen KM. Combined associations of prepregnancy body mass index and gestational weight gain with the outcome of pregnancy. *Am J Clin Nutr* 2008;**87**:1750–9.

6 Rizzo T, Metzger BE, Burns WJ, Burns K. Correlations between antepartum maternal metabolism and child intelligence. *N Engl J Med* 1991;**325**:911–6.

7 National Institute for Health and Clinical Excellence. *Diabetes in Pregnancy: Management of Diabetes and its Complications from Pre-conception to the Postnatal Period.* London: NICE, 2008. www.nice.org.uk/CG063

8 Institute of Medicine of the National Academies. *Influence of Pregnancy Weight on Maternal and Child Health: A Workshop Report.* Washington: Institute of Medicine, 2007. www.iom.edu/CMS/12552/31379/41424.aspx

9 Bonen A, Campagna P, Gilchrist L, Young DC, Beresford P. Substrate and endocrine responses during exercise at selected stages of pregnancy. *J Appl Physiol* 1992;**73**:134–42.

10 Robson SC, Hunter S, Boys RJ, Dunlop W. Serial changes in pulmonary haemodynamics during human pregnancy: a non-invasive study using Doppler echocardiography. *Clin Sci (Lond)* 1991;**80**:113–7.

11 Nelson-Piercy C. *Handbook of Obstetric Medicine.* Reading: Taylor & Francis, 2002.

12 Jensen D, Webb KA, Davies GA, O'Donnell DE. Mechanical ventilatory constraints during incremental cycle exercise in human pregnancy: implications for respiratory sensation. *J Physiol* 2008;**586**:4735–50.

13 Crowther CA, Hiller JE, Moss JR, McPhee AJ, Jeffries WS, Robinson JS. Effect of treatment of gestational diabetes mellitus on pregnancy outcomes. *N Engl J Med* 2005;**352**: 2477–86.

14 Brankston GN, Mitchell BF, Ryan EA, Okun NB. Resistance exercise decreases the need for insulin in overweight women with gestational diabetes mellitus. *Am J Obstet Gynecol* 2004;**190**:188–93.

15 Jovanovic-Peterson L, Durak EP, Peterson CM. Randomized trial of diet versus diet plus cardiovascular conditioning on glucose levels in gestational diabetes. *Am J Obstet Gynecol* 1989;**161**:415–9.

16 Lesser KB, Gruppuso PA, Terry RB, Carpenter MW. Exercise fails to improve postprandial glycemic excursion in women with gestational diabetes. *J Matern Fetal Neonatal Med* 1996;**5**:211–7.

17 Knowler WC, Barrett-Connor E, Fowler SE, *et al.* Reduction in the incidence of type 2 diabetes with lifestyle intervention or metformin. *N Engl J Med* 2002;**346**:393–403.

18 Report on Health and Social Subjects 41 *Dietary Reference Values (DRVs) for Food Energy and Nutrients for the UK,* Report of the Panel on DRVs of the Committee on Medical Aspects of Food Policy (COMA). London: The Stationary Office, 1991.

19 Jovanovic-Peterson L, Peterson CM, Reed GF, *et al.* Maternal postprandial glucose levels and infant birth weight: the Diabetes in Early Pregnancy Study. The National Institute of Child Health and Human Development – Diabetes in Early Pregnancy Study. *Am J Obstet Gynecol* 1991;**164**:103–11.

20 Parretti E, Mecacci F, Papini M, *et al.* Third-trimester maternal glucose levels from diurnal profiles in nondiabetic pregnancies: correlation with sonographic parameters of fetal growth. *Diabetes Care* 2001;**24**:1319–23.

21 Confidential Enquiry into Maternal and Child Health. *Pregnancy in Women with Type 1 and Type 2 Diabetes in 2002–03, England, Wales and Northern Ireland.* London: CEMACH, 2005.

22 Clapp JF, III. Maternal carbohydrate intake and pregnancy outcome. *Proc Nutr Soc* 2002;**61**:45–50.

23 Fraser RB. The effect of pregnancy on the normal range of the oral glucose tolerance in Africans. *East Afr Med J* 1981;**58**:90–4.

24 Fraser RB, Ford FA, Lawrence GF. Insulin sensitivity in third trimester pregnancy. A randomized study of dietary effects. *Br J Obstet Gynaecol* 1988;**95**:223–9.

25 Algert S, Shragg P, Hollingsworth DR. Moderate caloric restriction in obese women with gestational diabetes. *Obstet Gynecol* 1985;**65**:487–91.

26 Artal R, Catanzaro RB, Gavard JA, Mostello DJ, Friganza JC. A lifestyle intervention of weight-gain restriction: diet and exercise in obese women with gestational diabetes mellitus. *Appl Physiol Nutr Metab* 2007;**32**:596–601.

27 Dornhorst A, Nicholls JS, Probst F, *et al.* Calorie restriction for treatment of gestational diabetes. *Diabetes* 1991;**40** (Suppl 2):161–4.

28 Magee MS, Knopp RH, Benedetti TJ. Metabolic effects of 1200-kcal diet in obese pregnant women with gestational diabetes. *Diabetes* 1990;**39**:234–40.

29 Brown CJ, Dawson A, Dodds R, *et al.* Report of the Pregnancy and Neonatal Care Group. *Diabet Med* 1996; **13**:S43–S53.

30 Connor H, Annan F, Bunn E, *et al.* The implementation of nutritional advice for people with diabetes. *Diabet Med* 2003;**20**:786–807.

Section 4

Complications in pregnancy

14 Malformations and miscarriages in diabetes in pregnancy

Elisabeth R. Mathiesen & Peter Damm

Center for Pregnant Women with Diabetes, Departments of Obstetrics and Endocrinology, Rigshospitalet, University of Copenhagen, Faculty of Health Sciences, Copenhagen, Denmark

PRACTICE POINTS

- Women with Type 1 or Type 2 diabetes have a two- to five-fold increased risk of having a fetal congenital malformation.
- The increased rate of major malformations and miscarriages in women with diabetes prior to pregnancy is related to high glucose values during the first trimester of pregnancy.
- Self-monitored blood glucose and hemoglobin A1c (HbA1c) levels close to the normal range are recommended prior to and in early pregnancy to reduce the risk of malformations.
- A reduction in HbA1c by 1% reduces the risk of malformations by around 50%.
- Obesity is independently associated with an increased risk of malformations.
- Folic acid supplementation is recommended prior to pregnancy and during organogenesis to decrease the risk of a fetal neural tube defect, although there is no consensus regarding the appropriate dose (0.4–5 mg).
- Metformin and glyburide (glibenclamide) probably do not contribute to malformations.

CASE HISTORY

A 35-year-old woman with Type 2 diabetes for 5 years booked for antenatal care at 18 weeks of gestation with an unplanned pregnancy. She had had two uncomplicated pregnancies 9 and 12 years before. She had not been seen for prepregnancy counseling and was not taking folic acid. She had been treated with metformin and human insulin twice daily. Her initial HbA1c was 9.0%. An ultrasound scan demonstrated an anencephalic fetus. The couple were counseled regarding the possibility of terminating the pregnancy, but they decided to continue with the pregnancy. The pregnancy progressed without further complication, although she missed a number of her clinic appointments and blood glucose control remained above target. She went into labor spontaneously at term and an anencephalic baby girl was born,

who died shortly after birth. The woman went home the following day with arrangements made for her to return for a discussion about the pregnancy, her diabetes management, and the future, but she did not attend.

- How frequent is severe malformation in diabetic pregnancy?
- What is the role of metabolic control?
- Does antihypertensive treatment or other drugs increase the risk of malformations?
- Folic acid supplementation – does it have a role?
- What can in clinical practice be done to reduce the prevalence of severe malformed babies?

BACKGROUND

Large population-based investigations[1–4] have shown that Type 1 and Type 2 diabetes preceding pregnancy is associated with a two- to five-fold increased risk of major congenital malformations. This disappointing reality is in sharp contrast to the aspiration expressed in the 1989 St Vincent declaration,[5] which proposed as a 5-year target that the outcome of pregnancy complicated by diabetes should approximate that of the non-diabetic population. Optimal glycemic control before and during pregnancy in women with diabetes is critical to obtain a satisfactory maternal and neonatal outcome. As organogenesis is complete by 8 weeks, inadequate preconceptional glycemic control is associated with an increased risk of congenital abnormality.[6,7] Diabetes in pregnancy is also associated with an increased risk of miscarriage, which is also presumed to be secondary to poor glycemic control.[6,7] As expected, gestational diabetes developing in late pregnancy has not been associated with an increased risk of either congenital malformations or miscarriage.[4]

TYPES OF CONGENITAL MALFORMATIONS

Organogenesis takes place between 2 and 8 weeks of gestation and the malformations which are found with

A Practical Manual of Diabetes in Pregnancy, 1st Edition.
Edited by David R. McCance, Michael Maresh and David A. Sacks.
© 2010 Blackwell Publishing

Table 14.1 Detectable major congenital malformations in babies of women with pregestational diabetes. (Adapted from National Collaborating Centre for Women's and Children's Health[4].)

Group of malformations	Specific malformations	Prevalence (per 100 births)	Relative risk compared to women without diabetes
Cardiac	Transposition of the great arteries Ventricular septal defect Coarctation of the aorta Atrial septal defect Asymmetric septal hypertrophy	3.0–10.0	3–5
Caudal regression syndrome		0.2–0.5	200
Central nervous system	Neural tube defects (inc anencephaly) Microcephaly Isolated hydrocephalus	2.1	2–10
Gastrointestinal	Duodenal atresia Anorectal atresia Hypoplastic left colon	1.0	3
Musculoskeletal system	Talipes Arthrogryposis	0.8–2.4	2–20
Orofacial cleft		1.8	1.5
Urinary tract	Uretal duplication Cystic kidney Renal dysgenesis Hydronephrosis	1.7–3.0	2–5

increased frequency in association with maternal diabetes must have their origins in some type of insult occurring during this period.[8] Glycemic control in this time period is therefore of the utmost importance with regard to the possibility for the development of malformations.[7] All types of major malformations are more frequent in offspring of diabetic mothers (Table 14.1). Cardiac malformations, e.g. transposition of the great vessels, ventricular or atrial septum defects, and coarctation of the aorta are the most common.[1,4] However, malformations in the central nervous system (e.g. neural tube defects; Fig. 14.1) are also relatively common, as are renal and skeletal malformations, and duodenal and anal atresia. In addition, one type of malformation – caudal regression syndrome – is exceedingly rare outside of diabetes in pregnancy. Many infants demonstrate multiple major malformations. In one study of pregnant women who had Type 2 diabetes, the higher the initial maternal fasting glucose the more likely multiple, rather than single, fetal anomalies.[9] The increased frequency of major malformations is probably the reason for the increased risk of miscarriage in women with diabetes.

ROLE OF METABOLIC CONTROL IN MALFORMATIONS AND MISCARRIAGES

A recent systematic review[7] of 13 mainly observational studies found an overall three-fold increased risk of malformations in women with diabetes compared to the background population. The risk of major malformations was found to be increased five-fold and the risk of miscarriages three-fold when there was poor metabolic control. For each 1% reduction in HbA1c the risk of severe malformations was reduced by around 50%. Relating the percentage reduction in HbA1c to relative risk of adverse pregnancy events may be useful in motivating women to achieve optimal control prior to conception. Those diabetic women offered prepregnancy care and achieving HbA1c concentrations less than 7% before conception, have a considerably reduced risk of adverse outcomes, including malformations, compared to those pregnant women with diabetes who do not.[10] This is supported by results from a new large population-based Danish study,[11] which showed no clear threshold of HbA1c for the risk of congenital malformations, although the risk was not statistically increased when

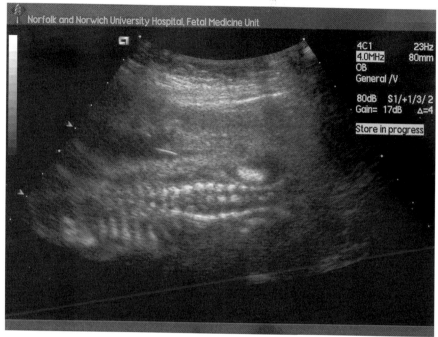

Fig. 14.1 Ultrasound scan showing neural tube defect with splaying of vertebra.

periconceptual HbA1c was below 7%, which corresponded to fewer that 3 SDs above the mean for the background population. Intensified glycemic control with average premeal capillary glucose values less than 6 mmol/L (<108 mg/dL) and 1-hour postprandial values less than 7.5 mmol/L (<135 mg/dL), commenced before and continuing during early pregnancy, was found to reduce malformation rates to a level approaching the background risk.[12]

The precise mechanism responsible for fetal teratogenesis in pregnancy complicated by diabetes is unclear. Freinkel[13] introduced the concept of "pregnancy as a tissue culture experience," proposing that the fetus develops in an "incubation medium" that is totally derived from maternal fuels. Experimental animal studies have suggested that the major teratogen in pregnancy is hyperglycemia, although other diabetes-related factors may adversely influence fetal outcome. Increased levels of ketone bodies or episodes of severe hypoglycemia may also be teratogenic.[12] Several possible teratologic pathways in embryogenic tissues have emerged, including alterations in the metabolism of inositol, arachidonic acid, and reactive oxygen species.

The embryonic formation of sorbitol, glycated proteins, the level of folic acid, and the maternal and fetal genotypes are also suggested to influence the complex teratologic events in diabetes in pregnancy. The subject has been extensively studied and reviewed by Eriksson *et al.*[14]

INFLUENCE OF OBESITY AND METABOLIC SYNDROME

Obesity *per se* is associated with menstrual irregularities, infertility, miscarriages, and other adverse pregnancy outcomes, and in many cases is part of the polycystic ovarian syndrome (PCOS).[15] A population-based study found that offspring with spina bifida, heart defects, anorectal atresia, hypospadias, limb reduction defects, diaphragmatic hernia, and omphalocele were significantly more likely to have had obese mothers than controls, with odds ratios ranging between 1.33 and 2.10.[16] The mechanisms underlying these associations are not yet understood, and whether they are related to undiagnosed diabetes or other metabolic changes associated with obesity[16] remains unanswered.

The possibility that the combination of maternal obesity and prepregnancy diabetes mellitus potentiates the risk for neural tube defects has been investigated.[17] The presence of one feature of the metabolic syndrome was associated with a two-fold increased risk for a neural tube defect and two or more features with a six-fold higher risk, although no allowance was made for glycemic control. Obesity and the metabolic syndrome might therefore add to the risk of congenital malformations seen with diabetes. This may explain the observation that women with Type 2 diabetes have similar rates of congenital malformations to those with Type 1 diabetes, despite HbA1c values in women who have Type 2 diabetes tending to be lower in the first trimester.[18]

ROLE OF FOLIC ACID

It is well established that the folate requirements increase during pregnancy and that supplementing 0.4 mg of folic acid/day to the general population reduces the risk of neural tube defects.[19] In addition, it has been reported that folic acid supplementation may prevent other birth defects, such as heart defects, cleft lip and palate, limb deficiency defects, and urinary tract abnormalities.[20] In animal models, folic acid supplementation reduces glucose-induced congenital malformations with a threshold effect.[21] Furthermore, mRNA expression of folic acid-binding protein, a folic acid transporter, is decreased in the diabetic state.[21]

In humans, the protection afforded by folic acid supplementation against diabetes-associated malformations is less clear. Multivitamin supplements have been reported to reduce the risk of congenital malformations,[22] but the compositions of the supplements were unknown and the benefit probably included that of overall prepregnancy care. In recent years several national bodies[4,23,24] have recommended high doses of folic acid (4–5 mg/day) to diabetic women before and during early pregnancy. However, the wisdom of this strategy has been questioned[25] since a high folate intake might be associated with promotion of neoplasia. Therefore, many centers around the world still advocate the use of 0.4 mg of folic acid/day supplementation. In a small series using the latter strategy, low rates of congenital malformations were reported.[26]

A consensus exists that all women with diabetes preparing for pregnancy are advised to take supplementary folic acid. Whether the dose should be 0.4, 1 or 5 mg/day remains unclear. Supplementation should be continued for the first 12 weeks of pregnancy.

ROLE OF ORAL AGENTS

Biguanides and sulfonylureas

The experience from Copenhagen and South Africa including almost 500 pregnant women with Type 2 diabetes does not suggest that either metformin or glyburide (glibenclamide) are teratogenic.[27,28] A meta-analysis of metformin-treated women in early pregnancy, most of whom had PCOS, found that metformin treatment in the first trimester may even protect against malformations.[29] However, since metformin crosses the placental barrier and no long-term follow-up of the offspring has occurred, potential long-term adverse effects of metformin cannot be excluded. Thus, many centers continue to change women on metformin to insulin either before pregnancy or when pregnancy is diagnosed. The subject is discussed in more detail in chapter 11

Antihypertensive drugs, aspirin, and statins

Angiotensin-converting enzyme inhibitors (ACE-I) and angiotensin receptor blockers (ARBs) are both frequently used in young diabetic women for treatment of hypertension and to prevent development or progression of diabetic nephropathy. For both drugs teratogenicity and fetotoxicity have been reported.[30–32] The relative risk of congenital malformations in offspring of 209 women taking ACE-I during organogenesis was 2.71 (95% CI 1.72–4.27) compared to women not taking antihypertensive drugs.[32] The relative risk of malformations in 202 women taking other types of antihypertensive drugs was 0.66 (95% CI 0.25–1.75). The most common malformations encountered were in the cardiovascular or central nervous system.[32] A change from an ACE-I or ARB to other types of antihypertensive prior to a planned pregnancy is therefore recommended. However, in women suffering from diabetic nephropathy, decisions must be made on an individual basis. The benefit has to be considered of either using drugs to inhibit the renin angiotensin system while the woman is trying to conceive, and then stopping treatment as soon the pregnancy is diagnosed,[33] or to have a period of indefinite duration without inhibition of the renin angiotensin system, which might lead to disease progression prior to pregnancy. These issues are further highlighted in chapters 15 and 16.

Cholesterol-lowering drugs, such as statins, modulate lipid synthesis and are contraindicated during pregnancy.[34] Aspirin is widely used in patients with diabetes to reduce the incidence of cardiovascular events. In addition, aspirin from 12 weeks of gestation might reduce the prevalence of pre-eclampsia in high-risk women.[35] Whether aspirin is associated with a slightly increased risk of malformations is a matter of debate.[36] Accordingly, the use of aspirin during organogenesis should be based on an individual risk–benefit assessment (see also chapter 15).

PRACTICAL ASPECTS OF PREPREGNANCY MANAGEMENT TO PREVENT MALFORMATIONS AND MISCARRIAGE (See also Chapter 8)

The importance of pregnancy planning should be an essential component of diabetes education, starting in puberty, for women with diabetes. Knowledge of methods of prevention of unplanned pregnancy should be made available to all reproductive-age women and adolescents who have diabetes.

Women with diabetes who are planning to become pregnant should be advised to increase the frequency of self-monitoring of blood glucose to include fasting and a mixture of pre- and 1-hour postprandial levels, and be offered monthly measurements of HbA1c, aiming for values as close to normal as possible (HbA1c < 6.1%), balanced against the risk of hypoglycemia. If it is safely achievable, women with diabetes should aim to keep fasting blood glucose between 3.5 and 5.9 mmol/L (63–106 mg/dL) and 1-hour postprandial blood glucose below 7.8 mmol/L (<140 mg/dL) before and during pregnancy.

Women with diabetes who are planning to become pregnant should be advised to take folic acid (at least 0.4 mg/day) until 12 weeks of gestation to reduce the risk of having a baby with a neural tube defect.

ACE-Is and ARBs should be discontinued before conception or as soon as pregnancy is confirmed. Alternative antihypertensive agents suitable for use during pregnancy should be substituted. Statins should be discontinued before pregnancy or as soon as pregnancy is confirmed.

PRACTICAL MANAGEMENT IN PREGNANCY FOR THE PREVENTION, SCREENING, DETECTION, AND MANAGEMENT OF MALFORMATIONS AND MISCARRIAGE

As soon as contact is made by any health professional with the diabetic woman, whether by telephone or in person, an immediate review of medication is required to ensure that she is taking folic acid and that any potentially teratogenic medication is stopped.

Between 7 and 9 weeks of gestation pregnancy viability and gestational age should be confirmed by ultrasound scanning. For non-viable pregnancies the use of drugs to cause a miscarriage is often considered preferable to surgical evacuation as the drug regimes are usually successful and this avoids the need for anesthesia.

Maternal diabetes is not associated with an increased risk of chromosomal anomalies and so Down syndrome screening should be offered as per normal practice. However, the levels of two serum markers, alpha-fetoprotein (AFP) and unconjugated estriol (uE3), appear to be about 8% and 6% lower, respectively, in maternal diabetes.[37] Human chorionic gonadotrophin and inhibin A do not appear to be significantly affected by maternal diabetes. A subsequent review[4] included data on another serum marker used to screen for Down syndrome, pregnancy-associated plasma protein-A (PAPP-A), and found no consensus as to whether the value of this marker was altered in diabetes. The same review recommends correction for the AFP and uE3 variation in diabetic pregnancy.[4] Ultrasound-determined nuchal translucency (NT) measurements may also be used in conjunction with the serum markers and appear to be unaffected by maternal diabetes. As women with diabetes have a chronic and potentially serious medical condition, the threshold for having an invasive diagnostic test may differ from the general population.

Ultrasound scanning at 11–13 weeks, even if not utilized for NT measurement, may still be considered, particularly in women with a very high risk of malformations (e.g. previous neural tube defect or a high glycosylated hemoglobin in the first trimester), as major abnormalities such as anencephaly should be detected at this stage.

Women with diabetes should be offered a fetal anomaly ultrasound scan at 18–20 weeks (Table 14.1). In view of the high risk of cardiac anomalies, fetal echocardiography is often considered. While this may not be readily available for all women with pregestational diabetes, as a minimum a four-chamber view of the fetal heart and outflow tracts should be obtained. In addition, because of the increased risk of neural tube and genitourinary tract anomalies, these systems should be very carefully assessed. As women with diabetes tend to be overweight, ultrasound visualization of the fetus may be suboptimal. One study highlighted that the ultrasound detection rate for anomalies is significantly lower in maternal diabetes in contrast with the lighter weight general population.[38]

Accordingly, women should be warned of the limitations of the ultrasound scan, particularly if their weight is excessive and imaging is unsatisfactory.

Women diagnosed as having a fetus with severe malformation must be offered non-directive counseling regarding terminating or continuing the pregnancy. Women who elect to continue with the pregnancy should, wherever possible, be offered consultations with specialists who will be involved in the care of the baby post delivery; for example, a pediatric cardiologist if there is a major cardiac anomaly. Delivery should be planned in a tertiary center with a neonatal intensive care unit and neonatal surgeons available if early surgery is likely to be required. For women who decide to terminate the pregnancy, management should be as for the woman without diabetes, but with additional specialist advice with regard to the care of her diabetes.

Postpregnancy counseling following the birth of a baby with a significant malformation can be difficult, particularly if it was clear that maternal diabetic control was poor in the first trimester. This should be discussed in a sensitive non-recriminatory manner as the mother will almost always feel guilty. It is important to support her and make her appreciate that it was not necessarily the diabetic control which was responsible, that the etiology of malformations is not fully understood, and that achieving perfect diabetic control, particularly during the first trimester, can be very difficult. It is also usually appropriate to attempt to ascertain future pregnancy intentions and to ensure that measures are put in place for diabetes follow-up and further discussion on the importance of contraception use and meticulous planning of any future pregnancy, with the anticipation that such an approach should result in a satisfactory pregnancy outcome. If the woman with a pregnancy loss is planning to conceive again soon, urgent arrangements must be made to ensure she has appropriate prepregnancy diabetes preparation and is using effective contraception in the interim.

SUMMARY AND FUTURE DIRECTIONS FOR RESEARCH

Congenital malformations and miscarriage are closely associated with glycemic control during organogenesis and unfortunately continue to present major problems. Hyperglycemia during the periconceptional period is probably the major teratogen, but obesity and other factors associated with the metabolic syndrome might also be of relevance.

Pregnancy planning including strict metabolic control with near-normal glucose values and supplementary folic acid is advocated to prevent malformations and miscarriages. Metformin seems safe with regard to the risk of malformations and miscarriages.

Future research needs to be directed at two areas. First, there are the social issues. These include a general need to increase knowledge on reproductive health of these women and to understand the reasons for them failing to attend for prepregnancy care, to allow the development of more appropriate facilities and methods which hopefully should improve uptake. These will vary between countries and cultures. Another social issue is trying to address the obesity epidemic which may not only increase the risk of malformations, but may also make their antenatal detection more difficult. The second area is for continuing basic research into the mechanisms causing defective organogenesis, which in turn may lead to strategies for prevention.

REFERENCES

1 Jensen DM, Damm P, Moelsted-Pederson L, *et al.* Outcomes in type 1 diabetic pregnancies: a nationwide, prospective study. *Diabetes Care* 2004;**27**:2819–23.
2 Evers IM, de Valk HW, Visser GHA. Risk of complications or pregnancy in women with type 1 diabetes: nationwide prospective study in the Netherlands. *BMJ* 2004;**328**:915–19.
3 Macintosh MCM, Fleming KM, Bailey JA, *et al.* Perinatal mortality and congenital anomalies in babies of women with type 1 and type 2 diabetes in England, Wales and Northern Ireland: population based study. *BMJ* 2006;**333**:177–80.
4 National Collaborating Centre for Women's and Children's Health. *Diabetes in Pregnancy: Management of Diabetes and its Complications from Preconception to the Postnatal Period.* London: RCOG, 2008.
5 Diabetes care and research in Europe: the Saint Vincent declaration. *Diabet Med* 1990;**360**:7.
6 Rosen B, Miodovnik M, Combs CA, Khoury J, Siddiqi TA. Glycaemic threshold for spontaneous abortion and congenital malformations in insulin dependent diabetes mellitus. *Obstet Gynecol* 1994;**84**:515–20.
7 Inkster ME, Fahey TP, Donnan PT, Leese GP, Mires GJ, Murphy DJ. Poor glycated haemoglobin control and pregnancy outcomes in type 1 and type 2 diabetes mellitus: Systematic review of observational studies. *BMC Pregnancy Childbirth* 2006;**6**:30 doi:10.1186/1471-2393-6-30.
8 Kucera J. Rate and type of congenital anomalies among offspring of diabetic women. *J Reprod Med* 1971;**7**:73–82.
9 Schaefer-Graf UM, Buchanan TA, Xiang A, Songster G, Montoro M, Kjos SL. Patterns of congenital anomalies

and relationship to initial maternal fasting glucose levels in pregnancies complicated by type 2 and gestational diabetes. *Am J Obstet Gynecol* 2000;**182**:313–20.

10 Pearson DW, Kernaghan D, Lee R, Penny GC, Scottish diabetes in pregnancy study group. The relationship between pre-pregnancy care and early pregnancy loss, major congenital anomaly or perinatal death in diabetes mellitus. *BJOG* 2007;**114**:104–7.

11 Jensen DM, Korsholm L, Ovesen P, *et al*. Peri-conceptional HbA1c and risk of serious adverse pregnancy outcome in 933 women with type 1 diabetes. *Diabetes Care* 2009;**32**:1046–8.

12 Kitzmiller JL, Jovanovic L, Brown F, Coustan D, Reader DM (eds). *Managing Preexisting Diabetes and Pregnancy: Technical Reviews and Consensus Recommendations for Care.* Alexandria, VA: American Diabetes Association, 2008.

13 Freinkel N. Banting lecture 1980. Of pregnancy and progeny. *Diabetes* 1980;**29**:1023–35.

14 Erikson UJ, Wentzel P, Hod M. Clinical and experimental advances in the understanding of diabetic embryopathy. In: Hod M, Jovanovic L, Di Renzo GC, Leiva A, Langer O (eds). *Textbook of Diabetes and Pregnancy.* London: Martin Dunitz, 2003:262–75.

15 Lilja A, Mathiesen ER. Polycystic ovary syndrome and metformin in pregnancy. *Acta Obstet Gynecol Scand* 2006;**85**:861–8.

16 Waller DK, Shaw G, Rasmussen SA, *et al*, for the birth defects prevention group. Prepregnancy obesity as a risk factor for structural birth defects. *Arch Pediatr Adolesc Med* 2007;**161**:745–50.

17 Ray JG, Thomson MD, Vermulen MJ, *et al*. Metabolic syndrome features and risk of neural tube defects. *BMC Pregnancy Childbirth* 2007;**7**:21.

18 Confidential Enquiry into Maternal and Child Health. *Pregnancy in Women with Type 1 and Type 2 Diabetes in 2002–03, England, Wales and Northern Ireland.* London: CEMACH, 2005. www.cemach.org.uk

19 MRC Vitamin study research group. Prevention of neural tube defects: results of the Medical Research Counsil Vitamin Study. *Lancet* 1991;**338**:131–7.

20 Botto LD, Mulinare J, Ericksons JD. Occurrence of congenital heart defects in relation to maternel multivitamin use. *Am J Epidemiol* 1996;**151**:878–84.

21 Wentzel P, Gareskog M, Eriksson UJ. Folic acid supplementation diminishes diabetes and glucose induced dysmorphogenesis in rat embryos in vivo and in vitro. *Diabetes* 2005;**54**:546–7.

22 Correa A, Botto L, Liu Y, Mulinare J, Erikson JD. Do multivitamin supplements attenuate the risk of diabetes associated birth defects? *Pediatrics* 2003;**111**:1146–51.

23 American College of Obstetricians and Gynecologists. ACOG Practice bulletin #44: Neural tube defects. *Obstet Gynecol* 2003;**102**:203–13.

24 Allen VM, Armson BA, Wilson RD, *et al*. Society of obstetricians and gynecologists of Canada. Teratogenecity associated with pre-existing and gestational diabetes. *J Obstet Gynecol Can* 2007;**29**:927–44.

25 Capel I, Corcoy R. What dose of folic acid should be used for pregnant diabetic women? *Diabetes Care* 2007;**30**:e63.

26 Nielsen LR, Pedersen-Bjerregaard U, Thorsteinsson B, Johansen M, Damm P, Mathiesen ER. Hypoglycaemia in pregnant women with type 1 diabetes: Predictors and role of metabolic control. *Diabetes Care* 2008;**31**:9–14.

27 Hellmuth E, Damm P, Mølsted-Petersen L, Bendtsen I. Prevalence of nocturnal hypoglycemia in first trimester of pregnancy in patients with insulin treated diabetes mellitus. *Acta Obstet Gynecol Scand* 2000;**79**:958–62.

28 Ekpeberg CO, Coetzee EJ, van der Merwe L, Levitt NS. A 10-year retrospective analysis of pregnancy outrcome in pregestational type 2 diabetees: comparison of insulin and oral glucose lowering agents. *Diabet Med* 2007;**24**:253–8.

29 Gilbert C, Valois M, Koren G. Pregnancy outcome after first trimester exposure to metformin: a meta-analysis. *Fertil Steril* 2006;**86**:658–63.

30 Shotan A, Widerhorn J, Hurst A, Elkayam U. Risks of angiotensin-converting enzyme inhibition during pregnancy: experimental and clinical evidence, potential mechanisms, and recommendations for use. *Am J Med* 1994;**96**:451–6.

31 Alwan S, Polifka JE, Friedman JM. Angiotensin II receptor antagonist treatment during pregnancy. *Birth Defects Res A Clin Mol Teratol* 2005;**73**:123–30.

32 Cooper WO, Hernandez-Diaz S, Arbogast PG, *et al*. Major congenital malformations after first-trimester exposure to ACE inhibitors. *N Engl J Med* 2006;**354**:2443–51.

33 Hod M, van Dijk DJ, Karp M, *et al*. Diabetic nephropathy and pregnancy: the effect of ACE inhibitors prior to pregnancy on fetomaternal outcome. *Nephrol Dial Transplant* 1995;**10**:2328–33.

34 Statins: beware during pregnancy. *Prescribe Int* 2006;**15**:18–9.

35 Ruano R, Fontes RS, Zugiab M. Prevention of preeclampsia with low-dose aspirin – a systematic review and meta-analysis of the main randomized controlled trials. *Clinics* 2005;**60**:407–14.

36 Norgard B, Puho E, Czeizel AE, Skriver MV, Sorensen HT. Aspirin use during early pregnancy and the risk of congenital abnormalities: a population-based case-control study. *Am J Obstet Gynecol* 2005;**192**:922–3.

37 Huttly W, Rudnicka A, Wald NJ. Second-trimester prenatal screening markers for Down syndrome in women with insulin-dependent diabetes mellitus. *Prenat Diagn* 2004;**24**:804–7.

38 Wong SF, Chan FY, Cincotta RB, *et al*. Routine ultrasound screening in diabetic pregnancies. *Ultrasound Obstet Gynecol* 2002;**19**:171–6.

15 Hypertension in diabetes in pregnancy

Elisabeth R. Mathiesen, Lene Ringholm Nielsen & Peter Damm

Center for Pregnant Women with Diabetes, Departments of Obstetric and Endocrinology, Rigshospitalet, Faculty of Health Sciences, University of Copenhagen, Denmark

PRACTICE POINTS

- The prevalence rates of chronic hypertension, gestational hypertension, pre-eclampsia, and superimposed pre-eclampsia are all more frequent in diabetic pregnancy compared to normal pregnancy.
- The presence of chronic hypertension, microalbuminuria or diabetic nephropathy in early pregnancy should be evaluated.
- All pregnant diabetic women should receive strict metabolic control and be closely monitored for development of pre-eclampsia.
- Blood pressure (BP) should be measured at booking and at each visit at approximately 1–2-week intervals.
- The goal for antihypertensive treatment in pregnant diabetic women with chronic hypertension is 110–139 mmHg for systolic and 65–89 mmHg for diastolic BP. Some centres strive for values below 135/85 mmHg or even below 130/80 mmHg. Strict antihypertensive treatment is important when microalbuminuria or diabetic nephropathy is present.
- BP medications that are safe for pregnancy should be added sequentially until target BP levels are achieved.
- Methyldopa, selected beta-adrenergic blockers (labetalol) and long-acting calcium blockers may be used during pregnancy.
- Angiotensin-convering enzyme inhibitors (ACE-Is) and angiotensin receptor blockers (ARBs) are contraindicated in pregnancy and should be substituted with drugs that are safe in pregnancy when planning pregnancy or in early pregnancy.
- Methyldopa, labetalol, captopril, and enalapril can be used during lactation.

CASE HISTORY

A 28-year-old woman with a 23-year history of Type 1 diabetes and a 2-year history of diabetic nephropathy presented in her first pregnancy. BP (114/75 mmHg) and serum creatinine were normal, but urinary albumin excretion was elevated at 941 mg/24 h on an ACE inhibitor and diuretic treatment. She was treated with a conservative antihypertensive strategy as follows: at the first pregnancy visit at 10 weeks of gestation she was changed from the ACE inhibitor to methyldopa 250 mg twice daily, while diuretic treatment with furosemide 40 mg twice daily was continued. When BP exceeded 140/90 mmHg at 29 weeks, methyldopa was gradually increased to 500 mg four times daily. Unfortunately, she progressed to pre-eclampsia with severe hypertension and proteinuria and was delivered at 32 weeks. The baby's birthweight was 1800 g.

A few years later she was again pregnant. The serum creatinine level had increased to 120 μmol/L (1.36 mg/dL) and the urinary albumin excretion to 3000 mg/24 h, with BP 108/68 mmHg controlled with ACE inhibition and diuretics. Again ACE inhibition was stopped, but in this pregnancy she was treated with an aggressive antihypertensive strategy and by 16 weeks of gestation was on the maximum dose of methyldopa, unchanged diuretics, and labetalol treatment was initiated and gradually increased to maximum dose. She continued to excrete nephrotic range proteinuria but BP remained below 130/80 mm/Hg. At 36 weeks she had no symptoms of pre-eclampsia but was delivered due to an increasing serum creatinine level. The baby's birthweight was 2584 g.

- Does the presence of proteinuria early in pregnancy affect pregnancy outcome?
- Why was the pregnancy outcome better in the second pregnancy?
- What type of antihypertensive can be used during pregnancy?

A Practical Manual of Diabetes in Pregnancy, 1st Edition.
Edited by David R. McCance, Michael Maresh and David A. Sacks.
© 2010 Blackwell Publishing

- What is the treatment goal for hypertension during pregnancy?
- What type of antihypertensive can be used during lactation?

HYPERTENSION IN THE NON-PREGNANT DIABETIC POPULATION

Outside of pregnancy hypertension is more common in diabetic women compared with the background population. The prevalence of hypertension defined as BP greater than 140/90 mmHg was reported as 12% and 22% in non-pregnant women with Type 1 diabetes aged 15–30 and 30–44 years, respectively.[1] Hypertension increases in the presence of microalbuminuria or diabetic nephropathy.[2] Among women with Type 2 diabetes, the prevalence of hypertension is probably even higher.[1]

The diagnostic cut-off level for a diagnosis of hypertension in diabetic patients is a matter of debate but a treatment goal of 130/80 mmHg is now widely accepted.[3]

The development of hypertension in diabetic subjects is often associated with a slightly elevated albumin excretion – microalbuminuria – or even frank proteinuria. Diabetic nephropathy is characterized by development of proteinuria, hypertension, edema, and decline in kidney function (see chapter 16).

In non-pregnant subjects with Type 1 diabetes, hypertension is closely associated with an increased risk of cardiovascular disease. Reduction of BP with antihypertensive drugs, particularly those affecting the renin angiotensin system, in diabetic patients with microalbuminuria or diabetic nephropathy is of utmost importance to prevent the progression of kidney disease, reduce cardiovascular morbidity, and improve survival.[3–5] Treatment with these drugs is indicated even in normotensive non-pregnant diabetic patients with microalbuminuria, the forerunner of overt diabetic nephropathy.

HYPERTENSIVE DISORDERS IN PREGNANCY

Hypertension is a very common medical disorder of pregnancy, being reported to complicate one in 10 pregnancies.[6] The prevalence is even higher in diabetic women,[1,7] mainly in women with Type 1 or Type 2 diabetes present before pregnancy, but also in women developing gestational diabetes. There are four major hypertensive disorders in pregnancy: (1) chronic hypertension, (2) gestational hypertension, (3) pre-eclampsia, and (4) pre-eclampsia superimposed on hypertension or diabetic nephropathy. Each of these conditions has unique pathophysiologic features that have implications for antihypertensive therapy (Table 15.1). All categories are more common in diabetic than in non-diabetic women.[1] The diagnostic criterion for diabetic women follows that of the normal population (≥140/90 mmHg),

Table 15.1 Hypertensive disorders in pregnancy.

Chronic hypertension	BP ≥ 140 mmHg systolic or ≥90 mmHg diastolic prior to pregnancy or before 20 weeks of gestation; or hypertension diagnosed for the first time during pregnancy that does not resolve postpartum.[1] (However, in diabetic women BP > 135/85 or even BP >130/80 mmHg may be classified as chronic hypertension in some centers[1,7])
Gestational hypertension	BP > 140 mmHg systolic or >90 mmHg diastolic first detected after 20 weeks of gestation without proteinuria. If increased blood pressure returns to normal by 12 weeks postpartum the diagnosis is retrospectively made as transient hypertension of pregnancy. If it persists, a diagnosis of chronic hypertension applies[6]
Pre-eclampsia	BP > 140 mmHg systolic or >90 mmHg diastolic and proteinuria (≥1+ on a dipstick or ≥300 mg/24 h) after 20 weeks of gestation[6]
Chronic hypertension with superimposed pre-eclampsia	In women with hypertension early in pregnancy developing new-onset proteinuria fulfilling the criteria for pre-eclampsia In women with diabetic nephropathy with proteinuria in early pregnancy, development of pre-eclampsia is defined as above if accompanied by a sudden increase of ≥15% in systolic or diastolic blood pressure[7] A sudden 2–3-fold increase in proteinuria and/or thrombocytopenia (platelets < 100 000) and/or an increase in aspartate aminotransferase or alanine aminotransferase above normal levels also indicates pre-eclampsia[1]

BP, blood pressure

Table 15.2 Blood pressure (mmHg) in normal pregnancy and in women with Type 1 diabetes.

		First trimester	Second trimester	Third trimester	Average
Napoli et al[10]*	48 controls,	114/68	117/69	114/69	
	71 diabetics	118/71	116/72	115/72	
Nielsen et al[7]**	25 controls				117 (102–128)/70 (56–78)
	86 diabetics				120 (101–138)/72 (62–82)

* Daytime ambulatory blood pressure monitoring, given as mean values
** Average of office blood pressure measured at least once in each trimester given as medians and range

however, as in the non-pregnant diabetic population, lower diagnostic levels for chronic hypertension have been suggested.[1,7] In Copenhagen, a diagnostic level of chronic hypertension in pregnancy of 135/85 mm/Hg has been used[7] and even lower levels of greater than or equal to 130/80 mmHg for chronic hypertension in diabetic pregnant women are suggested in the 2008 American Diabetes Association (ADA) guidelines.[1]

Chronic hypertension, i.e. present before pregnancy, is associated with an increased risk of mid-trimester fetal loss, superimposed pre-eclampsia, preterm birth, intrauterine fetal growth restriction, and neonatal morbidity.[8] In addition, women with chronic hypertension are at risk of developing severe hypertension (≥160/110 mmHg) and stroke during pregnancy.

Gestational hypertension is the onset of hypertension after 20 weeks of gestation and does not lead to pregnancy complications in mild cases. However, it may progress to pre-eclampsia in a substantial proportion of cases (10–50%) or to severe hypertension (≥160/110 mmHg) with a comparable risk of severe pregnancy complications as in women with pre-eclampsia.[8]

Pre-eclampsia presents clinically as development of hypertension later than 20 weeks of gestation accompanied by proteinuria: greater than or equal to 1+ on a sterile urinary dipstick or ≥300 mg/24 h. Pre-eclampsia is associated with a substantial risk of severe maternal and fetal complications, such as placental abruption, cerebral catastrophe, coagulation abnormalities, and even maternal death. Termination of pregnancy is the most effective treatment and, consequently, pre-eclampsia often leads to preterm delivery with all its sequelae. The prevalence (7–20%) of pre-eclampsia is increased in pregnant women with Type 1 diabetes.[1] In patients with chronic hypertension, superimposed pre-eclampsia often develops early in pregnancy and with a more severe clinical presentation.

In diabetic women with microalbuminuria or diabetic nephropathy, superimposed pre-eclampsia is also prevalent and often of early onset, leading to preterm delivery.[9] The prevalence of pre-eclampsia in Type 1 diabetes is 6–10% in women with normal urinary albumin excretion, but is increased to 42% in women with microalbuminuria and 64% in women with diabetic nephropathy.[7]

Normal blood pressure in diabetes in pregnancy

Knowledge of normal BP is relevant to setting targets for treatment of hypertensive diabetic pregnant women. Even in normotensive normoalbuminuric women, diabetes is associated with a slightly higher BP in pregnancy, but still well within the normal range (Table 15.2).[7,10]

PRACTICAL ASPECTS OF DETECTING HYPERTENSION IN PREGNANCY

At the first pregnancy visit, BP and urinary albumin excretion should be measured, as well as history of hypertension, microalbuminuria or diabetic nephropathy, and antihypertensive treatment recorded. The patient can thereafter be classified according to presence of hypertension, microalbuminuria or diabetic nephropathy. BP should be recorded at each visit. Home BP measurements might be applicable to women with hypertension in pregnancy, but 24-hour BP monitoring generally has not been useful. Normotensive normoalbuminuric patients should be tested for the presence of proteinuria by dipstix at each visit, while progression of urinary albumin excretion in women with microalbuminuria, hypertension or diabetic nephropathy should be followed at each visit with determinations of the 24-hour urinary albumin excretion or the albumin-to-creatinine ratio in a spot urine sample.

PRINCIPLES FOR TREATMENT OF HYPERTENSION IN PREGNANCY

Mild-to-moderate hypertension

The benefit of antihypertensive therapy for mild-to-moderate elevation of BP in non-diabetic pregnancy (140–160/90–110 mmHg) with either chronic or pregnancy-induced hypertension has not been demonstrated in clinical trials. A recent Cochrane review showed that antihypertensive treatment appeared to reduce the risk of developing severe hypertension, but no differences were observed in the rates of pre-eclampsia, neonatal death, preterm delivery, and small for gestational age infants.[11]

International guidelines for treatment of hypertension in pregnancy vary with respect to threshold for initiating treatment and target BP goals, but all are higher than National Committee guidelines[12] for treatment of hypertension outside pregnancy. In Canada, antihypertensive therapy is considered at greater than or equal to 140/90 mmHg, targeting a diastolic BP of 80–90 mmHg,[13] and in Australia, elevations of greater than or equal to 160/90 mmHg are treated.[14] In the US, the guidelines are very conservative, advocating therapy when BP is greater than or equal to 160/105 mmHg.[6]

A recent Consensus Recommendation for Care of pregnant diabetic women recommends treatment of chronic hypertension during pregnancy to a systolic BP of 110–129 mmHg and a diastolic BP of 65–80 mmHg in the interest of long-term maternal health and to reduce the risk of impaired fetal growth.[1] Published data of pregnancy outcome using this strategy are not available and many obstetricians still advocate a target BP of 110–139 mmHg systolic and 65–90 mmHg diastolic. Randomized clinical trials are urgently needed to establish the treatment goal for antihypertensive treatment in diabetic pregnancy.

In women with underlying renal dysfunction, it may be reasonable to choose a lower threshold for treatment and to focus on the level of albumin excretion.[7,15] Thus, patients with either microalbuminuria or diabetic nephropathy prior to pregnancy might benefit from targeting urinary albumin excretion levels irrespective of BP level.[7,15] Our group has aimed for urinary albumin excretion levels below 300 mg/24 h and BP below 135/85 mmHg in women with pregestational microalbuminuria or diabetic nephropathy.[7] In a recent study, 14% of women with Type 1 diabetes and normal urinary albumin excretion, 50% of women with microalbuminuria, and 100%

Table 15.3 Goals for antihypertensive treatment of diabetic women during pregnancy based on both blood pressure and urinary albumin excretion.[2,3]

	Blood pressure (mmHg)	Urinary albumin excretion (mg/24 h)
Chronic hypertension*	110–139/65–89	
Microalbuminuria*	110–139/65–89	<300
Diabetic nephropathy*	110–139/65–89	<300
Gestational hypertension	110–139/65–89	
Pre-eclampsia	110–139/65–89	<300

* Some centers aim for blood pressure below 135/85 or even below 130/80 mm/Hg.

of women with diabetic nephropathy received antihypertensive treatment during pregnancy.[7] Compared with older patient series,[9,15,16] this strategy with early and strict antihypertensive treatment appeared to be associated with improved pregnancy outcome and fewer preterm deliveries.[7]

New treatment goals, including both BP levels and the level of urinary albumin excretion, are therefore suggested in Table 15.3.

Severe hypertension

There is a consensus that severe hypertension in pregnancy, defined as greater than or equal to 160/110 mmHg, requires treatment, because these women are at increased risk of intracerebral hemorrhage, and treatment decreases the risk of maternal death.[6,8] When treating severe hypertension it is important to avoid hypotension, because placental blood flow autoregulation is limited and aggressive lowering of BP may thus cause fetal hypoxia.[1]

CHOICE OF ANTIHYPERTENSIVE DRUGS FOR USE BEFORE AND DURING PREGNANCY

Angiotensin-converting enzyme inhibitors (ACE-Is) and angiotensin receptor blockers (ARBs) are both frequently used to treat hypertension and microalbuminuria in young diabetic women. Teratogenicity and fetotoxicity have been reported with these drugs.[14,17,18] The relative risk of congenital malformations in offspring of 209 women taking an ACE-I during organogenesis was 2.7 compared with women not taking antihypertensive drugs.[18] The relative risk of malformations in 202 women taking other types of antihypertensive therapy was 0.66. The most common malformations were in the cardiovascular or central nervous systems.[18] In addition to congenital malformations, fetal and neonatal renal failure and oligohydramnios have been observed.[14,17] A change from an ACE-I or ARB to other types of antihypertensive drugs prior to a planned pregnancy is therefore recommended.[1] However, in women suffering from diabetic nephropathy, it is necessary to consider each case individually. In particular, the benefits of continuing drugs which inhibit the renin angiotensin system until pregnancy is confirmed[19,20] must be balanced against the risk of disease progression prior to pregnancy, particularly if conception is delayed, resulting in a protracted period of withdrawal of ACE-I/ARB therapy.

Diuretics are commonly prescribed in essential hypertension before conception and, given their apparent safety, the National High Blood Pressure Education Program Working Group on High Blood Pressure in Pregnancy concluded that these drugs may be continued throughout gestation (with an attempt to lower the dose or used in combination with other agents).[6] Hypertension in diabetic women with renal disease (microalbuminuria or diabetic nephropathy) is often very salt sensitive. In light of this, it may be more appropriate for subjects to continue these drugs to avoid the rebound hypertension associated with their discontinuation.[7,15] However, initiating diuretic treatment in women with pre-eclampsia might reduce placental flow and thereby cause fetal hypoxia.[11] The commencement of diuretic treatment in late pregnancy should therefore be avoided, except in carefully selected cases, and with close ultrasound monitoring of fetal growth, amniotic fluid, and Doppler blood flow profiles.

Methyldopa remains one of the most widely used drugs for the treatment of hypertension in pregnancy. It is a centrally acting alpha-adrenergic agonist not thought to be teratogenic based on limited data and over 40 years of use in pregnancy. It has been assessed in a number of trials in pregnant women compared with placebo and with other alternative antihypertensive drugs.[11] It does not appear to have an adverse effect on utero-placental or fetal hemodynamics, or on fetal well-being. In a follow-up study of offspring at 7 years of age exposed to methyldopa *in utero*, the children exhibited intelligence and cognitive development similar to control subjects.[11]

Beta-blockers have been used extensively in pregnancy with no reports of teratogenicity, but long-term use in pregnancy may result in lower birthweight.[21] Intravenous treatment with beta-blockers has also been associated with fetal bradycardia and hypoglycemia in the newborn.[21] In addition, beta-blockers reduce the adrenal symptoms of maternal hypoglycemia and might therefore increase the risk of hypoglycemic unawareness and severe hypoglycemia in diabetes in pregnancy. However, labetalol, a non-selective beta-blocker with vascular alpha-receptor blocking capabilities, has been extensively investigated during pregnancy and has also gained wide acceptance in diabetes in pregnancy. In the US, both intravenous hydralazine and labetalol are recommended for treatment of diastolic BP levels of 105–110 mmHg.[22]

Calcium channel antagonists are also commonly used to treat chronic hypertension and pre-eclampsia presenting in late gestation. Nifedipine, verapamil or other calcium antagonists have not been associated with teratogenicity. Nifedipine, the most extensively investigated calcium antagonist during pregnancy, does not seem to cause a detectable decrease in uterine blood flow.[23] Short-acting nifedipine, particularly when administered sublingually, should be used with caution because of its potential to induce a steep drop in BP, which has been associated with maternal myocardial infarction and fetal bradycardia and hypoxia. Slow-release nifedipine preparations do not have this side effect and may be used during pregnancy. Calcium antagonists, and other antihypertensive drugs, can be used together with magnesium sulfate, which is used to prevent seizures during pre-eclampsia, without increasing the risk of serious side effects.[23]

Hydralazine selectively relaxes arteriolar smooth muscle and has been extensively used for oral and parenteral treatment of severe hypertension in late pregnancy, but has been replaced by agents with less adverse effects.[23] However, rarely it may have a place in women resistant to other drugs. When given intravenously it may be associated with dramatic drops in BP, which may result in the maternal and fetal effects mentioned above.

The remaining classes of antihypertensive drugs are rarely used in pregnancy.

STATINS

Cholesterol-lowering drugs such as statins are often used in non-pregnant diabetic women with hypertension to modulate lipid synthesis. They are contraindicated during pregnancy due to the possible effect on brain and nerve development.[24]

ASPIRIN

Aspirin is widely used in patients with diabetes to reduce the incidence of cardiovascular events. From the 12th week of gestation, aspirin may reduce the prevalence of pre-eclampsia in high-risk women.[25] Although it has been widely used in the first trimester, it is a matter of debate whether aspirin is associated with a slightly increased risk of malformations.[26] Use of aspirin during organogenesis is therefore not routine and should be based on an individual risk–benefit assessment. A woman already on aspirin treatment due to increased risk of cardiovascular events might therefore continue with aspirin during organogenesis.

ANTIHYPERTENSIVE DRUGS DURING BREASTFEEDING

Neonatal exposure to methyldopa via nursing is low and is generally considered safe. Atenolol and metropolol are concentrated in breast milk, possibly to levels that may affect the infant. In contrast, exposure to labetalol and propranolol seems low. Although milk concentrations of diuretics are low and considered safe, these agents can reduce milk production significantly.[23] Both captopril and enalapril are excreted in insignificant amounts in breast milk[27,28] and the American Academy of Pediatrics deemed these drugs to be compatible with breastfeeding. There are currently insufficient data regarding other ACE-Is or ARBs.

FUTURE DIRECTIONS

Randomized controlled trials determining the treatment goal for BP in pregnant women with diabetes and hypertension are needed with a special focus on patients with microalbuminuria, chronic hypertension or diabetic nephropathy. Those comparing the beneficial effects and side effects of different types of antihypertensive drugs, i.e. methyldopa *versus* calcium blockers, during pregnancy are also required. The Diabetes and Pre-eclampsia Intervention Trial[29] is a large multicenter trial investigating the role of antioxidants to prevent pre-eclampsia in Type 1 diabetes in pregnancy and is due to publish shortly. This study will also provide data on the prevalence rates and outcome of pregnancies complicated by microalbuminuria and diabetic nephropathy.

REFERENCES

1 Kitzmiller JL, Jovanovic L, Brown F, Coustan D, Reader DM (eds). *Managing Preexisting Diabetes and Pregnancy: Technical Reviews and Consensus Recommendations for Care*. Alexandria, VA: American Diabetes Association, 2008.
2 Nørgård K, Feldt Rasmussen B, Borch-Johnsen K, Saelan H, Deckert T. Prevalence of hypertension in type 1 diabetes mellitus. *Diabetologia* 1990;**33**:407–10.
3 American Diabetes Association. Standards of medical care in diabetes – 2008 position statements. *Diabetes Care* 2008;**31** (Suppl 1):s12–s54.
4 UK Prospective Diabetes Study Group. Efficacy of atenolol and captopril in reducing risk of macrovascular and microvascular complications in type 2 diabetes. *BMJ* 1998;**317**: 713–20.
5 Hansson L, Zanchetti A, Carruthers SG, *et al*. Effects of intensive blood-pressure lowering and low-dose aspirin in patients with hypertension: principal results of the Hypertension Optimal Treatment (HOT) randomised trial. HOT Study Group. *Lancet* 1998;**351**:1755–62.
6 Report of the National High Blood Pressure Education Program Working Group on High Blood Pressure in Pregnancy. *Am J Obstet Gynecol* 2000;**183**:S1–S22.
7 Nielsen LR, Damm P, Mathiesen ER. Improved pregnancy outcome in type 1 diabetes with microalbuminuria or diabetic nephropathy – Effect of intensified antihypertensive treatment? *Diabetes Care* 2009;**32**:38–44.
8 Sibai BM. Chronic hypertension in pregnancy. *Obstet Gynecol* 2002;**100**:369–77.
9 Ekbom P, Damm P, Feldt-Rasmussen B, Feldt-Rasmussen U, Molvig J, Mathiesen ER. Pregnancy outcome in type 1 diabetic women with microalbuminuria. *Diabetes Care* 2001;**24**:1739–44.
10 Napoli A, Sabbatini A, Di BN, Marceca M, Colatrella A, Fallucca F. Twenty-four-hour blood pressure monitoring in normoalbuminuric normotensive type 1 diabetic women during pregnancy. *J Diabet Complicat* 2003;**17**:292–6.
11 Abalos E, Duley L, Steyn D, Henderson-Smart D. Antihypertensive drug therapy for mild to moderate hypertension in pregnancy. *Cochrane Database Syst Rev* 2006, Issue 4:CD002252.
12 American Diabetes Association. Standards of Medical Care in Diabetes. Clinical Practice Recommendations. *Diabetes Care* 2008;**31** (Suppl 1):S3–S110.
13 Helewa ME, Burrows RF, Smith J, Williams K, Brain P, Rabkin SW. Report of the Canadian Hypertensive Society consensus conference: Definitions, evaluation and classification of hypertensive disorders of pregnancy. *CMAJ* 1997;**157**:715–25.
14 Brown MA, Hague WM, Higgins J, *et al*. The detection, investigation and management of hypertension in pregnancy: full consensus statement. *Aust N Z J Obstet Gynaecol* 2000;**40**:139–55.

15 Nielsen LR, Muller C, Damm P, Mathiesen ER. Reduced prevalence of early preterm delivery in women with Type 1 diabetes and microalbuminuria–possible effect of early anti-hypertensive treatment during pregnancy. *Diabet Med* 2006;**23**:426–31.

16 Carr DB, Koontz GL, Gardella C, *et al*. Diabetic nephropathy in pregnancy: suboptimal hypertensive control associated with preterm delivery. *Am J Hypertens* 2006;**19**:513–19.

17 Shotan A, Widerhorn J, Hurst A, Elkayam U. Risks of angiotensin-converting enzyme inhibition during pregnancy: experimental and clinical evidence, potential mechanisms, and recommendations for use. *Am J Med* 1994;**96**:451–6.

18 Alwan S, Polifka JE, Friedman JM. Angiotensin II receptor antagonist treatment during pregnancy. *Birth Defects Res A Clin Mol Teratol* 2005;**73**:123–30.

19 Cooper WO, Hernandez-Diaz S, Arbogast PG, *et al*. Major congenital malformations after first-trimester exposure to ACE inhibitors. *N Engl J Med* 2006;**354**:2443–51.

20 Hod M, van Dijk DJ, Karp M, *et al*. Diabetic nephropathy and pregnancy: the effect of ACE inhibitors prior to pregnancy on fetomaternal outcome. *Nephrol Dial Transplant* 1995;**10**:2328–33.

21 Magee LA, Duley L. Oral betablockers for mild to moderate hypertension during pregnancy. *Cochrane Database Syst Rev* 2004, Issue 1: CD002863.

22 American College of Obstetricians and Gynecologists. Diagnosis and Management of Preeclampsia and Eclampsia. ACOG Practice Bulletin #33. Washington, DC: ACOG, 2002.

23 Podymow T, August P. Hypertension in pregnancy. *Adv Chronic Kidney Dis* 2007;**14**:178–90.

24 Kazmin A, Garcia-Bournissen F, Koren G. Risk of statin use during pregnancy: a systematic review. *J Obstet Gynaecol Can* 2007:**29**:906–8.

25 Ruano R, Fontes RS, Zugiab M. Prevention of preeclampsia with low-dose aspirin – a systematic review and meta-analysis of the main randomized controlled trials. *Clinics* (Sao Paulo) 2005;**60**:407–14.

26 Norgard B, Puho E, Czeizel AE, Skriver MV, Sorensen HT. Aspirin use during early pregnancy and the risk of congenital abnormalities: a population-based case-control study. *Am J Obstet Gynecol* 2005;**192**:922–3.

27 Devlin RG, Fleiss PM. Captopril in human blood and breast-milk. *J Clin Pharmacol* 1981;**21**:110–3.

28 Rush JE, Snyder DL, Barrish A, Hichens M. Comment on Huttunen K, Gronhagen-Riska C, Fyhrquist F. Enalapril treatment of a nursing mother with slightly impaired renal function. *Clin Nephrol* 1989;**31**:278. *Clin Nephrol* 1991;**35**:234.

29 Holmes VA, Young IS, Maresh MJA, Pearson DWM, Walker JD, McCance DR on behalf of the DAPIT Study Group. The Diabetes and Pre eclampsia Intervention Trial. *Int J Obstet Gynecol* 2004;**87**:66–71.–23

16 Diabetic nephropathy in pregnancy

Baha M. Sibai

Department of Obstetrics & Gynecology, University of Cincinnati College of Medicine, Cincinnati, OH, USA

PRACTICE POINTS

- Tight control of blood glucose and blood pressure (BP) prior to conception and throughout gestation are the key to improved perinatal outcome.
- Patients with moderate-to-severe renal insufficiency and uncontrolled hypertension prior to conception and/or early in pregnancy are at increased risk for accelerated progression to endstage renal disease.
- Perinatal survival is greater than 95% in patients with minimal (serum creatinine < 125 μmol/L [<1.4 mg/dL]) renal dysfunction; however, pre-eclampsia and preterm delivery are common.
- Angiotensin-converting enzyme inhibitors (ACE-Is) and angiotensin receptor blockers (ARBs) should not be used during pregnancy.
- Pregnant patients with diabetes and renal transplant have pregnancy outcomes similar to those with nephropathy.

CASE HISTORY

A 25-year-old woman with a 15-year history of poorly controlled Type 1 diabetes presented at 8 weeks of gestation in her third pregnancy. Her past obstetric history included two early first trimester miscarriages. She had recently undergone laser treatment for proliferative diabetic retinopathy. Diabetic nephropathy had been diagnosed 5 years previously for which she had been commenced on an ACE-I. At presentation her BP was 140/90 mmHg, hemoglobin A1c (HbA1c) 8.5%, and serum creatinine 110 μmol/L (1.2 mg/dL). Urinalysis showed 3+ protein and 24-hour urinary protein was 0.6 g. Her ACE-I was stopped and methyldopa substi-

A Practical Manual of Diabetes in Pregnancy, 1st Edition.
Edited by David R. McCance, Michael Maresh and David A. Sacks.
© 2010 Blackwell Publishing

tuted. Urgent ophthalmologic referral revealed stable retinopathy. By 20 weeks her BP was 144/92 mmHg despite maximal doses of methyldopa and a calcium antagonist was added. At 32 weeks she required laser treatment for further new vessel development. At this time, her BP had risen to 150/94 mmHg, there was evidence of 3+ edema, urinary protein was 2.4 g/24 h, and serum creatinine 150 μmol/L (1.7 mg/dL). By 35 weeks, her BP had risen to 160/100 mmHg and she was admitted for bedrest. She came to elective cesarean at 36 weeks because of rising BP and poor fetal growth, giving birth to an infant weighing 2.5 kg. The baby was bottle fed. At her 6-week follow-up visit, her BP was 144/90 mmHg and serum creatinine 120 μmol/L (1.4 mg/dL). Her antihypertensive treatment was revised with recommencement of her ACE-I. She was referred to family planning and for ongoing ophthalmologic, diabetic, and renal follow-up. She was advised about the possible risks of any future pregnancy to herself and the baby, and of the critical need to use regular contraception.

- What is the effect of diabetes on pregnancy and *vice versa*?
- How should diabetic nephropathy be evaluated and managed before and during pregnancy?
- What are the risks and benefits of using ACE-Is and other antihypertensive agents during pregnancy?
- What are the maternal and perinatal outcomes in pregnancies complicated by vascular disease and nephropathy?

BACKGROUND

Diabetic nephropathy during pregnancy has been defined as a total urinary protein excretion of greater than or equal to 300 mg/24 h measured prior to pregnancy or greater than or equal to 300–500 mg/24 h measured prior to 20 weeks of gestation.[1–6] Diabetic nephropathy is also defined as microalbuminuria (urinary albumin excretion of 30–299 mg/24 h) either prior to pregnancy or early in gestation.[6–8] Incipient diabetic nephropathy is defined as either microalbuminuria (urinary albumin excretion of 30–299 mg/24 h)[7–10] or total protein excretion of 190–499 mg/24 h prior to 20 weeks of gestation.[1,5] These differences in definitions (use of albuminuria or proteinuria) reflect the variation in methods used to measure protein excretion.

The term diabetic nephropathy during pregnancy also refers to an heterogenous group of women with either Type 1 or Type 2 diabetes with or without significant derangement in renal function (creatinine clearance, serum creatinine, level of proteinuria) and a wide spectrum of BP values (normal, mild, moderate or severe hypertension). Thus, pregnant women with diabetic nephropathy may encompass subjects who have normal renal function (serum creatinine and creatinine clearance) and normal BP to those with endstage renal disease with severe hypertension, proliferative retinopathy, and ischemic cardiac changes.[1–15] Consequently, pregnancy outcome as well as long-term prognosis will vary because of confusing terminology and nomenclature, as well as differing stages of nephropathy.

PREVALENCE

In the US, the prevalence of diabetic nephropathy in women is increasing because of the trend of increasing prevalence of Type 2 diabetes.[3,16] The exact prevalence of diabetic nephropathy in pregnant women with diabetes is unknown. However, reports range from 5% to 10% of pregnancies complicated by diabetes mellitus.[3,13] Prevalence rates vary with the diagnostic criteria used (depending on whether proteinuria or albuminuria was present prior to pregnancy or whether it was measured before 20 weeks of gestation).

PATHOPHYSIOLOGY

Diabetic nephropathy is one of the most common microvascular complications of diabetes and is the leading cause of renal failure in developed countries.[17–19] Nephropathy due to Type 2 diabetes accounts for the majority of patients with renal failure.[17–19] The exact mechanisms by which diabetes induces nephropathy remain unclear; however, it has been suggested that diabetic nephropathy results from the interaction between genetic predisposi-

tion and certain environmental insults (both metabolic and hemodynamic abnormalities) related to the diabetic state.[17–19] Overt diabetic nephropathy is usually preceded by a long silent phase of glomerular changes (hypertrophy–hyperfunction, increased intraglomerular pressure) that is followed by incipient nephropathy with microalbuminuria. It has been reported that the natural course of diabetic nephropathy has five stages which correlate with specific changes in glomerular anatomy, physiology, and renal function. In order of development these include:

1 Glomerular hypertrophy with increased intraglomerular pressure (stage 1)
2 Increased glomerular basement membrane thickness with mesangial proliferation (stage 2)
3 A decrease in the number and density of podocytes (glomerular epithelial cells), including changes in podocyte foot process (stage 3)
4 Glomerulosclerosis and tubulointerstitial fibrosis (stages 4 and 5).

These structural changes in the glomeruli ultimately occur concurrently with the renal functional changes described in Table 16.1.[19]

The natural history of nephropathy differs between patients with Type 1 and Type 2 diabetes. At the time of presentation, patients with Type 2 diabetes exhibit an increased glomerular filtration rate (GFR) and glomerular hypertrophy. Microalbuminuria is unusual during the first 5 years following diagnosis of Type 1 diabetes, whereas it is more likely to be present at diagnosis in Type 2 diabetes. However, approximately 20% of patients with Type 1 diabetes will develop microalbuminuria after 5–10 years. Overt nephropathy will subsequently develop within 5–10 years after the onset of microalbuminuria.[6,16] This phase is usually characterized by a decrease in GFR, and a slight increase in serum creatinine and BP. The final stages are frequently associated with a progressive decline in renal function, severe hypertension, and ultimately development of endstage renal disease. It is important to emphasize that retinopathy is almost always present in patients with overt nephropathy, and is proliferative in 60–70% of cases.[3,6]

There are several factors that increase the risk of progression of nephropathy.[17–19] Some of the factors studied include increased hyperfiltration, poor glycemic control, and hypertension. Consequently, several observational studies and randomized trials have evaluated the benefits of tight blood glucose control with insulin and diet and the use of medications that lower BP and intraglomerular pressure, such as ACE-Is and ARBs in ameliorating or

Table 16.1 Stages of diabetic nephropathy. (Adapted from Jermendy & Ruggenenti,[19] with permission.)

Estimated GFR*		Albuminuria	Serum creatinine (μmol/L) [mg/dL]	Blood pressure (mmHg)	Renal structural changes
I stage	≥90	Normoalbuminuria	Normal (<100 [<1.1])	Normal < 130/80	Glomerular hypertrophy
II stage	60–89	Intermittent microalbuminuria	Normal	Normal < 130/80	Increased glomerular basement membrane thickness
III stage	30–59	Persistent microalbuminuria	100–124 [1.1–1.4]	Slightly elevated (130–139)	Decrease in and changes in glomerular epithelial cells
IV stage	15–29	Macroalbuminuria (≥300 mg/24 h)	Moderately increased (azotemia)	Moderately increased (140–159)	Glomerulosclerosis and tubulointerstitial fibrosis
V stage	<15 or dialysis	Macroalbuminuria (can decrease, pseudonormalization)	Markedly increased (uremia)	Markedly increased (≥160/110)	

*Glomerular filtration ratio estimated as ml/min/m²

preventing the development of nephropathy in patients with Type 1 and Type 2 diabetes. In general, these studies suggest that therapeutic intervention with ACE-Is for preventing diabetic nephropathy should ideally begin prior to the development of microalbuminuria.[3,16–19] In addition, they suggest that ACE-Is and ARBs are the drugs of choice to prevent and/or reduce the risks of progressive diabetic nephropathy.[6,16–19]

SCREENING FOR NEPHROPATHY PRIOR TO CONCEPTION AND/OR IN EARLY PREGNANCY

Screening for microalbuminuria should ideally be performed in all women with Type 1 and Type 2 diabetes prior to conception. There is no consensus regarding the method to be used for detecting microalbuminuria. Urinary excretion of albumin can be measured either by estimation of albumin-to-creatinine ratio in a random sample or a 24-hour urinary timed sample. There is a large intraindividual day-to-day variation in albumin excretion in diabetic patients. Therefore, repeated measurements are important to establish albuminuria. Although dipstick measurements of albuminuria are useful for screening purposes, they are not recommended to detect the presence or absence of microalbuminuria.[19]

Pregnancy in non-diabetic women is characterized by an increase in GFR and renal plasma flow. The increase in GFR begins very early in the first trimester,[3]

and thus may be confused with stage 1 diabetic nephropathy. As a result, serum creatinine values tend to be lower in normal pregnant women compared with non-pregnant values. The renovascular changes during pregnancy in patients with diabetic nephropathy are similar to those in patients with pre-existing renal disease. These changes will depend on the level of renal insufficiency prior to conception or early in pregnancy. Normal pregnancy is characterized by increased GFR, reaching about 50% above pre-pregnancy values by 18 weeks of gestation, a state of hyperfiltration and reduced serum creatinine (usually <71 μmol/L [<0.8 mg/dL]). In addition, there is an increase in protein excretion with advanced gestation; however, total protein excretion remains below 300 mg/24 h.[3] Several studies have compared the value of urinary dipstick protein values and protein-to-creatinine ratios in random urine samples with 24-hour protein measurements in normotensive and hypertensive pregnancies. A recent systematic review suggested that in normal pregnancy urinary protein dipstick measurements did not correlate with quantitative timed collections.[20] In addition, a systematic review of studies using protein-to-creatinine ratios to measure proteinuria also found that values of less than 130–150 mg of protein/g of creatinine were reliably able to rule out significant proteinuria (>300 mg/24 h), but values above this level were not able to quantitate proteinuria.[21] Therefore, in pregnant women with Type 1 and Type 2 diabetes, 24-hour timed collections should be used to establish the presence of micro- and macro-albuminuria and for the serial evaluation of protein excretion during pregnancy.

PREGNANCY OUTCOMES

There are numerous studies that have described pregnancy outcomes in patients with diabetic nephropathy. However, many of these have methodologic limitations. First, the majority of these studies are retrospective in design, of small sample size, usually performed at a single institution over a long period of time, and frequently there is inadequate control for confounding variables. Second, many of the studies lack detail about the presence or absence of associated comorbid conditions, as well as the degree of blood glucose and BP control prior to conception and during pregnancy. Third, in many of these reports, the diabetic patients under study are heterogenous with various degrees of renal impairment, protein excretion, and hypertension at the time of inclusion. Finally, the definition of maternal clinical outcomes, such as pre-eclampsia, deterioration in renal function, and fetal outcomes (congenital malformations, perinatal death, and preterm delivery) frequently differ among studies.

Nonetheless, the available literature clearly indicates the importance of maternal renal function and vascular status prior to conception in counseling these patients about the acute and long-term effects of pregnancy on maternal outcome.[2–6,22] In addition, it emphasizes the importance of strict glycemic control and aggressive control of maternal hypertension on overall maternal and perinatal outcome.[2–6,13,22]

Incipient nephropathy

The rubric of incipient nephropathy in pregnancies complicated by diabetes with onset prior to conception and/or early in gestation (before 20 weeks) includes women who had a normal serum creatinine and either micro-albuminuria (30–300 mg/24 h) or proteinuria (190–499 mg/24 h) before 20 weeks of gestation. Overall, those pregnancies associated with incipient nephropathy have increased rates of both pre-eclampsia and preterm delivery (Table 16.2).[1,5,7–9] Data on pre-eclampsia need to be interpreted with caution (see below).

Overt nephropathy

During the past decade, there has been a significant improvement in maternal and perinatal outcomes of pregnancies complicated by diabetic nephropathy. This improved outcome has resulted from advances in BP control, intensive fetal monitoring, early hospitalization for control of pregnancy complications, timely delivery,[3,22] and advances in neonatal care. Nevertheless, pregnancies complicated by diabetic nephropathy are still associated with increased rates of cesarean section, pre-eclampsia, preterm delivery, fetal growth restriction (FGR), and perinatal mortality. The magnitude of these risks will depend on the appropriateness of management prior to conception and during pregnancy, the degree of

Table 16.2 Rate of pre-eclampsia and preterm delivery in women with incipient nephropathy.

Authors	No. of women	Pre-eclampsia No. (%)	Preterm delivery No. (%)
Miodovnik et al (1993)[4*]			
<190 mg/24 h	204	20 (10)	47 (23)
190-499 mg/24 h	45	18 (40)	23 (51)
How et al (2004)[5*]			
<190 mg/24 h	94	16 (17)	12 (13)*
190–499 mg/24 h	35	7 (20)	5 (14)[†]
Ekbom et al**			
16–278 mg/24 h (2000)[7]	26	11 (42)	16 (62)
30–300 mg/24 h (2001)[8]	30	13 (43)	NR
Schroder et al (2000)[9]	13	6 (46)	NR

* These studies used total proteinuria
** This study used albuminuria
[†] Delivery < 34 weeks
NR, not reported

abnormalities in renal function (serum creatinine, creatinine clearance, amount of proteinuria), and the presence or absence of associated vascular involvement (hypertension, retinopathy, cardiovascular dysfunction).[3,22,23] In general, pregnancy outcome is usually favorable in patients with normal to minimal elevations in serum creatinine less than 124 μmol/L (1.4 mg/dL), and/or proteinuria of less than 1 g/24 h, and/or normal BP, and/or absent proliferative retinopathy prior to conception or early in pregnancy.[2–6,11–14] In contrast, maternal and perinatal outcomes are usually poor in patients with serum creatinine above 124 μmol/L (>1.4 mg/dL) and/or in those with severe hypertension, and/or nephrotic range proteinuria (≥3 g/24 h), and those with pre-existing cardiovascular disease.[3,4,22,23]

Pre-eclampsia is one of the most important and the major obstetric complication in patients with overt nephropathy. The diagnosis of pre-eclampsia can be difficult to make in the diabetic patient with pre-existing hypertension and proteinuria. General guidelines include:

- Pre-eclampsia in the woman with pregestational diabetes who is normotensive and non-proteinuric can be diagnosed after 20 weeks of gestation by a BP of greater than 140/90 mmHg associated with proteinuria of at least 300 mg/24 h[11]
- In diabetic women with hypertension but without baseline proteinuria, pre-eclampsia is diagnosed by the new onset of proteinuria (>300 mg/24 h)[11]
- If the patient is normotensive, but has proteinuria in early pregnancy, pre-eclampsia is diagnosed by the onset of hypertension or thrombocytopenia. In those diabetic patients with both proteinuria and hypertension prior to pregnancy or before 20 weeks of gestation, the presence of pre-eclampsia can be determined by new onset of thrombocytopenia, and/or a severe exacerbation of hypertension (systolic BP ≥ 160 and/or diastolic BP ≥ 110 mmHg) with exacerbation of proteinuria or symptoms (cerebral or visual).[11]

The above criteria are based on expert consensus opinion and were recommended by the National Working Group on Hypertension in Pregnancy as well as the American College of Obstetricians and Gynecologists.[11] The rate of pre-eclampsia in recently reported studies has ranged from 32 to 65% (Table 16.3).[2,4,5,8,11–15,24] This variation in rate is likely due to differences in the study population demographics, presence and degree of nephropathy, sample size, as well as differences in criteria used to diagnose pre-eclampsia. Glycemic control is also thought to play a role in the development of pre-eclampsia. It is

Table 16.3 Rate of pre-eclampsia in women with overt diabetic nephropathy.

Authors	No. of women	Pre-eclampsia No. (%)
Reece et al[33]	31	11 (35)
Gordon et al[2]	45	24 (53)
Miodovnik et al[4]	46	30 (65)
How et al[5]	65	21 (32)
Khoury et al[14]	60	24 (40)
Sibai et al[11]	48	17 (36)
Ekbom et al[8]	11	7 (65)
Diabetes and Pregnancy Group[12]	41	21 (51)
Bagg et al[15]	24	8 (33)
Carr et al[13]	43	15 (35)
Dunne et al[24]	21	11 (50)

hypothesized that poor glycemic control leads to a restriction of the proliferation of cytotrophoblasts during the first trimester and to the decreased conversion of maternal spiral arteries to large sinusoidal vessels (see chapter 3). When this occurs, insufficient utero-placental circulation results. There are other adverse pregnancy outcomes in patients with diabetic nephropathy (Table 16.4).[8,11,13–15,24] Again, the rate of these complications will depend on the degree of renal dysfunction and presence of associated comorbidities prior to conception.

RISK ASSESSMENT AND PRECONCEPTION COUNSELING AND CARE

The first step in the management of a patient with diabetic nephropathy is to evaluate potential risk factors for adverse maternal and perinatal outcome. Several risk factors are recognized prior to conception that have been associated with an increased risk for poor outcome (Table 16.5). The magnitude of this risk will depend on the specific medical condition and its severity prior to conception. The presence of one or more of these risk factors will increase the likelihood that the patient will have superimposed pre-eclampsia, preterm delivery, FGR, abruptio placentae, congenital malformations, perinatal death, and accelerated deterioration in renal function leading to endstage renal disease. Therefore, a comprehensive evaluation prior to conception or early in pregnancy will help in appropriate counseling and in many instances, will allow for the implementation of targeted strategies to reduce the development of some of these complications.

Table 16.4 Perinatal outcome in diabetic nephropathy.

Perinatal outcome	Dunne et al[24] (n = 21) No. (%)	Ekbom et al[8] (n = 11) No. (%)	Sibai et al[11] (n = 58) No. (%)	Bagg et al[15] (n =24) No (%)	Carr et al[13] (n = 43) No. (%)	Khoury et al[14] (n = 60) No (%)
Preterm delivery < 37 weeks	12 (57)	10 (91)	36 (62)	NR	NR	NR
<35 weeks	NR	5 (45)	21 (36)	11 (46)	9 (21)*	9 (15)*
Birth weight < 10th percentile	3 (14)	5 (45)	6 (11)	NR	8 (19)	7 (12)
Major anomalies	1 (5)	1 (9)	1 (2)	3 (12)	NR	4 (6.7)
Perinatal death	2 (9.5)	0	1 (2)	0	4 (9)	3 (5)

* Delivery < 32 weeks
NR, not reported

Table 16.5 Preconception factors for poor pregnancy outcome in diabetic nephropathy.

- Serum creatinine ≥124 µmol/L (≥1.4 mg/dL)
- Proteinuria >3 g/24 h
- Chronic hypertension >5 years
- Left ventricular dysfunction by echocardiogram (ECG)
- Ischemic changes on ECG
- Poor compliance with insulin and/or antihypertensive therapy
- Poor outcome in a previous pregnancy

Patients presenting for preconception care should undergo a detailed evaluation of their renal and cardiovascular status, metabolic profile (glucose control, serum lipids, HbA1c), and current medication. In addition, the past obstetric history (if appropriate) should be reviewed. Following this assessment, patients should be counseled about the impact of their condition on pregnancy and the potential effects of pregnancy on their medical condition. In addition, a detailed management plan for care before and during pregnancy should be discussed. If the patient elects to proceed with pregnancy, preconception care should focus on the treatment of any maternal conditions to improve pregnancy outcome. This includes tight glucose control with insulin therapy using frequent pre- and post-prandial self-blood glucose monitoring, and aiming to achieve a target HbA1c of less than 1% above normal at least 3 months prior to conception.[22] In addition, if possible, BP should be kept below 130/80 mmHg. Folic acid supplementation (5 mg/day) should be prescribed since it can reduce the risk of congenital malformations[25] and may reduce the risk of preterm delivery.[26]

There is convincing evidence that tight glucose control and the use of ACE-Is in non-pregnant patients with Type 1 and Type 2 diabetes will reduce the risks of their developing microalbuminuria and progression to overt nephropathy and/or endstage renal disease.[6,17–19] However, there are limited data regarding such benefit when used preconception. In a small number of subjects with diabetic nephropathy, Jovanovic et al[27] reported that normalization of glucose levels and BP before and during pregnancy was associated with improvement in creatinine clearance in the first trimester and later in gestation. Hod et al[28] in a study of eight class R/F diabetic women reported that strict glucose control and administration of ACE-Is for at least 6 months prior to conception resulted in a significant decrease in the amount of proteinuria at the time of conception. Similar findings were also reported by Bar et al.[29] These benefits continued despite the fact that ACE-Is were discontinued at the time of conception. These findings suggest that ACE-Is should be used concomitantly with intensive insulin management in patients with diabetic nephropathy attempting to conceive. These studies also suggest that ACE-Is should be discontinued at the time of conception. However, this recommendation is based on a limited number of study subjects. In addition, it may result in patients being exposed to these agents early in pregnancy since some women may become pregnant while on treatment.

PREGNANCY MANAGEMENT AND CARE IN DIABETIC NEPHROPATHY

Care should be conducted by a multidisciplinary team experienced in managing women with diabetic nephropathy. Frequent prenatal visits, tight glycemic control, and aggressive management of BP are the keys to improved pregnancy outcome. These patients should have intensive insulin therapy, frequent self-monitoring of blood glucose, and serial evaluation of HbA1c levels.

Fetal evaluation with serial ultrasound is required with more intensive monitoring if there is concern about growth or maternal deterioration, and consideration of early delivery. The following sections concentrate on issues directly relating to BP and renal function.

Blood pressure management

ACE-I and ARBs should be discontinued at the time of conception because of their potential teratogenic and fetal–neonatal effects.[30,31] Following their discontinuation, other agents that have similar proven beneficial effects on renal function and BP control should be utilized. Methyldopa has been viewed as the drug of choice in treating hypertension in pregnancy, primarily because of its lack of teratogenicity, but it is associated with side effects, particularly at increased doses. Several trials have compared the effects of ACE-Is with calcium channel blockers in non-pregnant diabetic patients. Overall, these studies suggest similar efficacy in preserving renal function in diabetic nephropathy.[6,16–19,32] There are no prospective observational studies or randomized trials evaluating the benefits of various antihypertensive drugs in pregnant women with diabetic nephropathy. However, because of the proven benefits of treating mild degrees of hypertension in non-pregnant diabetic subjects, there is general agreement that maternal BP should be aggressively treated to levels below 130/80 mmHg (both systolic and diastolic) in pregnant women with diabetic nephropathy.[2,6,13] Most patients will require at least two antihypertensive drugs. These

type of data have led some to consider a calcium channel blocker such as diltiazem or nifedipine as the drug of first choice. If an additional agent is needed, a diuretic or a combined beta- and alpha-blocker, such as labetalol, may be used. A recent retrospective study of perinatal outcome in 43 patients with diabetic nephropathy found that aggressive control of maternal BP (target mean arterial pressure < 100 mmHg) was associated with lower rates of preterm delivery compared with treatment to a target mean arterial pressure greater than or equal to 100 mmHg.[13] Table 16.6 summarizes the initial and maximum doses of the various antihypertensive medications to be used to control BP in such women.

Monitoring and management of renal function

Several retrospective studies have analyzed the influence of pregnancy on reno-vascular function in patients with various stages of diabetic nephropathy.[2,3,6,14,24,33–38] All studies found increased levels of proteinuria from the first trimester to term, returning to prepregnant levels postpartum. In addition, these studies found that more than 50% of patients had protein excretion values exceeding nephrotic range proteinuria during pregnancy.[2,3,14,24,33–38] Renal function (24-hour urine protein and creatinine clearance) should be measured at least once in every trimester. More frequent measurements are indicated in those with an initial serum creatinine greater than or equal to 124 μmol/L (>1.4 mg/dL) and in those who show deterioration with advanced gestation. It is

Table 16.6 Recommended drugs to be used in treatment of hypertension in diabetic nephropathy in pregnancy.*

Drug	Daily dose (mg)	Side effects
Methyldopa	750–3000	Drowsiness, hemolytic anemia, elevated liver enzymes
Nifedipine (short acting)	60–120	Tachycardia, headaches
Nifedipine (long acting)	60–120	Tachycardia, headaches
Nifedipine (sustained release)	60–240	Headaches
Diltiazem (extended release)	180–420	
Labetalol	400–2400	Bronchospasm
Thiazide diuretics	2.5–50	Avoid in case of pre-eclampsia
Atenolol	50–100	Fetal growth restriction
Hydralazine	25–100	Lupus-like syndrome, neonatal thrombocytopenia

* Most patients will require a combination of at least three drugs to achieve the target blood pressure range

important to emphasize that estimated glomerular filtration rate (EGFR) measurements using the modification of diet in renal disease (MDRD) formula are not reliable during pregnancy since they tend to underestimate the actual clearance values.[39] In addition, dipstick and urine protein-to-creatinine ratio measurements in random urine samples are not reliable to quantify the amount of proteinuria during pregnancy. In some patients with overt nephropathy, protein excretion may exceed 10 g/day during the late second or third trimester. Some of these women can develop severe vulvar edema, particularly when serum albumin values drop below 2.0 g/L (<20 mg/dL). In such cases, treatment with intravenous (IV) albumin and/or a loop diuretic may be beneficial. It is recommended to infuse the drugs together (e.g. 40 mg of frusemide premixed with 6 g of salt-poor albumin). In some refractory cases, it is suggested that 300 ml of 15% albumin be infused over 45 minutes followed by a bolus injection of 40 mg of IV frusemide. It is important to monitor such patients for the development of pulmonary edema.

In patients who have diabetic nephropathy and who are normotensive prior to pregnancy and/or during the first trimester, approximately 25% will develop new-onset hypertension. In those with pre-existing hypertension, the BP is likely to rise to a significant degree, particularly in the third trimester. The rates of new-onset hypertension as well as worsening of hypertension during pregnancy will increase with increased severity of renal dysfunction prior to conception. Consequently, patients who conceive with serum creatinine levels above 124 μmol/L (>1.4 mg/dL) usually require several antihypertensive medications to achieve the target BP value during pregnancy. Because of the expected changes in protein excretion and exacerbation of BP during pregnancy, the diagnosis of pre-eclampsia is usually difficult to make in such patients. Thus, it is important to include changes in platelet count and liver enzymes, and in presence of maternal symptoms to confirm the diagnosis in such patients.[11] A completed blood count and liver function test should be obtained once every 4 weeks, starting at 24 weeks of gestation. In addition, they should be obtained in all patients who develop new symptoms of pre-eclampsia and/or if pre-eclampsia is suspected.

In general, serum creatinine values remain stable during pregnancy in patients who have minimal-to-mild renal dysfunction (serum creatinine <124 μmol/L [<1.4 mg/dL]) prior to conception or early in pregnancy. In contrast, patients with serum creatinine levels greater than or equal to 124 μmol/L (>1.4 mg/dL) are more likely to demonstrate a greater increase in serum creatinine with profound deterioration in renal function early in the third trimester.[2,3,14,24,33–38]

In general, with the onset of pregnancy, creatinine clearance values do not demonstrate the expected increase seen in normal pregnancy, even though the data are not consistent among published studies.[2,6,14,24,27,28,33–36] It is important to emphasize that serum creatinine and creatinine clearance will be influenced by the presence or absence of hypertension, development of pre-eclampsia, as well as by the degree of glucose control during gestation.

LONG-TERM OUTCOME IN PREGNANT WOMEN WITH DIABETIC NEPHROPATHY

Maternal outcome

An important question is whether pregnancy increases the risk for development and progression of diabetic nephropathy. There are several reasons why this should be, including increased GFR leading to glomerular hyperfiltration, increased dietary protein intake, development of gestational hypertension or pre-eclampsia, and withholding ACE-Is and ARBs during pregnancy. For ethical reasons, randomized trials are not available to answer this question. Consequently, all available data have been generated from observational studies, retrospective studies, and a few case–control studies.[2–4,14,15,24,32–38,40–41]

Two large multicenter, prospective cohort studies examined the effects of pregnancy on microvascular complications in women with Type 1 diabetes.[40,41] The Diabetes Control and Complications Trial (DCCT)[40] included 180 women with 270 pregnancies and revealed that pregnancy did not increase the long-term risk of albumin excretion (microalbuminuria). The EURO-DIAB prospective complications study[41] included 163 diabetic women who became pregnant during the follow-up period (which averaged 7.3 years) and showed that pregnancy was not a risk factor for progression to microalbuminuria.

Several other studies have addressed the impact of pregnancy on long-term progression of renal disease in patients with overt nephropathy. The results of these studies are inconsistent because of differences in study populations, sample size, and duration of follow-up after pregnancy.[2–4,6,14–16,32–38] Nevertheless, the following conclusions can be made. In women with mild renal dysfunction (serum creatinine <124 μmol/L [<1.4 mg/dL], creatinine clearance ≥ 80 ml/min, and proteinuria <3 g/24 h), pregnancy does not seem to worsen long-term renal outcome.[2–4] In contrast, in women with moderate-to-severe renal dysfunction at conception (serum creatinine $\geq 133\,\mu$mol/L [≥ 1.5 mg/dL], proteinuria ≥ 3 g/24 h), limited data suggest that pregnancy may accelerate deterioration in renal function, resulting in endstage renal disease and the need for dialysis within a short period after pregnancy.[2,14,33–38] It is important to note the accelerated deterioration in renal function in these studies was usually associated with poor glycemic control, and the development of either accelerated hypertension or pre-eclampsia.

Neonatal and childhood outcome

The long-term outcome of infants born to patients with diabetic nephropathy is related to the obstetric complications mentioned previously, such as hypoxia from pre-eclampsia and/or abruptio placentae, preterm delivery at less than 37 or less than 34 weeks of gestation, low birthweight, FGR, and diabetic ketoacidosis. Consequently, long-term outcome in these infants will depend on the neonatal condition and gestational age at delivery. It might be anticipated that these infants would have higher rates of motor and cognitive delays, as well as cerebral palsy and learning disabilities. Unfortunately, there are only two studies with a limited number of infants that have evaluated long-term outcome in infants of pregnancies complicated by diabetic nephropathy.[36,37] Both of these studies reported that the adverse neonatal effects (cerebral palsy and neurologic delay) were related to gestational age and birthweight at delivery.

PREGNANCY IN DIABETIC WOMEN WITH RENAL TRANSPLANT

New-onset diabetes mellitus is a well-recognized complication of solid organ transplantation attributable to the use of immunosuppressive drugs, such as corticosteroids, and calcineurin inhibitors, such as tacrolimus and cyclosporin,[42] each of which may provoke hyperglycemia. In addition, endstage renal disease secondary to diabetes may be the indication for renal transplant in women with renal and/or pancreatic transplant. There are limited data describing the course of pregnancy in diabetic women after renal transplant. Consequently, most of the available literature addresses pregnancy outcome in women with renal transplant secondary to all forms of renal disease, and not just diabetes.[43–48]

The reported incidence of diabetes during pregnancy in patients with renal transplant ranges from 5% to 12%. In addition, the reported rate of hypertension prior to pregnancy and early in pregnancy following renal transplant ranges from 40% to 72%. These high rates are due either to the pre-existing conditions leading to transplant and/or to the side effects of the required immunosuppressive drugs.[43–47]

There are several reviews reporting pregnancy outcome in women with renal transplant and these make consistent observations.[43–48] Pregnancy should be delayed for at least 1 year following transplant, at which time the patient is more likely to be on maintenance doses of immunosuppressive agents and to have stable graft function (serum creatinine <133 μmol/L [<1.5 mg/dL], minimal proteinuria ≤ 500 mg/24 h). These women should be managed by a multidisciplinary team, including a transplant surgeon, a nephrologist, and an obstetrician skilled in the management of such patients. Perinatal survival in these patients is almost 75%, but a large percentage of pregnancies will be associated with increased maternal and perinatal complications (Table 16.7). It is important to emphasize that the diagnosis of superimposed pre-eclampsia may again be difficult to make in such patients because of the pre-existing hypertension, the increased levels of uric acid secondary to calcineurin inhibitor treatment, and the progressive increase in proteinuria.[43–47] In addition, the clinical findings of pre-eclampsia may mimic those of acute graft rejection.

The management of the patient with diabetes and renal transplant is similar to that in patients with diabetic nephropathy. Preconception care, early and frequent perinatal care, tight glycemic and BP control, intensive fetal testing and timely delivery are the keys to successful pregnancy outcome. In addition to the risks seen in diabetic nephropathy, these patients are at increased risk of bacterial infections (all forms of urinary tract), viral

Table 16.7 Pregnancy outcome in renal transplant.

	Percentage
Miscarriage	15–20
Pre-eclampsia	30–35
Preterm delivery	50–55
Urinary tract infection	2–5
Fetal growth restriction	5–10
Rejection during pregnancy	35–40
Graft rejection within 2 years of delivery	30–50

infections (hepatitis C and herpes simplex), and toxo-plasmosis.[45–47] Therefore, these patients should have frequent monitoring for these infections and be managed accordingly if the results are positive. Acute graft rejection occurs in approximately 5–10% of patients. Rejection must be distinguished from pre-eclampsia and pyelonephritis because of their similar clinical and laboratory manifestations. In cases of uncertainty, the diagnosis should be confirmed by renal biopsy, which can be done safely under ultrasound guidance during pregnancy.

PREGNANCY IN PATIENTS ON CHRONIC DIALYSIS

The incidence of pregnancy in patients on chronic dialysis is 1–7%.[49–52] There is no information on pregnant patients with diabetes on chronic dialysis. Perinatal outcome has improved in the past decade, but the data on pregnancy outcome in patients on dialysis are limited and are usually described as case reports or case series.[49–52] A recent study described the outcome in 13 pregnancies (10 on hemodialysis and three on peritoneal dialysis), and included a review of previous studies (117 on hemodialysis and 14 on peritoneal dialysis).[52] In this review, the authors reported a perinatal survival rate of 50% (five of 10 women) among those who elected to continue with their pregnancy. In contrast, among the reviewed case series, the perinatal survival was 71% in those on hemodialysis and 64% in those on peritoneal dialysis. In general, 90% ended in preterm delivery with 50% delivering at 30–32 weeks of gestation. The rate of hypertension or pre-eclampsia was 40%. Thirty-four percent developed polyhydramnios. In addition, adverse pregnancy outcome is usually higher in women who conceive after dialysis has been initiated, compared with those who start dialysis during pregnancy.[52]

Management of patients on dialysis requires a multidisciplinary team approach. Dialysis should be performed at least six times per week, with each session lasting at least 4 hours and aiming to keep maternal blood urea nitrogen (BUN) values below 17.9 mmol/L (<50 mg/dL). Erythopoetin (EPO) is safe to use during pregnancy and an increase of 50–100% compared with prepregnancy levels may be required to keep the hemoglobin level above 1 g/L (10 g/dL). These patients require close monitoring of their ferritin levels. Oral iron supplements will not help in improving hemoglobin levels. In addition, it is important to monitor nutritional requirements carefully as well as changes in electrolytes during dialysis.

CONCLUSIONS AND FUTURE DIRECTIONS

During the past decade there has been a significant improvement in maternal and perinatal outcome in pregnancies complicated by diabetic nephropathy. This improvement has been achieved using multidisciplinary programs that focus on preconception counseling and aggressive control of blood sugars and BP, as well as early detection and control of associated complications. None the less, management of such women continues to be based on expert opinion with limited information from randomized trials.

It remains unclear as to whether ACE-Is or ARBs should be continued up to conception in women desiring pregnancy. At present, recommendations are to switch to either methyldopa, calcium channel blockers or beta-blockers. There is an urgent need for randomized trials to evaluate the safety and efficacy of such recommendations. In addition, there are no randomized trials which have evaluated the safety and efficacy of various antihypertensive drugs to treat hypertension in diabetic women. Moreover, there are no data to support the target BPs to achieve during therapy. Finally, there are no standardized criteria to define pre-eclampsia in women with diabetic nephropathy. Future studies are needed to answer these questions.

REFERENCES

1 Combs CA, Rosenn B, Kitzmiller JL, *et al*. Early pregnancy proteinuria in diabetes related to preeclampsia. *Obstet Gynecol* 1993;**82**:802–7.

2 Gordon M, Landon MB, Samuels P, *et al*. Perinatal outcome and long-term follow-up associated with modern management of diabetic nephropathy. *Obstet Gynecol* 1996;**87**: 401–9.

3 Landon ML. Diabetic nephropathy and pregnancy. *Clin Obstet Gynecol* 2007;**50**:998–1006.

4 Miodovnik M, Rosenn BM, Khoury JC, *et al*. Does pregnancy increase the risk for development and progression of diabetic nephropathy? *Am J Obstet Gynecol* 1996;**174**: 1180–91.

5 How H, Sibai B, Lindheimer M, Caritis S, et al. Is early pregnancy proteinuria associated with an increased rate of pre eclampsia in women with pregestational diabetes mellitus? *Am J Obstet Gynecol* 2004;**190**:775–8.

6 Leguizamon G, Reece EA. Effect of medical therapy on progressive nephropathy: Influence of pregnancy, diabetes and hypertension. *J Matern Fetal Neonatal Med* 2000;**9**:70–8.

7 Ekbom P, Danne P, Norgaard K, *et al*. Urinary albumin excretion and 24-hour blood pressure as predictors of

pre-eclampsia in type 1 diabetes. *Diabetologia* 2000;**43**: 927–31.

8 Ekbom P, Danne P, Feldt-Rasmussen B, *et al*. Pregnancy outcome in type 1 diabetic women with micro-albuminuria. *Diabetes Care* 2001;**24**:1739–44.

9 Schroder W, Heyl W, Hill-Grasshoff B, Rath W. Clinical value of detecting microalbuminuria as a risk factor for pregnancy-induced hypertension in insulin-treated diabetic pregnancies. *Eur J Obstet Gynecol Reprod Biol* 2000;**91**: 155–8.

10 Lauszus FF, Rasmussen OW, Lousen T, *et al*. Ambulatory blood pressure as predictor of preeclampsia in diabetic pregnancies with respect to urinary albumin excretion rate and glycemic regulation. *Acta Obstet Gynecol Scand* 2001;**80**: 1096–103.

11 Sibai BM, Caritis S, Hauth J, Lindheimer M, et al. Risks of preeclampsia and adverse neonatal outcomes among women with pregestational diabetes mellitus. *Am J Obstet Gynecol* 2000;**182**:364–9.

12 Diabetes and Pregnancy Group, France. French multicentric survey of outcome of pregnancy in women with pregestational diabetes. *Diabetes Care* 2003;**26**:2990–93.

13 Carr DB, Koontz GL, Gardella C, *et al*. Diabetic nephropathy in pregnancy: Suboptimal hypertensive control associated with preterm delivery. *Am J Hypertens* 2006;**19**:513–9.

14 Khoury JC, Miodovnik M, LeMasters G, Sibai BM. Pregnancy outcome and progression of diabetic nephropathy. What's next? *J Matern Fetal Neonatal Med* 2002;**11**:238–44.

15 Bagg W, Neale L, Henley P, *et al*. Long-term maternal outcome after pregnancy in women with diabetic nephropathy. *N Z Med J* 2003;**116**:1180.

16 How HY, Sibai BM. Use of angiotensin-converting enzyme inhibitors in patients with diabetic nephropathy. *J Matern Fetal Neonatal Med* 2002;**12**:402–7.

17 Giunti S, Barit D, Cooper ME. Mechanisms of diabetic nephropathy: Role of hypertension. *Hypertension* 2006;**48**: 519–26.

18 Ritz E, Dikow R. Hypertension and antihypertensive treatment of diabetic nephropathy. Nature Clinical Practice. *Nephrology* 2006;**2**:562–7.

19 Jermendy G, Ruggenenti P. Preventing microalbuminuria in patients with type 2 diabetes. *Diabetes Metab Res Rev* 2007;**23**:100–10.

20 Waugh JJ, Clark TJ, Divakram TG, *et al*. Accuracy of urinalysis dipstick techniques in predicting significant proteinuria in pregnancy. *Obstet Gynecol* 2004;**103**:769–77.

21 Papnna R, Mann LK, Kouides RW, Glantz JC. Protein/creatinine ratios in preeclampsia. A systematic review. *Obstet Gynecol* 2009;**112**:135–44.

22 Gabbe SG, Graves CR. Management of diabetes mellitus complicating pregnancy. *Obstet Gynecol* 2003;**102**:857–68.

23 Gordon MC, Landon MB, Boyle J, Stewart K, Gabbe SG. Coronary artery disease in insulin dependent diabetes mellitus of pregnancy (class H). A review of the literature. *Obstet Gynecol Surv* 1996;**51**:437–44.

24 Dunne FP, Chowdhury TA, Hartland A, *et al*. Pregnancy outcome in women with insulin-dependent diabetes mellitus complicated by nephropathy. *Q J Med* 1999;**92**:451–4.

25 Pearson DWM, Kernaghan D, Lee R, *et al*. The relationship between pre-pregnancy care and early pregnancy loss, major congenital anomaly or perinatal death in type 1 diabetes mellitus. *BJOG* 2007;**114**:104–7.

26 Bukowski R, Malone FD, Porter F, *et al*. Preconceptional folate prevents preterm delivery. *Am J Obstet Gynecol* 2007;**197** (Suppl 10):S5.

27 Jovanovic R, Jovanovic L. Obstetric management when normoglycemia is maintained in diabetic pregnant women with vascular compromise. *Am J Obstet Gynecol* 1984;**149**:617–23.

28 Hod M, Van Kijk DJ, Karp M, *et al*. Diabetic nephropathy and pregnancy: the effect of ACE inhibitors prior to pregnancy on maternal outcome. *Nephrol Diab Transplant* 1995;**10**:2328–33.

29 Bar J, Chen R, Schoenfeld A, *et al*. Pregnancy outcome in patients with insulin dependent diabetes mellitus and diabetic nephropathy treated with ACE inhibitors before pregnancy. *J Pediatr Endocrine Metab* 1999;**12**:659–65.

30 Cooper WO, Hernandez-Diaz S, Arbogast PG, *et al*. Major congenital malformations after first-trimester exposure to ACE inhibitors. *N Engl J Med* 2006;**354**:2443–51.

31 Velazquez-Armenta EY, Han JY, *et al*. Angiotensin II receptor blockers in pregnancy: A case report and systematic review of the literature. *Hypertens Pregnancy* 2007;**26**: 51–66.

32 Tobe S, Epstein M. The use of calcium antagonists in the treatment of hypertensive persons with kidney disease. *Curr Hypertens Rep* 2002;**4**:191–4.

33 Reece EA, Leguizamon G, Homko C. Pregnancy performance and outcomes associated with diabetic nephropathy. *Am J Perinatol* 1998;**15**:413–21.

34 Purdy LP, Hantsch CE, Molitch ME, *et al*. Effect of pregnancy on renal function in patients with moderate to severe diabetic renal insufficiency. *Diabetes Care* 1996;**19**: 1067–74.

35 Biesenbach G, Grafinger P, Stoger H, *et al*. How pregnancy influences renal function in nephropathic type 1 diabetic women depends on their pre-conception creatinine clearance. *J Nephrol* 1999;**12**:41–6.

36 Kimmerle R, Zass RP, Cupisti S, *et al*. Pregnancies in women with diabetic nephropathy: long-term outcome for mother an child. *Diabetologia* 1995;**38**:227–35.

37 Biesenbach G, Grafinger P, Zagornik J, *et al*. Perinatal complications and three-year follow-up of infants of diabetic mothers with diabetic nephropathy stage IV. *Ren Fail* 2000;**22**:573–80.

38 Rosing K, Jacobson P, Homuel E, *et al*. Pregnancy and progression of diabetic nephropathy. *Diabetologia* 2002;**45**: 36–41.

39 Smith MC, Moran P, Ward MK, Davison JM. Assessment of glomerular filtration rate during pregnancy using the MDRD formula. *BJOG* 2008;**115**:109–12.

40 The Diabetes Control and Complications Trial Research Group. Effect of pregnancy on microvascular complications in the Diabetes Control and Complications Trial. *Diabetes Care* 2000;**23**:1084–91.

41 Verier-Mine O, Chaturvedi N, Webb D, Fuller JH, and the EURODIAB Prospective Complications Study Group. Is pregnancy a risk factor for microvascular complications? The EURODIAB prospective complications study. *Diabet Med* 2005;**22**:1503–9.

42 Wilkinson A, Davidson J, Dotta F, *et al.* Guidelines for the treatment and management of new-onset diabetes after transplantation. *Clin Transplant* 2005;**19**:291–8.

43 Armenti VT, Radomski JS, Morit MJ, *et al.* Report from the National Transplantation Pregnancy Registry (NTPR): Outcomes of pregnancy after transplantation. *Clin Transplant* 2005;69–83.

44 McKay DB, Josephson MA. Pregnancy in recipients of solid organs – Effects on mother and child. *N Engl J Med* 2006;**354**:1281–93.

45 Josephson MA, McKay DA. Considerations in the medical management of pregnancy in transplant recipients. *Adv Chronic Kidney Dis* 2007;**14**:156–67.

46 de Mar Colon M, Hibbard JU. Obstetric considerations in the management of pregnancy in kidney transplant recipients. *Adv Chronic Kidney Dis* 2007;**14**:168–77.

47 Fucho KM, Wu D, Ebcioglu Z. Pregnancy in renal transplant recipients. *Semin Perinatol* 2007;**31**:339–47.

48 Kurata A, Matsuda Y, Tanabe K, *et al.* Risk factors of preterm delivery at less than 35 weeks in patients with renal transplant. *Eur J Obstet Gynecol Reprod Biol* 2006;**128**:64–8.

49 Tan L-K, Kanagalingam D, Tan H-K, Choong H-L. Obstetric outcomes in women with end-stage renal failure requiring renal dialysis. *Int J Gynecol Obstet* 2006;**94**:17–22.

50 Holley JL, Reddy SS. Pregnancy in dialysis patients: A review of outcomes, complications, and management. *Semin Dialysis* 2003;**16**:384–88.

51 Reddy SS, Holley JL. Management of the pregnancy chronic dialysis patient. *Adv Chronic Kidney Dis* 2007;**14**:146–55.

52 Chou C-Y, Ting I-W, Lin T-H, Lee C-N. Pregnancy in patients on chronic dialysis: A single center experience and combined analysis of reported results. *Eur J Obstet Gynecol Reprod Biol* 2008;**136**:165–70.

17 Retinopathy in diabetes in pregnancy

Catherine B. Meyerle & Emily Y. Chew

National Eye Institute of National Institutes of Health, Bethesda, MA, USA

PRACTICE POINTS

- Diabetic retinopathy, a microvascular complication of diabetes, remains a leading cause of acquired blindness in young and middle-aged adults.
- Pregnancy, with its hormonal, hemodynamic, metabolic, and immunologic changes, is a risk factor for progression of diabetic retinopathy.
- The etiology of retinopathy acceleration during pregnancy is unknown, although proposed mechanisms involve rapid improvement in glycemic control, altered hemodynamic properties, and immunoinflammatory processes.
- Visual loss from diabetic retinopathy aggravated by pregnancy is usually preventable if a patient has optimal systemic and ocular management prior to conception and during pregnancy.
- Dilated ocular examinations should be performed prior to pregnancy and then at least on one further occasion during pregnancy (or more often at the discretion of the ophthalmologist, depending on the retinopathy status).

CASE HISTORY

A 27-year-old woman with Type 1 diabetes for 20 years presented for ophthalmic monitoring during pregnancy. During the first trimester, she was 20/20 in both eyes and had minimal non-proliferative diabetic retinopathy on dilated examination (Fig. 17.1A and B). Upon institution of tighter metabolic control, her glycosylated hemoglobin (HbA1c) fell from 8.6% to 7% during early pregnancy. On second trimester examination, her vision was 20/25 in both eyes and her retinopathy had progressed to severe non-proliferative diabetic retinopathy (Fig. 17.1C and D). During the third trimester, her vision declined to 20/60 in the right eye and 20/80 in the left eye due to

A Practical Manual of Diabetes in Pregnancy, 1st Edition.
Edited by David R. McCance, Michael Maresh and David A. Sacks.
© 2010 Blackwell Publishing

clinically significant macular edema (Fig. 17.1E and F). After treatment, her macular edema resolved and vision partially recovered to 20/40 in both eyes.

- What are the putative mechanisms and risk factors for progression of retinopathy during pregnancy?
- What is the relevance of intensification of glycemic control to retinopathy progression? Is this a transient phenomenon?
- How often should the fundi be examined during pregnancy?

First, we will briefly review diabetic retinopathy in general and then focus on how the unique state of pregnancy affects retinopathy progression.

BACKGROUND

Diabetic retinopathy prevalence at baseline

Diabetic retinopathy, a microvascular complication of diabetes, remains a leading cause of acquired blindness in young and middle-aged adults.[1] Currently, the estimated general population prevalence rates for retinopathy and vision-threatening retinopathy in the US are 3.4% (4.1 million persons) and 0.75% (899 000 persons), respectively.[2] These pooled data focus almost exclusively on Type 2 diabetes.[1] An epidemiologic study of subjects with Type 1 diabetes based on data from the New Jersey 725 Study and Wisconsin Epidemiologic Study of Diabetic Retinopathy, estimated prevalence rates of retinopathy at 1 per 300 persons aged 18 years and older and rates of vision-threatening retinopathy at 1 per 600 persons.[3] Specifically, of the estimated 889 000 persons with Type 1 diabetes diagnosed before age 30 years in the US, 767 000 (86.4%) have some degree of retinopathy

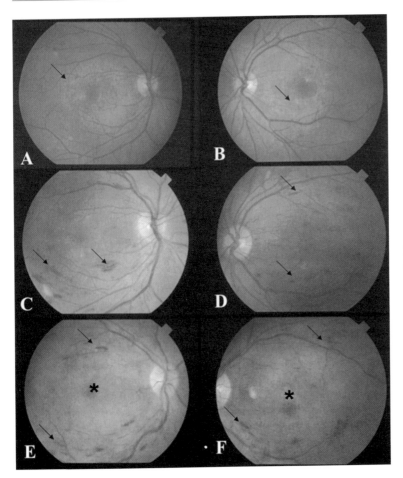

Fig. 17.1 During the first trimester, dilated examination of the (A) right and (B) left eye reveals occasional intraretinal hemorrhages (arrows) consistent with minimal non-proliferative diabetic retinopathy. (C and D) After institution of rapid glycemic control, the patient developed increasing intraretinal hemorrhages (arrows) indicative of severe non-proliferative diabetic retinopathy during the second trimester. (E and F) In the third trimester, examination revealed further retinopathy progression (arrows) with the development of clinically significant macular edema (*).

and 376 000 (42.1%) have vision-threatening retinopathy.[3] These prevalence rates of diabetic retinopathy are particularly concerning given the increasing prevalence of diabetes mellitus.[1]

Pregnancy as a risk factor for worsening retinopathy

Pregnancy, with its hormonal, hemodynamic, metabolic, and immunologic changes, is a risk factor for progression of diabetic retinopathy. While the landmark studies focused on worsening retinopathy in pregnant Type 1 diabetic women,[4–6] the findings of these studies can be extrapolated to pregnant women with Type 2 diabetes as the retinopathy seen in the two groups is essentially similar. Gestational diabetes, however, is not a risk factor

for the development of retinopathy during pregnancy, but may be suggestive of a genetic risk for subsequent diabetes mellitus.[7]

OVERVIEW OF DIABETIC RETINOPATHY CLASSIFICATION

Diabetic retinopathy in both Type 1 and Type 2 diabetes is broadly classified as either non-proliferative or proliferative (Table 17.1). Non-proliferative diabetic retinopathy occurs when there are only intraretinal microvascular changes, such as microaneurysms and retinal hemorrhages (Fig. 17.2). In advanced non-proliferative diabetic retinopathy, progressive capillary non-perfusion of the retina may develop and lead to increasing ischemia, which results in the more severe proliferative phase. Pro-

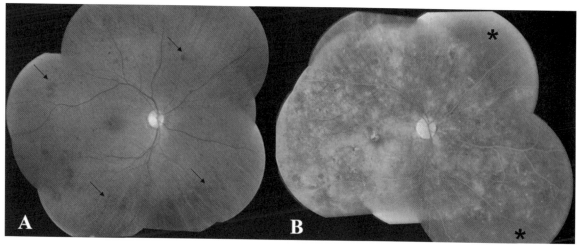

Fig. 17.2 (A) Fundus photograph of the right eye reveals dot-blot intraretinal hemorrhages in all four quadrants (arrows), consistent with severe non-proliferative diabetic retinopathy. (B) Fluorescein angiograghy shows patches of non-perfusion in the peripheral retina (*), indicative of the severe nature of the non-proliferative retinal changes.

Table 17.1 Classification of diabetic retinopathy.

Classification	Lesions present
No retinopathy	No lesions present
Non-proliferative retinopathy	Intraretinal microvasculature changes only
Mild	Mild levels of microaneurysms and intraretinal hemorrhage
Moderate	Moderate levels of microaneurysms and intraretinal hemorrhage
Severe	Presence of one of the following features (4:2:1 rule): • Severe intraretinal hemorrhage in all four quadrants • Venous beading in two or more quadrants • Moderate intraretinal microvascular anomaly (IRMA) in at least one quadrant
Proliferative retinopathy	Neovascularization on the retinal surface

liferative diabetic retinopathy (Fig. 17.3) is characterized by new vessels on the retinal surface or optic disc that can bleed and result in the vision-threatening complications of vitreous hemorrhage, fibrotic scarring, and fractional retinal detachment. In both non-proliferative and proliferative diabetic retinopathy, increased retinal vascular permeability can result in accumulation of fluid in the

retinal area serving central vision. This retinal thickening, known as macular edema (Fig. 17.4), is a leading cause of visual loss in diabetic patients.

RISK FACTORS FOR PROGRESSION OF DIABETIC RETINOPATHY

Diabetic retinopathy, a microvascular complication, is an end-organ response to a systemic disease. Concomitant systemic factors, therefore, influence the development and progression of diabetic retinopathy.[8] A thorough understanding of diabetic retinopathy is necessary to discuss the specific retinal changes found in the diabetic pregnant patient. To do this, landmark studies regarding diabetic retinopathy in non-pregnant individuals will first be examined followed by a review of the specific studies focusing on diabetic retinopathy during pregnancy. A number of risk factors have been identified in large epidemiologic studies that are relevant to both pregnant and non-pregnant diabetic patients, although their role in the dynamic physiologic state of pregnancy is unique.

Glycemic control

Chronic hyperglycemia instigates a cascade of events leading to microvascular complications in diabetes. The landmark studies investigating glycemic control and its effects on diabetic complications include the Diabetes

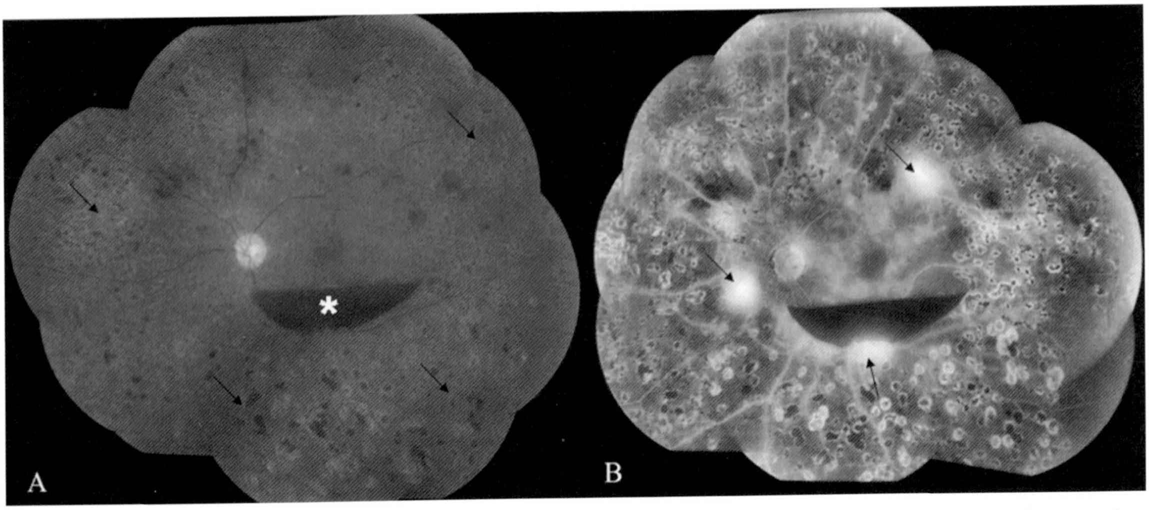

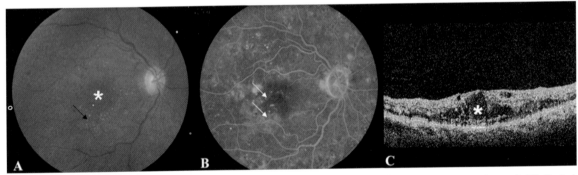

Fig. 17.3 (A) Fundus photograph of the left eye shows preretinal hemorrhage overlying the macula (*). The peripheral retina has many laser photocoagulation scars (arrows) indicative of previous treatment for proliferative diabetic retinopathy. (B) Fluorescein angiogram shows patches of bright hyperfluorescence (arrows) corresponding to areas of leaking neovascularization consistent with proliferative diabetic retinopathy.

Fig. 17.4 (A) Fundus photograph of the right eye shows macular fluid (*) and lipid (arrow) consistent with clinically significant macular edema. (B) Fluorescein angiography reveals multiple leaking microaneurysms (arrows). (C) Optical coherence tomography confirms the presence of cystic fluid changes in the macula (*).

Control and Complications Trial (DCCT) and the United Kingdom Prospective Diabetes Study (UKPDS). Both of these clinical trials demonstrated the beneficial effects of intensive glycemic control in reducing the complications of diabetes.

Diabetes Control and Complications Trial
The DCCT was a randomized, multicenter, prospective trial designed to determine if intensive glucose control, with the goal of near-normal HbA1c levels, would affect the development and progression of diabetic complica-

tions in Type 1 diabetes. The 1441 participants were randomly assigned to either conventional or intensive treatment for glucose control and followed for a mean duration of 6.5 years.[9–13] The mean HbA1c was 7.2% in the intensive treatment group and 9.1% in the conventional control cohort. Intensive treatment resulted in a decreased risk of either the development or progression of diabetic retinopathy. One of the adverse effects of intensive therapy included initial worsening of retinopathy; however, this reversed after 18 months. In patients without any visible retinopathy when enrolled in the

DCCT, the 3-year risk of developing retinopathy was reduced by 75% in the intensive treatment group compared with the standard treatment group. The benefit of the strict control was also evident in patients with existing retinopathy. There was a 50% reduction in the rate of progression of retinopathy compared with controls. When the DCCT results were stratified by HbA1c levels, there was a 35–40% reduction in the risk of retinopathy progression for every 10% decrease in HbA1c (e.g. from 8% to 7.2%).

United Kingdom Prospective Diabetes Study

The UKPDS,[14] the largest and longest study of patients with Type 2 diabetes to date, was designed to evaluate the effect of conventional *versus* intensive glucose management on diabetic complications in 3867 subjects with newly diagnosed diabetes. The study confirmed that the beneficial effects of tight glycemic control on the incidence and progression of diabetic retinopathy also apply to patients with Type 2 diabetes. During a 9-year follow-up, the UKPDS showed a 25% reduction in the risk of the "any diabetes-related microvascular end point," including the need for retinal photocoagulation, in the intensive treatment group compared with the conventional treatment group. For every percentage point decrease in HbA1c (e.g. 9% to 8%), there was a 35% reduction in the risk of microvascular complications.

Concomitant hypertension

Multiple studies have suggested that diabetic patients with concomitant hypertension are at increased risk for the development and progression of diabetic retinopathy, although the data are conflicting. Hypertension is thought to exacerbate diabetic retinopathy through mechanical stretching of endothelial cells, resulting in increased release of vascular endothelial growth factor (VEGF).[15] Large studies correlating tight blood pressure control with reduced risk of retinopathy progression include the Wisconsin Epidemiology Study of Diabetes Retinopathy (WESDR), the UKPDS, and the Appropriate Blood Pressure Control in Diabetes (ABCD) trials.

Wisconsin Epidemiology Study of Diabetic Retinopathy

The WESDR was a 14-year population-based cohort study in southern Wisconsin assessing the prevalence and risk of diabetic retinopathy among 634 subjects with Type 1 diabetes, diagnosed before age 30 years.[16] In addition to higher HbA1c and greater severity of retinopathy

at baseline, hypertension was demonstrated to be a risk factor for the development of proliferative diabetic retinopathy. Furthermore, participants in the lowest quartile of systolic and diastolic blood pressure had significantly lower rates of progression to proliferative diabetic retinopathy compared with the highest quartile. These findings were independent of glycosylated hemoglobin.[16]

United Kingdom Prospective Diabetes Study

Of the 3867 Type 2 diabetic subjects in the UKPDS, a cohort of 1148 hypertensive subjects were selected of whom 758 were allocated to tight blood pressure control (defined as a blood pressure <150/85 mmHg) and 390 to less tight control, with a median follow-up of 8.4 years.[17] There was a 34% reduction in a two-step progression of retinopathy and a 47% reduction in the risk of moderate vision loss (≥15 letters) in the tight control group compared with the conventional group. The vision data, although not controlled for glycosylated hemoglobin, suggest that tight blood pressure control reduced the risk of diabetic macular edema, the primary cause of visual loss in Type 2 diabetes.

Appropriate Blood Pressure Control in Diabetes Trial

The ABCD trial also showed a correlation between tight blood pressure control and decreased risk of retinopathy.[18–20] In the normotensive cohort of 480 subjects with Type 2 diabetes, there were no significant differences in glycosylated hemoglobin levels between patients randomly allocated to intensive or moderate antihypertensive therapy. For the last 4 years of follow-up, the mean blood pressure was 128/75 mmHg in the intensive treatment arm and 137/81 mmHg in the moderate group.[19] During a 5-year follow-up period, there was less progression of diabetic retinopathy in the intensive blood pressure therapy group (34% in the intensive group compared with 46% in the moderate control group; p = 0.019).

Elevated serum lipid levels

Although the association between elevated serum lipids and diabetic retinopathy is uncertain, both the WESDR and Early Treatment Diabetic Retinopathy Study (ETDRS) found that elevated levels of serum lipids were associated with increased severity of retinal hard exudates.[21,22] In the ETDRS, patients with total serum cholesterol levels of 6.21 mmol/L (240 mg/dL) or more were twice as likely to have hard exudates as those with levels less than 5.17 mmol/L (<200 mg/dL). Low density lipoprotein (LDL) cholesterol levels paralleled the total serum cholesterol results, with subjects having almost twice the risk of developing hard exudates when serum LDL levels were 4.14 mmol/L (160 mg/dL) or more compared with levels less than 3.36 mmol/L (<130 mg/dL). Hard exudates are significant because their severity at baseline in the ETDRS was associated with decreased visual acuity independent of accompanying macular edema. In fact, the strongest risk factor for the development of vision-threatening subretinal fibrosis in the ETDRS patients with diabetic macular edema was the presence of severe hard exudates.[23] Of the 264 eyes with multiple hard exudates at baseline or during follow-up, subretinal fibrosis developed in 30.7%. In contrast, this complication only developed in 0.05% of the 5498 eyes with clinically significant macular edema but no severe hard exudates.[23]

Renal disease

Renal disease is a risk factor for retinopathy just as retinopathy is a risk factor for renal disease. In the WESDR, gross proteinuria was shown to be a risk factor for proliferative diabetic retinopathy.[24] The study demonstrated that subjects taking insulin with gross proteinuria at baseline had approximately twice the risk of developing proliferative retinopathy over 4 years of follow-up compared with those without gross baseline proteinuria. Additionally, microalbuminuria is a marker for the risk of proliferative retinopathy. A cross-sectional examination of the WESDR data showed that younger-onset diabetic subjects (diagnosed before 30 years of age) and older-onset subjects (diagnosed aged 30 years of age or older) were both more likely to have retinopathy than those without microalbuminuria. This relationship remained true even after controlling for glycemia, hypertension, and duration of diabetes.[25]

RISK FACTORS FOR PROGRESSION OF DIABETIC RETINOPATHY DURING PREGNANCY

Early case–control studies reported that pregnancy is a risk factor for the progression of diabetic retinopathy,[26,27] although these changes often regress postpartum.[26] Several larger studies have since confirmed the transient progression of diabetic retinopathy during pregnancy without increased long-term risk.[4,5] The mechanism of retinopathy acceleration is unknown, although multiple theories exist related to the hormonal, hemodynamic,

metabolic, and immunologic changes associated with pregnancy. Reported risk factors for retinopathy progression in pregnant diabetic patients are described below.

Glycemic control

Diabetes in Early Pregnancy study

The Diabetes in Early Pregnancy (DIEP) study[6] was a prospective cohort study of 155 diabetic women followed from the periconceptional period to 1 month postpartum. Acceleration of retinopathy was observed in 10.3% of patients with no retinopathy, 21.1% of those with microaneurysms only, and 18.8% of those with mild non-proliferative diabetic retinopathy. However, the greatest progression was noted in patients with moderate-to-severe non-proliferative diabetic retinopathy at baseline of whom 54.8% experienced a worsening of retinopathy. Proliferative diabetic retinopathy developed in 6.3% with mild and 29% with moderate-to-severe baseline retinopathy. Unlike earlier studies,[26] the DIEP found that changes in metabolic control were more important then duration of diabetes in predicting retinopathy progression. Women in this study with the poorest pre-pregnancy glycemic control and the greatest reduction in HbA1c during the first trimester were at higher risk for retinopathy progression. While the DIEP study did not elucidate the mechanism for worsening retinopathy, it did indicate the clinical importance of optimizing metabolic control before conception to reduce the risk of retinopathy progression.

Diabetes Control and Complications Trial ancillary study

An ancillary study of the DCCT[5] evaluated the role of pregnancy on diabetic retinopathy progression. Similar to the DIEP study,[6] the DCCT study emphasized the importance of optimal glycemic control prior to pregnancy. In this study of 680 diabetic women, 180 women became pregnant. These pregnant women had a higher risk of retinopathy progression compared with the 500 non-pregnant study participants. In addition, the women in the conventional treatment group who did not have tight control prior to conception had a 2.48-fold greater risk of retinopathy acceleration during pregnancy compared with the non-pregnant group. By contrast, women in the intensive therapy arm who had tight control prior to pregnancy had only a 1.63-fold greater risk of retinopathy progression during pregnancy compared with the non-pregnant women. Therefore, tight metabolic control prior to conception is the ideal.

Hypertension

Hypertension during pregnancy is a risk factor for retinopathy progression. A prospective study of 154 diabetic women found that 55% of women with chronic or gestational hypertension suffered a deterioration in retinopathy compared with 25% of the pregnant diabetic women without hypertension.[28] Another prospective study by Klein *et al* indicated that elevated diastolic blood pressure was a risk factor for progression of retinopathy, although not as strong a risk factor as glycemic control.[27]

Serum lipids

Although dyslipidemia has been associated with increasing macular exudates that can lead to the vision-threatening complication of subretinal fibrosis in general diabetic studies,[21,22] the role of increased serum lipids in pregnant diabetic women has not been studied extensively. Nevertheless, because of the general health benefits of lipid control, optimizing cholesterol and lipids prior to pregnancy is recommended as this could reduce the risk of macular exudates.

Renal disease

As with serum lipid levels, renal disease indicated by proteinuria or microalbuminuria has not been examined in a controlled fashion in pregnant diabetic subjects. However, since microalbuminuria has been identified as a risk factor for retinopathy development in the general diabetic population, careful renal monitoring in pregnancy is prudent.[24,25]

POSSIBLE MECHANISMS OF DIABETIC RETINOPATHY PROGRESSION DURING PREGNANCY

Metabolic theory

The metabolic theory simply states that the rapid normalization of glycemia during pregnancy promotes acceleration of diabetic retinopathy. Pregnancy is a state where aggressive control of serum glucose has been routinely instituted, even prior to the results of the DCCT.[6,28,29] The concept of rapid glycemic control resulting in a transient deterioration of retinopathy had previously been noted in non-pregnant diabetic patients.[30–32] While some studies suggest that pregnancy itself may be a risk factor for retinopathy progression after adjusting for HbA1c levels, the common practice of instituting tight control at the onset of pregnancy confounds our ability to conclude that pregnancy itself is the cause of retinopathy acceleration.[27]

Hormonal theory

Beyond the rapid glycemic normalization in pregnancy, hormonal changes are suspected to exacerbate diabetic retinopathy. The characteristic progesterone surge of pregnancy may upregulate intraocular VEGF[33] and result in increased retinal capillary leakage and neovascularization. Additionally, placental hormones create a physiologically adaptive insulin-resistant state to ensure an adequate supply of maternal glucose to the fetus to optimize intrauterine growth. A key factor is human placental growth hormone which appears to regulate the maternal levels of insulin-like growth factor-1 (IGF-1). Like human placental growth factor, IGF-1 increases after 20 weeks of pregnancy. Transgenic mice studies have demonstrated that human placental growth hormone can cause an insulin-resistant state, although the precise mechanism is unknown.[34] Additionally, increasing serum IGF-1 levels may promote retinal neovascularization by supporting vascular endothelial growth factor induction of endothelial cell proliferation.[35]

Hemodynamic theory

Altered retinal hemodynamics may also play a role in retinopathy exacerbation. Pregnancy is noteworthy for extensive hemodynamic and cardiovascular changes. Blood volume increases on average about 45% above non-pregnancy levels, cardiac output is increased, and peripheral vascular resistance is decreased.[34] This increased blood flow, coupled with an impaired retinal vascular autoregulatory response in diabetes, may result in a hyperdynamic retinal capillary blood flow that exacerbates diabetic retinopathy via increased sheer on the vascular endothelium and a resultant net increase in fluid leaving the capillaries.[36] Some studies have demonstrated increased flow in the retinal circulation and hyperperfusion in all pregnant diabetic subjects compared with non-diabetic pregnant women,[37] while others have shown increased retinal blood flow only in pregnant women with pre-existing[36] or progressive diabetic retinopathy.[38] Another small study showed a fall in retinal volumetric blood flow in pregnant diabetic subjects and a more profound decrease in retinal venous diameter in the diabetic subjects compared with non-diabetic pregnant controls.[39] The contradictory results of these studies may be explained by different patient populations or differing methods of assessment of the retinal circulation.

Immunoinflammatory theory

Another theory involves proinflammatory factors. Diabetic retinopathy has been suggested to be a low-grade inflammatory disease, with leukocyte adhesion to the retinal vasculature possibly resulting in retinal vascular dysfunction.[40,41] During pregnancy, increased inflammation has been implicated in patients who develop gestational diabetes.[42] A prospective study examining the relation of maternal cytokine levels with diabetic retinopathy showed that although the proinflammatory factors interleukin-6, c-reactive protein, and vascular cell adhesion molecule-1 were similar in the diabetic pregnant patients and non-diabetic controls, c-reactive protein levels were higher in pregnant women with retinopathy progression and worse glycemic control compared with their pregnant counterparts with stable retinopathy and tighter metabolic control. Another study examined glycodelin, an anti-inflammatory serum marker secreted from the endometrial glands during pregnancy, and found that low levels were associated with retinopathy progression in pregnant diabetic women.[43]

CLINICAL MANAGEMENT OF RETINOPATHY BEFORE AND DURING PREGNANCY

Preconceptional care is essential to reduce the risk of retinopathy progression during pregnancy. Both systemic and ocular care play an instrumental role.

Systemic management

Systemically, optimal metabolic control prior to pregnancy is essential. Rather than the aggressive tightening of glycemic control once the patient is pregnant, a gradual optimization of glycemic control prior to pregnancy avoids the rapid drop in HbA1c during pregnancy which has been associated with retinopathy progression.

Optimizing glycemic control prepregnancy is also essential for the health of the fetus. Multiple studies have demonstrated that the risk of fetal abnormalities increases with poor glycemic control.[5,44–47] In a prospective cohort study of 301 Type 1 diabetic subjects with 573 pregnancies followed from 1985 to 2003,[44] the prevalence of adverse outcomes varied six-fold from 12% in the lowest HbA1c quintile to 79% in the highest quintile group. Specifically, when HbA1c levels were above 7%, there was an almost linear relationship between HbA1c level and risk of adverse fetal outcome. For every 1% increase in HbA1c level above 7%, the risk of adverse fetal outcome rose by 5.5%. Additionally, hypertension and elevated serum lipids should be controlled to reduce the risk of retinal changes. Such management not only reduces the risk of retinopathy progression, but is also important for the systemic health of the mother and fetus.

Ocular management and scheduling of dilated examinations

From an ocular perspective, all diabetic patients should have a dilated ophthalmic examination by an ophthalmologist or optometrist experienced in retinal evaluation prior to pregnancy and again during the first trimester of pregnancy. Depending on the individual patient's findings, additional imaging such as retinal photography, optical coherence tomography, and fluorescein angiography may be performed at the discretion of the examiner. The official guidelines for retinal care of pregnant women with Type 1 and Type 2 diabetes established by the American Academy of Ophthalmology are as follows:[48]

1 First dilated examination should be preconception or early in the first trimester

2 If the patient has no retinopathy or mild-to-moderate non-proliferative retinopathy, follow-up examinations should be scheduled every 3–12 months

3 If the patient has severe non-proliferative or proliferative retinopathy, follow-up examinations should be scheduled every 1–3 months.

These recommendations are broadly similar to the pregnancy guidelines recently published by the UK National Institute for Health and Clinical Excellence (NICE),[49] which state that, "Retinopathy with digital photography should be carried out when pregnancy is detected (if not performed in the past 12 months), following the first antenatal clinic appointment, at 28 weeks if there is no diabetic retinopathy at the baseline examination or at 16–20 weeks if any diabetic retinopathy was present on initial screening, and any women with diabetic retinopathy during pregnancy should have ophthalmic follow-up for at least 6 months postpartum".

Both of these sets of guidelines are merely general recommendations for the pattern of practice and not for the care of the individual patient. Therefore, subsequent follow-up examinations vary depending on the retinal findings, but are usually performed in each trimester, particularly if there is any evidence of retinopathy at conception.

Occasionally patients will need a fluorescein angiogram to assess the retinal perfusion status and vasculature pattern. Although fluorescein dye has been used safely during pregnancy,[7] it crosses the placenta and most retinal specialists instead rely on the results of dilated examination and non-invasive imaging/photography to determine the stage of retinopathy to guide their management.

If a patient has evidence of severe non-proliferative or proliferative retinopathy prior to pregnancy, scatter or panretinal photocoagulation should be instituted according to the Diabetic Retinopathy Study guidelines.[50] Similarly, focal laser treatment should be initiated for clinically significant macular edema. If the patient develops new retinal changes during pregnancy that meet the criteria for laser treatment, this should be performed as such treatment is equally effective and safe in pregnant as in non-pregnant patients.[51]

Despite the recognized regression of retinopathy postpartum in many cases, conservative observation may be harmful as the patient could lose vision during pregnancy due to complications of proliferative changes or severe macular edema. Occasionally, retinopathy can progress after pregnancy so a dilated examination 2 months postpartum is recommended.

CONCLUSIONS

As systemic and ocular management of diabetes has progressed since the original studies on diabetic retinopathy in pregnancy, vision loss from diabetic retinopathy aggravated by pregnancy is usually preventable. Optimal systemic management of blood glucose, hypertension, and serum lipids prior to pregnancy is essential. Similarly, timely and appropriate intervention for retinopathy progression prior to or during pregnancy is critical to prevent visual loss. With greater physician and patient awareness of the importance of both systemic and ocular care, the outlook for pregnant diabetic women is optimistic.

REFERENCES

1 Klein BE. Overview of epidemiologic studies of diabetic retinopathy. *Ophthalmic Epidemiol* 2007;**14**:179–83.

2 Kempen JH, O'Colmain BJ, Leske MC, *et al.* The prevalence of diabetic retinopathy among adults in the United States. *Arch Ophthalmol* 2004;**122**:552–63.

3 Roy MS, Klein R, O'Colmain BJ, *et al.* The prevalence of diabetic retinopathy among adult type 1 diabetic persons in the United States. *Arch Ophthalmol* 2004;**122**:546–51.

4 Vérier-Mine O, Chaturvedi N, Webb D, *et al.* Is pregnancy a risk factor for microvascular complications? The EURO-DIAB Prospective Complications Study. *Diabet Med* 2005;**22**:1503–9.

5 Diabetes Control and Complications Trial Research Group. Effect of pregnancy on microvascular complications in the diabetes control and complications trial. *Diabetes Care* 2000;**23**:1084–91.

6 Chew EY, Mills JL, Metzger BE, *et al.* Metabolic control and progression of retinopathy. The Diabetes in Early Pregnancy Study. National Institute of Child Health and Human Development Diabetes in Early Pregnancy Study. *Diabetes Care* 1995;**18**:631–7.

7 Soubrane G, Canivet J, Coscas G. Influence of pregnancy on the evolution of background retinopathy. Preliminary results of a prospective fluorescein angiography study. *Int Ophthalmol* 1985;**8**:249–55.

8 Aiello LP, Cahill MT, Wong JS. Systemic considerations in the management of diabetic retinopathy. *Am J Ophthalmol* 2001;**132**:760–76.

9 Diabetes Control and Complications Trial Research Group. The effect of intensive treatment of diabetes on the development and progression of long-term complications in insulin-dependent diabetes mellitus. *N Engl J Med* 1993;**329**:977–86.

10 Diabetes Control and Complications Trial Research Group. The effect of intensive diabetes treatment on the progression of diabetic retinopathy in insulin-dependent diabetes mellitus. *Arch Ophthalmol* 1995;**113**:36–51.

11 Diabetes Control and Complications Trial Research Group. The relationship of glycemic exposures (HbA_{1c}) to the risk of development and progression of retinopathy in the Diabetes Control and Complications Trial. *Diabetes* 1995;**44**:968–83.

12 Diabetes Control and Complications Trial Research Group. Perspectives in diabetes: the absence of a glycemic threshold for the development of long-term complications: the perspective of the Diabetes Control and Complications Trial. *Diabetes* 1996;**45**:1289–98.

13 Reichard P, Nilsson BY, Rosenqvist U. The effect of long-term intensified insulin treatment on the development of microvascular complications of diabetes mellitus. *N Engl J Med* 1993;**329**:304–9.

14 UK Prospective Diabetes Study Group. Intensive blood-glucose control with sulphonylureas or insulin compared with conventional treatment and risk of complications in patients with type 2 diabetes (UKPDS 33). *Lancet* 1988;**352**:837–53.

15 Suzuma I, Hata Y, Clermont A, *et al.* Cyclic stretch and hypertension induce retinal expression of vascular endothelial growth factor and vascular endothelial growth factor receptor-2: potential mechanisms for exacerbation of diabetic retinopathy by hypertension. *Diabetes* 2001;**50**:444–54.

16 Klein R, Klein BE, Moss SE, *et al.* The Wisconsin Epidemiologic Study of Diabetic Retinopathy: XVII. The 14-year incidence and progression of diabetic retinopathy and associated risk factors in type 1 diabetes. *Ophthalmology* 1998;**105**:1801–15.

17 UK Prospective Diabetes Study Group. Tight blood pressure control and risk of macrovascular and microvascular complications in type 2 diabetes (UKPDS 38). *Br Med J* 1998;**317**:703–13.

18 Yam JC, Kwok AK. Update on the treatment of diabetic retinopathy. *Hong Kong Med J* 2007;**13**:46–60.

19 Schrier RW, Estacio RP, Esler A, Mehler P. Effects of aggressive blood pressure control in normotensive type 2 diabetic patients on albuminuria, retinopathy and strokes. *Kidney Int* 2002;**61**:1086–97.

20 Schrier RW, Estacio RO, Mehler PS, Hiatt WR. Appropriate blood pressure control in hypertensive and normotensive type 2 diabetes mellitus: a summary of the ABCD trial. *Nat Clin Pract Nephrol* 2007;**3**:428–38.

21 Chew EY, Klein ML, Ferris FL III, *et al*, for the Early Treatment Diabetic Retinopathy Study Research Group: Association of elevated serum lipid levels with retinal hard exudates in diabetic retinopathy. *Arch Ophthalmol* 1996;**114**:1079–84.

22 Klein BEK, Moss SE, Klein R, Surawicz TS. The Wisconsin Epidemiologic Study of Diabetic Retinopathy. XIII. Relationship of serum cholesterol to retinopathy and hard exudates. *Ophthalmology* 1991;**98**:1261–5.

23 Fong DS, Segal PP, Myers F, Ferris FL, Hubbard LD, Davis MD. Subretinal fibrosis in diabetic macular edema. ETDRS report no 23. *Arch Ophthalmol* 1997;**115**:873–7.

24 Klein R, Moss SE, Klein BE. Is gross proteinuria a risk factor for the incidence of proliferative diabetic retinopathy? *Ophthalmology* 1993;**100**:1140–6.

25 Cruickshanks KJ, Ritter LL, Klein R, *et al.* The association of microalbuminuria with diabetic retinopathy. The Wisconsin Epidemiologic Study of Diabetic Retinopathy. *Ophthalmology* 1993;**100**:862–7.

26 Moloney JB, Drury MI. The effect of pregnancy on the natural course of diabetic retinopathy. *Am J Ophthalmol* 1982;**93**:745–56.

27 Klein BE, Moss SE, Klein R. Effect of pregnancy on progression of diabetic retinopathy. *Diabetes Care* 1990;**13**:34–40.

28 Rosenn B, Miodovnik M, Kranias G, *et al.* Progression of diabetic retinopathy in pregnancy: association with hypertension in pregnancy. *Am J Obstet Gynecol* 1992;**166**:1214–8.

29 Diabetes Control and Complications Trial Research Group. The effect of intensive treatment of diabetes on the development and progression of long-term complications in insu-

lin-dependent diabetes mellitus. *N Engl J Med* 1993;**329**:977–86.

30 Jørgensen K, Brinchmann-Hansen O, Hanssen KF, *et al.* Rapid tightening of blood glucose control leads to transient deterioration of retinopathy in insulin dependent diabetes mellitus: the Oslo study. *Br Med J (Clin Res Ed)* 1985;**290**:811–5.

31 The Kroc Collaborative Study Group. Blood glucose control and the evolution of diabetic retinopathy and albuminuria. A preliminary multicenter trial. *N Engl J Med* 1984;**311**:365–72.

32 Lauritzen T, Frost-Larsen K, Larsen HW, *et al.* Effect of 1 year of near-normal blood glucose levels on retinopathy in insulin-dependent diabetics. *Lancet* 1983;**1**:200–4.

33 Sone H, Okuda Y, Kawakami Y, *et al.* Progesterone induces vascular endothelial growth factor on retinal pigment epithelial cells in culture. *Life Sci* 1996;**59**:21–5.

34 Barbour LA, Shao J, Qiao L, *et al.* Human placental growth hormone causes severe insulin resistance in transgenic mice. *Am J Obstet Gynecol* 2002;**186**:512–17.

35 Smith L, Shen W, Perruzzi C, *et al.* Regulation of vascular endothelial growth factor-dependent retinal neovascularization by insulin-like growth factor-1 receptor. *Nat Med* 1999;**5**:1390–5.

36 Patel V, Rassam S, Newsom R, *et al.* Retinal blood flow in diabetic retinopathy. *BMJ* 1992;**305**:678–83.

37 Loukovaara S, Harju M, Kaaja R, *et al.* Retinal capillary blood flow in diabetic and nondiabetic women during pregnancy and postpartum period. *Invest Ophthalmol Vis Sci* 2003;**44**:1486–91.

38 Chen HC, Newsom RS, Patel V, *et al.* Retinal blood flow changes during pregnancy in women with diabetes. *Invest Ophthalmol Vis Sci* 1994;**35**:3199–208.

39 Schocket LS, Grunwald JE, Tsang AF, *et al.* The effect of pregnancy on retinal hemodynamics in diabetic versus nondiabetic mothers. *Am J Ophthalmol* 1999;**128**:477–84.

40 Adamis AP. Is diabetic retinopathy an inflammatory disease? *Br J Ophthalmol* 2002;**86**:363–5.

41 Gardner TW, Antonetti DA, Barber AJ, *et al.* Diabetic retinopathy: more than meets the eye. *Surv Ophthalmol* 2002;**47** (Suppl 2):S253–62.

42 Wolf M, Sandler L, Hsu K, *et al.* First-trimester C-reactive protein and subsequent gestational diabetes. *Diabetes Care* 2003;**26**:819–24.

43 Loukovaara S, Immonen IR, Loukovaara MJ, *et al.* Glycodelin: a novel serum anti-inflammatory marker in type 1 diabetic retinopathy during pregnancy. *Acta Ophthalmol Scand* 2007;**85**:46–9.

44 Nielsen GL, Moller M, Sorensen HT. HbA$_{1c}$ in early diabetic pregnancy and pregnancy outcomes: a Danish population-based cohort study of 573 pregnancies in women with type 1 diabetes. *Diabetes Care* 2006;**29**:2612–16.

45 DCCT Research Group. Pregnancy outcomes in the Diabetes Control and Complications Trial. *Am J Obstet Gynecol* 1996;**174**:1343–53.

46 Hanson U, Persson B, Thunell S. Relationship between hae-moglobin A1C in early type 1 (insulin-dependent) diabetic pregnancy and the occurrence of spontaneous abortion and fetal malformation in Sweden. *Diabetologia* 1990;**33**:100–4.

47 Hod M, Jovanovic L. Improving outcomes in pregnant women with type 1 diabetes. *Diabetes Care* 2007;**30**:e62.

48 American Academy of Ophthalmology Retina Panel. *Preferred Practice Pattern: Diabetic Retinopathy*. San Francisco: American Academy of Ophthalmology, 2003.

49 National Institute of Health and Clinical Excellence. *Pregnancy Guidelines*, March 2008. www.nice.org.uk/CG063

50 The Diabetic Retinopathy Study Research Group. Four risk factors for severe visual loss in diabetic retinopathy. The third report from the Diabetic Retinopathy Study. *Arch Ophthalmol* 1979;**97**:654–5.

51 Horvat M, Maclean H, Goldberg L, *et al*. Diabetic retinopathy in pregnancy: a 12-year prospective survey. *Br J Ophthalmol* 1980;**64**:398–403.

18 Autonomic neuropathy in diabetes in pregnancy

Maternal & Fetal Health Research Centre, St Mary's Hospital, Manchester, UK

PRACTICE POINTS

- Diabetic neuropathy is common, affecting both Type 1 and Type 2 diabetic patients.
- Diabetic autonomic neuropathy (DAN) can affect any organ with autonomic innervation, causing cardiovascular, gastrointestinal, genitourinary, pupillomotor, and sudomotor disturbances.
- One of the commonest symptoms of DAN is vomiting secondary to delayed gastric emptying (gastroparesis); this may deteriorate significantly in pregnancy and may confound and compound nausea and vomiting of pregnancy.
- Cardiovascular disturbances include reduced heart rate variability, postural hypotension, and attenuated cardiovascular adaptation to pregnancy.
- Hypoglycemic unawareness is a common feature of DAN, which may be exacerbated in pregnancy.
- Diabetic women with autonomic dysfunction may exhibit labile blood pressure. Hypotension caused by sympathetic blockade after regional anesthesia may be severely exaggerated.

CASE HISTORY

A 29-year-old woman with a 22-year history of Type 1 diabetes, complicated by bilateral retinopathy and nephropathy, presented to the combined diabetes antenatal clinic following successful *in-vitro* fertilization (IVF) treatment. By 12 weeks of gestation, she had developed significant proteinuria (5.8 g/24 h), but was normotensive with excellent glycemic control (HbA1c 5.9%). She remained well and had a normal fetal anomaly ultrasound scan at 20 weeks of gestation.

At 25 weeks of gestation she was admitted with a progressive 7-day history of vomiting. On admission she was

unable to tolerate fluids and was dehydrated with ketonuria. Electrolytes and renal function were normal and thyrotoxicosis was excluded. She was treated with intravenous (IV) insulin and fluids. Various parenteral antiemetics were tried, including ondansetron and ranitidine, but with minimal improvement. In view of maternal pyrexia and loin pain she was also treated with IV antibiotics. She became increasingly oedematous secondary to severe hypoalbuminemia and developed bilateral pleural effusions. In view of her rapid clinical deterioration, IV hydrocortisone (50 mg four times daily) was commenced empirically and she was transferred to the intensive care unit where she received albumin infusions and parenteral nutrition via a central venous line. Intensified glycemic control was also necessary because of steroid-induced hyperglycemia.

Forty-eight hours later, her clinical condition had markedly improved, and diet and oral medication were gradually reintroduced. IV hydrocortisone was replaced with oral prednisolone (30 mg/day) in addition to oral ondansetron, erythromycin (a prokinetic agent), and frequent courses of antibiotics. She was transferred back to a subcutaneous insulin regime, which was adjusted daily as necessary. The oral prednisolone dose was gradually decreased, but doses below 10 mg daily were associated with a symptomatic relapse and recurrence of vomiting on several occasions. Fetal well-being was closely monitored and fetal growth remained satisfactory.

She remained in hospital until 32 weeks and thereafter was seen regularly at the antenatal clinic. She was delivered by emergency cesarean section at 36 weeks following an admission with severe right-sided abdominal pain, which was found to be secondary to an ovarian torsion. At delivery of a live male infant (2.6 kg), the right ovary was restored to its normal anatomic position. She made a good postnatal recovery and was discharged on her prepregnancy insulin regime.

A Practical Manual of Diabetes in Pregnancy, 1st Edition.
Edited by David R. McCance, Michael Maresh and David A. Sacks.
© 2010 Blackwell Publishing

176

- How frequent is autonomic neuropathy during pregnancy?
- What are the common manifestations?
- What problems may arise from this condition?
- What are the available therapeutic options?

BACKGROUND

Diabetic neuropathy is one of the commonest long-term complications of diabetes. The prevalence of neuropathy increases with age and duration of diabetes, and may be the presenting feature of Type 2 diabetes. The diabetic neuropathies are diverse, affecting different parts of the nervous system and presenting with various clinical manifestations. Most common among the neuropathies are a chronic sensorimotor distal symmetric polyneuropathy (DPN) and the autonomic neuropathies. Central to the development of all diabetic complications is poor glycemic control. The presence of neuropathy is frequently coexistent with other diabetic complications. Other forms of neuropathy, including chronic inflammatory demyelinating polyneuropathy, B12 deficiency, hypothyroidism, and uremia can occur more frequently in diabetic patients and should always be excluded.

Diabetic neuropathies can be classified into:[1]
- Generalized symmetric polyneuropathies:
  - Acute sensory: characterized by the acute onset of severe sensory symptoms; rare and may follow periods of poor metabolic control (e.g., ketoacidosis)
  - Chronic sensorimotor: characterized by aching or burning pain, electrical or stabbing sensations, paresthesia and hyperesthesia, typically worse at night; the symptoms are most commonly experienced in the feet and lower limbs
  - Autonomic: cardiovascular, gastrointestinal, urinary, sweating, and metabolic disturbances
- Focal and multifocal neuropathies:
  - Cranial
  - Truncal
  - Focal limb
  - Proximal motor (amyotrophy).

PATHOPHYSIOLOGY OF NEUROPATHY

Hypotheses concerning the multiple etiologies of diabetic neuropathy include a metabolic insult to nerve fibers, neurovascular insufficiency, autoimmune damage, and neurohormonal growth factor deficiency.[2] Several different factors have been implicated in this pathogenic process. Hyperglycemic activation of the polyol pathway has been shown to lead to an accumulation of sorbitol and potential changes in the NAD:NADH ratio. This may lead to direct neuronal damage and/or decreased nerve blood flow.[3] Increased oxidative stress, and the resultant increase in free radical production, may lead to vascular endothelial damage and reduced nitric oxide bioavailability.[4] Alternatively, excess nitric oxide production may result in the formation of peroxynitrite with damage to endothelium and neurons.[5] Other investigators have proposed that autoimmune mechanisms play a role in some diabetic subjects.[6] The result of this multifactorial process may be activation of polyADP ribosylation depletion of ATP, resulting in cell necrosis and activation of genes involved in neuronal damage.[7]

DIABETIC AUTONOMIC NEUROPATHY

The American Diabetes Association has defined DAN as: "A neuropathic disorder associated with diabetes that includes manifestations in the peripheral components of the autonomic nervous system".[1]

DAN is one of the least familiar and most poorly studied complications of diabetes despite being common and having a significant negative impact on survival and quality of life in people with diabetes.[2] As highlighted above, diabetic autonomic neuropathy is a subtype of the *generalized symmetric polyneuropathies* that can accompany diabetes and can involve the entire autonomic nervous system. The autonomic nervous system has vasomotor, visceromotor, and sensory fibers which innervate every organ. Alterations in this innervation result in dysfunction in one or more organ systems (e.g. cardiovascular, gastrointestinal, genitourinary, sudomotor or ocular), which can be either clinical or subclinical.[1] Most organs have dual innervation and receive fibers from both the parasympathetic and sympathetic parts of the autonomic nervous system (ANS). As the vagus nerve (the longest of the ANS nerves) accounts for approximately 75% of all parasympathetic activity, and as DAN appears to affect longer nerves more quickly than shorter nerves, even early effects of DAN are widespread.[1] The onset of DAN is variable and often symptoms, or subclinical alterations in organ function, are not apparent until long after the onset of diabetes. However, as with most other microvascular complications of diabetes, which are almost invariably present simultaneously, DAN appears to be more intimately related to glycemic control than duration of diabetes *per se.*[8,9] Subclinical autonomic dysfunction can occur within a year of diagnosis in patients with Type 2 diabetes and within 2 years of onset in Type 1 diabetes.[10]

Prevalence

The prevalence of DAN in the general diabetic population ranges from 1.6% to 90%, depending on the diagnostic tests used, population examined and the type and stage of disease.[1] Low *et al*[11] reported a prevalence of mild autonomic impairment (defined as a composite autonomic severity score of ≤3 using a validated self-report instrument [Autonomic Symptom Profile]) in 54% of patients with Type 1 and 73% in patients with Type 2 diabetes. Cardiovascular autonomic neuropathy (CAN) is the most clinically important and well-studied form of DAN because of its association with a variety of adverse outcomes, including cardiovascular death. Relatively low prevalence rates of CAN (7.7%) were reported among newly diagnosed patients with Type 1 diabetes, when strict diagnostic criteria were used;[12] however, in patients awaiting pancreatic transplants, prevalence rates were as high as 90%.[13] Gastrointestinal features of DAN appear to be more common. Cross-sectional studies have suggested that approximately 50% of diabetic outpatients with long duration of diabetes have delayed gastric emptying and up to 76% have one or more gastrointestinal symptoms, the most common of which is constipation.[14,15] Bladder dysfunction has been reported in 43–87% of individuals with Type 1 diabetes. Diabetic women have a five-fold higher risk of unrecognized voiding difficulty compared with non-diabetic women.[1]

Problems associated with diabetic autonomic neuropathy

DAN can affect several organs, resulting in cardiovascular, gastrointestinal, urinary, sweating, pupillary, and metabolic disturbances. As many of these symptoms are common both during and outwith pregnancy, autonomic neuropathy may go unnoticed by both the patient and her doctors. A summary of the symptoms, diagnostic tests, and possible treatment options for DAN is shown in Table 18.1.

Gastrointestinal features
The gastrointestinal features are as follows:
- Esophageal enteropathy: disordered peristalsis, abnormal lower esophageal sphincter function

- Gastroparesis diabeticorum: non-obstructive impairment of gastric propulsive activity, associated with vomiting and early satiety
- Diarrhea: impaired motility of the small bowel (bacterial overgrowth syndrome), increased motility and secretory activity (pseudocholeretic diarrhea)
- Constipation (dysfunction of intrinsic and extrinsic intestinal neurons, decreased or absent gastrocolic reflex)
- Fecal incontinence: abnormal internal anal sphincter tone, impaired rectal sensation, abnormal external sphincter.

Gastroparesis
Gastroparesis is very common among diabetic subjects and can be associated with both Type 1 and Type 2 diabetes. Prevalence rates of 30–50% have been reported. Gastrointestinal symptoms are very common in pregnancy, especially in the first trimester, among women both with and without diabetes. In diabetic women these symptoms, particularly vomiting, may be exacerbated by DAN.

Clinical features of gastroparesis include early satiety, anorexia, nausea, vomiting, epigastric discomfort, and bloating. Episodes of nausea or vomiting may last days to months or occur in cycles.[16] Gastric emptying largely depends on vagus nerve function, which can be severely disrupted in DAN. Radiographic gastric emptying studies can establish definitively the diagnosis of gastroparesis, but are not practical in pregnancy. A pragmatic approach during pregnancy is therefore to attempt to exclude other known causes of vomiting, e.g. hyperemesis gravidarum, gastro-oesophageal reflux, infection or peptic ulceration. Diabetic gastroparesis during pregnancy can exacerbate nausea and vomiting, cause nutritional problems, alter the absorption of pharmacologic agents and create difficulty with glucose control. Therefore, in pregnant diabetic women with severe nausea and vomiting and/or erratic blood glucose control, gastroparesis should always be suspected.

As highlighted above, nausea and vomiting are very common in pregnancy, ranging from mild to severe and unremitting with dehydration and weight loss. In a woman with diabetes, gastroparesis may contribute to the etiology of intractable vomiting. Gastroparesis may be exacerbated by pregnancy with catastrophic consequences. In addition to the case presented above, several others have been reported describing the severe impact of gastroparesis on pregnancy management and outcome.[17–19] Hare reported a case of severe nausea and

Table 18.1 Summary of symptoms associated with diabetic autonomic neuropathy, potential diagnostic tests, and therapeutic options in pregnancy.

Symptom	Diagnostic tests	Treatment options
Gastrointestinal		
Gastroparesis, erratic glucose control	Gastric emptying study, barium study (investigations outside pregnancy)	Frequent small meals, prokinetic agents (metoclopramide, domperidone, erythromycin)
Abdominal pain or discomfort, early satiety, nausea, vomiting, belching, bloating	Exclude metabolic disorders: thyroid function, celiac profile, B12 and folate, serum cortisol, autoimmune screen (gastric parietal cell and adrenal antibodies) may be considered) Endoscopy may be considered	Antibiotics, antiemetics, bulking agents, tricyclic antidepressants, pancreatic enzyme supplements, enteral feeding
Constipation		High-fiber diet and bulking agents, osmotic laxatives, prokinetic agents
Diarrhea, often nocturnal alternating with constipation and incontinence		Soluble fiber, gluten and lactose restriction, cholestyramine, antibiotics, pancreatic enzyme supplements
Cardiovascular		
Exercise intolerance, early fatigue and weakness with exercise	ECG, HRV (see Table 18.2)	Graded supervised exercise, beta-blockers
Postural hypotension, dizziness, light headedness, weakness, fatigue, syncope	HRV, standing and supine blood pressure (see Table 18.2), catecholamines	Mechanical measures, fludrocortisone, clonidine,* octreotide*
Bladder dysfunction		
Frequency, urgency, nocturia, urinary retention, incontinence	Urinalysis and culture, consider urodynamics	Bethanechol,* intermittent catheterization
Hypoglycaemic unawareness		
Failure to recognize early symptoms of hypoglycemia leading to more frequent episodes of severe hypoglycemia		Rational plan of insulin therapy, including the appropriate use of the short-acting insulin analogs, frequent blood glucose monitoring, individualized blood glucose targets and education programs
Pupillomotor		
Visual blurring, impaired adaptation to ambient light	Pupillometry, HRV	Care with driving at night

* FDA Category C – no safety data available for pregnancy/breastfeeding. Some reports of use in pregnancy without harmful effects
ECG, echocardiogram; HRV, heart rate variation

vomiting which complicated pregnancy in a diabetic woman with DAN, resulting in a stillborn fetus in the third trimester.[19] Two further cases of symptomatic autonomic neuropathy complicated by vomiting secondary to gastroparesis were described by Steel.[17] The author also highlighted the high morbidity and mortality associated with these cases and with two additional cases who died in their 30s of cardiopulmonary arrest secondary to CAN.

Severe nausea and vomiting in a pregnant woman with diabetes is problematic. In addition to the enormous psychologic impact, these symptoms may also cause significant difficulties in achieving metabolic control and affect the nutritional status of the mother and baby. Treatment must therefore be aimed not only at symptom control, but also in providing nutritional support. Improvement of symptoms has been observed following the administration of parenteral nutrition,[18] which may be due to the provision of essential nutrients but also as a result of psychologic reassurance.

Treatment with prokinetic agents such as metoclopramide, domperidone, and erythromycin can be tried in pregnancy, along with H2-receptor antagonists, such as ranitidine,[20] and antiemetics, such as chlorpromazine and ondansetron. The treatment of gastroparesis with glucocorticoids, as described in the case above, was empirical, but resulted in a dramatic improvement in symptomatology. Moreover, relapses were associated with dose reduction. Although steroids cannot be considered as standard practice, anecdotally we have also noted a transient improvement in gastric symptoms following the administration of large doses of steroids to improve fetal lung maturity in women where preterm delivery was contemplated. In these cases, steroid treatment for purposes of alleviating gastric symptoms was continued. Interestingly, in the cases discussed by Steel,[17] two women with severe autonomic neuropathy responded to treatment with fludrocortisone, which improved both their postural hypotension and symptoms of nausea and vomiting. The antiemetic properties of steroids have been well documented and they are widely used in the treatment of postoperative nausea, chemotherapy-induced vomiting and hyperemesis gravidarum. The exact mechanism by which glucocorticoids exert their antiemetic effect is unknown. They have been shown to have various effects on the central nervous system and may influence the regulation of the nausea and vomiting reflex. Alternatively, their benefit may be secondary to the correction of relative adrenal insufficiency, which should always be considered in such cases. The use of steroids in the management of vomiting secondary to gastroparesis requires rigorous testing before it is considered as standard practice. Close monitoring of maternal glucose concentrations and frequent adjustment of insulin doses is mandatory following steroid administration.

Constipation

Constipation is the most common lower gastrointestinal symptom, and it can alternate with episodes of diarrhea. Bacterial overgrowth due to stasis of the bowel may contribute to diarrhea, in which case broad-spectrum antibiotics (e.g. metronidazole) are useful. Treatment of diarrhea with or without constipation should always involve the use of a prokinetic agent rather than constipating agents that create vicious cycles of constipation and diarrhea. Fecal incontinence due to poor sphincter tone is common in individuals with diabetes[21] and may be associated with severe paroxysmal diarrhea or consti-

tute an independent disorder of anorectal dysfunction. This is obviously particularly important for women at increased risk of sustaining anal sphincter trauma during delivery, such as those with macrosomic fetuses.

Cardiovascular autonomic neuropathy

Outside of pregnancy, CAN is perhaps one of the most overlooked of all the complications of diabetes.[2] It is believed to arise secondary to damage to the autonomic nerve fibers that innervate the heart and blood vessels, resulting in abnormalities in heart rate control and vascular dynamics.[22] Importantly, the presence of autonomic neuropathy may limit an individual's exercise capacity and increase the risk of an adverse cardiovascular event during exercise. Of particular relevance to pregnancy is the hypotension and hypertension due to CAN, which are more likely to occur after vigorous exercise. Because thermoregulation may be affected, pregnant diabetic women suspected of having CAN should be advised to avoid vigorous exercise in hot or cold environments and to be vigilant about adequate hydration.

The clinical features of CAN in non-pregnant patients include:

- Resting tachycardia >100 bpm
- Postural hypotension (a fall in systolic blood pressure of $\geq$ 20–30 mmHg upon standing after 2 minutes)
- Loss of beat-to-beat variation in heart rate. This is one of the earliest objective signs of CAN. Cyclical heart rate variation, which depends on vagal innervation, is reduced, and is the basis of one of the tests of cardiovascular reflex function (Table 18.2).

There is very limited data on CAN in diabetic pregnant subjects. The normal hemodynamic adjustments of pregnancy are impaired in women with Type 1 diabetes.[23] This has been attributed to changes in cardiovascular function secondary to subclinical autonomic neuropathy. The increase in heart rate, a primary cardiovascular adjustment to pregnancy, was found to be blunted in diabetic pregnant women, but no significant differences were observed in the other measures of autonomic cardiovascular function.[24] In 1998, Lapolla *et al* studied cardiovascular autonomic function in 16 women who had Type 1 diabetes and did not find any cardiovascular functional abnormalities.[25] In addition, pregnancy did not appear to have an adverse effect on autonomic function. In a study of 100 consecutive women with Type 1 diabetes, Airaksinen *et al* investigated the influence of autonomic neuropathy on pregnancy outcome. Although there was no statistically significant increase in individual pregnancy complications (pre-eclampsia, congenital

Table 18.2 Tests of autonomic dysfunction.*

Beat-to-beat heart rate variation (HRV)	With the patient at rest, the supine heart rate is monitored by echocardiography (ECG) or autonomic instrument while the patient performs six cycles of maximal inspiration and expiration at a rate of six breaths/min, paced by a metronome or similar device. The difference between the maximum and minimum heart rate during each breath is measured, and the mean is used to reflect the heart rate variation during deep breathing. A difference in heart rate of >15 bpm is normal; <10 bpm is abnormal
Systolic blood pressure response to standing	Systolic blood pressure is measured in the supine subject. The patient stands, and the systolic blood pressure is measured after 2 min. Normal response is a fall of <10 mmHg, borderline is a fall of 10–29 mmHg, and abnormal is a fall of >30 mmHg with symptoms

* NB These tests are not routinely performed in pregnancy and therefore have not been validated for diagnostic purposes in pregnancy

malformations, diabetic ketoacidosis, hypoglycemic accidents) in the group with objective evidence of cardiovascular autonomic neuropathy (n = 21), the frequency of pregnancies with at least one of these complications was much higher (52% *vs* 23%) compared to the group with no objective evidence of CAN.[26] This increase was independent of glycemic control and duration of disease. Symptoms secondary to CAN are uncommon in pregnant women and only occasional cases have been reported. For example, the symptomatic and objective correction of severe postural hypotension, secondary to autonomic neuropathy, was described in a patient after she became pregnant.[27] This was thought to be secondary to the blood volume expansion which occurs in pregnancy. Interestingly, the debilitating postural hypotension returned within days of delivery.

Other problems
Hypoglycemic unawareness
Reduced awareness of hypoglycemia is presumed to be secondary to reduced catecholamine production in

response to low blood glucose levels. Studies outside of pregnancy found little overlap between decreased hypoglycemic awareness and objective evidence of DAN, as measured by cardiovascular testing.[28,29] In contrast, more recent data have suggested that autonomic neuropathy further attenuates the catecholamine response to hypoglycemia in diabetic individuals after recent hypoglycemic exposure.[30] The phenomenon of reduced counter-regulatory hormone responses and reduced perception of hypoglycemia due to decreased ANS activation after recent antecedent hypoglycemia has been termed "hypoglycemia-induced autonomic failure".[31] Hypoglycemia-induced autonomic failure leads to a vicious cycle of hypoglycemia unawareness that induces a further decrease in hormone responses to hypoglycemia. This vicious cycle occurs commonly in diabetic individuals with strict glycemic control but can also occur in the absence of DAN as measured by standard tests of autonomic function.[31] Most evidence suggests that autonomic neuropathy further attenuates the catecholamine response to hypoglycemia in diabetic subjects after recent hypoglycemic exposure[30] and that individuals with abnormal autonomic function have a greater risk of severe hypoglycemia.[32]

Again, little data exist in pregnant women. Airaksinen *et al* observed that despite comparable glycemic control during late pregnancy, there was no significant increase in the frequency of hypoglycemic accidents in women with proven autonomic cardiovascular neuropathy,[26] although the study was not powered to evaluate this outcome. The "tight" glycemic control expected of pregnant women is frequently accompanied by recurrent, potentially life-threatening hypoglycemia.[33] An abnormal counter-regulatory hormonal response to hypoglycemia has been reported during pregnancy in women with and without diabetes.[34,35] The magnitude of the catecholamine response among Type 1 diabetic women was significantly less than that among non-diabetic women. Thus, the impaired counter-regulatory response to hypoglycemia, which appears to be a normal concomitant of pregnancy, is likely to be exacerbated in women with DAN. Especially in regions where heavy reliance for transportation is placed on automobile travel, hypoglycemic unawareness in pregnant diabetic drivers has been associated with vehicular accidents.[36]

Other symptoms
Other symptoms such as heat intolerance, sweating disturbances, and visual blurring secondary to pupillomotor dysfunction are unlikely to cause significant medical

problems in diabetic pregnancies. The presence of these symptoms should alert healthcare professionals to the possibility of other features of DAN and of the need to screen for the development of complications.

Anesthetic considerations

Diabetic women with autonomic and/or peripheral neuropathy present some additional challenges to obstetric anesthetists. Patients with autonomic dysfunction can exhibit labile blood pressure. Hypotension, caused by sympathetic blockade after regional anesthesia, may be severely exaggerated. Severe hypotension during the induction of general anesthesia in the diabetic patient has also been observed.[26] As a result these women frequently require vasopressors for the treatment of hypotension. However, unlike pregnant women who do not have DAN, the response to vasopressors may be significantly blunted in these women. Prophylactic hydration, prompt use of vasopressors, and strict avoidance of aortocaval compression may minimize the severity and duration of hypotension.

Peripheral neuropathy may manifest as extensive sensory and motor deficits involving the distal extremities. Clear documentation of the extent and severity of the condition in the anesthetic record is therefore vital to avoid the wrong implication of regional anesthesia in the event of any neurologic defects developing in the postpartum period. Proper lithotomy positioning and careful padding of lower extremities is important during vaginal delivery. Similar attention to proper positioning and padding is important during cesarean section to avoid superficial nerve injuries.[37]

Effect of pregnancy

Among women with no or only mild diabetic neuropathy prior to pregnancy, there is no evidence of a significant deleterious effect of pregnancy.

SUMMARY

Hemodynamic and metabolic abnormalities associated with diabetic autonomic neuropathy are clinically important in pregnancy. Whilst most women with DAN have mild, asymptomatic abnormalities in autonomic function, those women with symptomatic features are at a significantly increased risk of developing complications during pregnancy. Detection of symptoms suspected to have an autonomic basis should prompt careful screening for other microvascular complications. The presence

of DAN should be taken into account when counseling women preconceptionally regarding pregnancy.

REFERENCES

1 Boulton AJ, Vinik AI, Arezzo JC, et al. Diabetic neuropathies: a statement by the American Diabetes Association. *Diabetes Care* 2005;**28**:956–62.
2 Vinik AI, Maser RE, Mitchell BD, Freeman R. Diabetic autonomic neuropathy. *Diabetes Care* 2003;**26**:1553–79.
3 Greene DA, Lattimer SA, Sima AA. Are disturbances of sorbitol, phosphoinositide, and Na+-K+-ATPase regulation involved in pathogenesis of diabetic neuropathy? *Diabetes* 1988;**37**:688–93.
4 Low PA, Nickander KK, Tritschler HJ. The roles of oxidative stress and antioxidant treatment in experimental diabetic neuropathy. *Diabetes* 1997;**46** (Suppl 2):S38–42.
5 Hoeldtke RD, Bryner KD, McNeill DR, et al. Nitrosative stress, uric acid, and peripheral nerve function in early type 1 diabetes. *Diabetes* 2002;**51**:2817–25.
6 Sundkvist G, Lind P, Bergstrom B, Lilja B, Rabinowe SL. Autonomic nerve antibodies and autonomic nerve function in type 1 and type 2 diabetic patients. *J Intern Med* 1991;**229**:505–10.
7 Pacher P, Liaudet L, Soriano FG, Mabley JG, Szabo E, Szabo C. The role of poly(ADP-ribose) polymerase activation in the development of myocardial and endothelial dysfunction in diabetes. *Diabetes* 2002;**51**:514–21.
8 Larsen JR, Sjoholm H, Berg TJ, et al. Eighteen years of fair glycemic control preserves cardiac autonomic function in type 1 diabetes. *Diabetes Care* 2004;**27**:963–6.
9 Reichard P, Jensen-Urstad K, Ericsson M, Jensen-Urstad M, Lindblad LE. Autonomic neuropathy – a complication less pronounced in patients with Type 1 diabetes mellitus who have lower blood glucose levels. *Diabet Med* 2000;**17**:860–6.
10 Pfeifer MA, Weinberg CR, Cook DL, et al. Autonomic neural dysfunction in recently diagnosed diabetic subjects. *Diabetes Care* 1984;**7**:447–53.
11 Low PA, Benrud-Larson LM, Sletten DM, et al. Autonomic symptoms and diabetic neuropathy: a population-based study. *Diabetes Care* 2004;**27**:2942–7.
12 Ziegler D, Gries FA, Spuler M, Lessmann F. The epidemiology of diabetic neuropathy. Diabetic Cardiovascular Autonomic Neuropathy Multicenter Study Group. *J Diabet Comp* 1992;**6**:49–57.
13 Kennedy WR, Navarro X, Sutherland DE. Neuropathy profile of diabetic patients in a pancreas transplantation program. *Neurology* 1995;**45**:773–80.
14 Maleki D, Locke GR 3rd, Camilleri M, et al. Gastrointestinal tract symptoms among persons with diabetes mellitus in the community. *Arch Intern Med* 2000;**160**:2808–16.
15 Bytzer P, Talley NJ, Leemon M, Young LJ, Jones MP, Horowitz M. Prevalence of gastrointestinal symptoms asso-

ciated with diabetes mellitus: a population-based survey of 15,000 adults. *Arch Intern Med* 2001;**161**:1989–96.

16 Horowitz M, Edelbroek M, Fraser R, Maddox A, Wishart J. Disordered gastric motor function in diabetes mellitus. Recent insights into prevalence, pathophysiology, clinical relevance, and treatment. *Scand J Gastroenterol* 1991;**26**: 673–84.

17 Steel JM. Autonomic neuropathy in pregnancy. *Diabetes Care* 1989;**12**:170–1.

18 Macleod AF, Smith SA, Sonksen PH, Lowy C. The problem of autonomic neuropathy in diabetic pregnancy. *Diabet Med* 1990;**7**:80–2.

19 Hare J. Diabetic neuropathy and coronary heart disease. In: Greece E, Coustan D (eds). *Diabetes Mellitus in Pregnancy: Principles and Practice.* 1988, New York: Churchill Livingstone, 1988:517–8.

20 Garner P. Type I diabetes mellitus and pregnancy. *Lancet* 1995;**346**:157–61.

21 Schiller LR, Santa Ana CA, Schmulen AC, Hendler RS, Harford WV, Fordtran JS. Pathogenesis of fecal incontinence in diabetes mellitus: evidence for internal-anal-sphincter dysfunction. *N Engl J Med* 1982;**307**:1666–71.

22 Maser RE, Lenhard MJ. Cardiovascular autonomic neuropathy due to diabetes mellitus: clinical manifestations, consequences, and treatment. *J Clin Endocrinol Metab* 2005; **90**:5896–903.

23 Airaksinen KE, Ikaheimo MJ, Salmela PI, Kirkinen P, Linnaluoto MK, Takkunen JT. Impaired cardiac adjustment to pregnancy in type I diabetes. *Diabetes Care* 1986;**9**: 376–83.

24 Airaksinen KE, Salmela PI, Ikaheimo MJ, Kirkinen P, Linnaluoto MK, Takkunen JT. Effect of pregnancy on autonomic nervous function and heart rate in diabetic and nondiabetic women. *Diabetes Care* 1987;**10**:748–51.

25 Lapolla A, Cardone C, Negrin P, *et al.* Pregnancy does not induce or worsen retinal and peripheral nerve dysfunction in insulin-dependent diabetic women. *J Diabet Comp* 1998;**12**:74–80.

26 Airaksinen KE, Anttila LM, Linnaluoto MK, Jouppila PI, Takkunen JT, Salmela PI. Autonomic influence on pregnancy outcome in IDDM. *Diabetes Care* 1990;**13**:756–61.

27 Scott AR, Tattersall RB, McPherson M. Improvement of postural hypotension and severe diabetic autonomic neuropathy during pregnancy. *Diabetes Care* 1988;**11**:369–70.

28 Hepburn DA, Patrick AW, Eadington DW, Ewing DJ, Frier BM. Unawareness of hypoglycaemia in insulin-treated diabetic patients: prevalence and relationship to autonomic neuropathy. *Diabet Med* 1990;**7**:711–7.

29 Ryder RE, Owens DR, Hayes TM, Ghatei MA, Bloom SR. Unawareness of hypoglycaemia and inadequate hypoglycaemic counterregulation: no causal relation with diabetic autonomic neuropathy. *BMJ* 1990;**301**:783–7.

30 Bottini P, Boschetti E, Pampanelli S, *et al.* Contribution of autonomic neuropathy to reduced plasma adrenaline responses to hypoglycemia in IDDM: evidence for a nonselective defect. *Diabetes* 1997;**46**:814–23.

31 Dagogo-Jack SE, Craft S, Cryer PE. Hypoglycemia-associated autonomic failure in insulin-dependent diabetes mellitus. Recent antecedent hypoglycemia reduces autonomic responses to, symptoms of, and defence against subsequent hypoglycemia. *J Clin Invest* 1993;**91**:819–28.

32 Stephenson JM, Kempler P, Perin PC, Fuller JH. Is autonomic neuropathy a risk factor for severe hypoglycaemia? The EURODIAB IDDM Complications Study. *Diabetologia* 1996;**39**:1372–6.

33 Evers IM, ter Braak EW, de Valk HW, van Der Schoot B, Janssen N, Visser GH. Risk indicators predictive for severe hypoglycemia during the first trimester of type 1 diabetic pregnancy. *Diabetes Care* 2002;**25**:554–9.

34 Rosenn BM, Miodovnik M, Khoury JC, Siddiqi TA. Counterregulatory hormonal responses to hypoglycemia during pregnancy. *Obstet Gynecol* 1996;**87**:568–74.

35 Diamond MP, Reece EA, Caprio S, *et al.* Impairment of counterregulatory hormone responses to hypoglycemia in pregnant women with insulin-dependent diabetes mellitus. *Am J Obstet Gynecol* 1992;**166**:70–7.

36 Rosenn BM, Miodovnik M, Holcberg G, Khoury JC, Siddiqi TA. Hypoglycemia: the price of intensive insulin therapy for pregnant women with insulin-dependent diabetes mellitus. *Obstet Gynecol* 1995;**85**:417–22.

37 Ramanathan J, Ivester T. Diabetes Mellitus in Pregnancy: Pathophysiology and Obstetric and Anesthetic Management. *Semin Anesth Periop Med Pain* 2002;**21**:26–34.

19 Ketoacidosis in diabetes in pregnancy

Bob Young

Diabetes Centre, Salford Royal Hospital, Salford, UK

PRACTICE POINTS

- Diabetic ketoacidosis (DKA) is a very serious complication of pregnancy that threatens the mother's life and the health and viability of the fetus.
- DKA only occurs in situations of severe insulin deficiency combined with increases in catabolic hormones. The metabolic physiology of pregnancy predisposes to DKA.
- Patients present with weakness, hypotension, vomiting, and abdominal pain. The diagnosis is confirmed if there is hyperglycemia, ketonemia, and anion gap acidosis.
- To prevent hypovolemic shock, aspiration, cardiac dysrhythmias, thromboembolism or cerebral edema, prompt management, including fluid and electrolyte replacement, insulin, airway protection, heparin and rigorous monitoring are essential.
- DKA in pregnancy is preventable if monitoring is intensive and corrective action prompt.

CASE HISTORY

A 19-year-old woman with an 11-year history of Type 1 diabetes presented as an emergency with 12 hours of vomiting progressing to drowsiness and collapse. She was at 28 weeks of gestation in her first pregnancy. The pregnancy had been confirmed at 8 weeks of gestation at which time the hemoglobin A1c (HbA1c) was 10.8%. The pregnancy was not planned and it was 2½ years since she had last attended anywhere for diabetes review. Her insulin had immediately been changed from twice daily fixed mix to basal bolus and with the help of an intensive re-education program and several times weekly support from the diabetes specialist nurse and midwife, glucose control improved. By the time of the 20-week anomaly scan, which was normal, self-monitoring results were

mostly close to target and HbA1c was 6.6%. However, after that visit she failed to attend for her scheduled joint diabetes antenatal clinic review appointments and could not be contacted by the diabetes specialist midwife or her family doctor.

On initial assessment her pulse was 118 bpm, blood pressure 76/42 mmHg, respiratory rate 26 breaths/min, and Glasgow coma score (GCS) 8. There were no pointers to infection. Emergency bloods revealed blood glucose 33.2 mmol/L (603.6 mg/dL), urea 24.2 mmol/L (67.8 mg/dL), creatinine 186 μmol/L (2.10 mg/dL), sodium 146 mmol/L (146 mEq/L), potassium 5.1 mmol/L (5.1 mEq/L), hemoglobin 13.4 g/L (1.34 g/dL), white cell count (WCC) '19.7 × 10⁶/mL, pH 6.94, venous bicarbonate 4 mmol/L (4 mM), base excess -24, pO₂ 25 kPa (on high-flow oxygen), and pCO₂ 2.3 kPa. The friend who accompanied her to A & E reported that she had been depressed, had stopped testing her blood glucose, and had been taking her insulin only erratically.

A nasogastric tube was passed and 1.5 L of gastric content drained. One liter of plasma expander was infused over 30 minutes. Blood pressure rose to 90/48 mmHg and pulse reduced to 110 bpm. Urinary catheterization released 200 mL of concentrated urine containing ketones +++.

She was commenced on a standardized DKA protocol involving fluid, insulin, and electrolyte replacement with frequent biochemical monitoring. Tinzaparin 4500 U was started subcutaneously (SC) once daily. By 12 hours from admission GCS was 15, nasogastric drainage had ceased, her pulse rate was 90–100 bpm, and blood pressure 100–110/60–70 mmHg. Bedside capillary blood glucose was consistently in the range 5–8 mmol/L (90–145 mg/dL), venous pH was 7.32, and creatinine normal.

The first dose of basal insulin was then administered while the nasogastric tube and urinary catheter were withdrawn. Intravenous (IV) fluids and insulin were con-

A Practical Manual of Diabetes in Pregnancy, 1st Edition.
Edited by David R. McCance, Michael Maresh and David A. Sacks.
© 2010 Blackwell Publishing

tinued for a further 24 hours alongside restitution of basal bolus SC insulin and normal eating until the urine was free of ketones.

During the period in which the mother was being resuscitated, fetal movements and heart rate were monitored intensively. An ultrasound scan showed the head circumference to be on the 50th centile and abdominal circumference on the 95th centile. There were occasional heart rate decelerations but none was sustained. On day 3 after admission it was planned to administer betamethasone to induce fetal surfactant. However, before this was given, fetal movements ceased and severe decelerations were suddenly recorded. An emergency lower segment cesarean section was performed but the baby was dead on delivery.

- What clinical symptoms and signs suggested DKA?
- What biochemical findings confirmed DKA?
- Why did DKA develop?
- Could DKA have been prevented?
- Why was a nasogastric tube inserted?
- Why was tinzaparin given?
- Why was there a leukocytosis?
- Why did the baby die?

BACKGROUND

DKA is one of a very small number of critical illnesses that occur with any regularity in pregnant women. However, although the frequency of pregnancy in women with diabetes preceding pregnancy is increasing, it is still uncommon and a large portion of the increase is due to the rise of Type 2 diabetes in women of reproductive age. Historically, DKA has been reported to occur in 1–3% of women with diabetes preceding pregnancy,[1,2] but these studies were in an era when almost all diabetes preceding pregnancy was Type 1 and insulin management was less intensive. So, since treatment has become more intensive, and as DKA occurs much more rarely in Type 2 diabetes than in Type 1 diabetes (particularly when diabetes duration is short), it is probable that the incidence is now much lower.

DKA occurs when profound insulin deficiency is combined with increased catabolic hormone concentrations. In consequence there is over production from the liver of both glucose and ketone bodies. This over production then combines with progressively decreasing tissue and renal clearance of glucose and ketoacids to produce an accelerating spiral of worsening hyperglycemia, hyperketonemia, and acidosis, the classical triad of DKA.[3–5]

ETIOLOGY

Infection is a classical precipitant of DKA because it induces a release of catabolic hormones such as epinephrine, cortisol, glucagon, and growth hormone. More common causes, however, include management errors, omission of insulin, and new cases of undiagnosed diabetes. Because DKA occurs only in the context of severe insulin deficiency, the majority of patients have Type 1 diabetes. However, ketoacidosis can sometimes be precipitated in Type 2 diabetes. Furthermore subtypes of Type 2 diabetes occur in certain ethnic groups in whom the development of ketoacidosis seems to occur more readily.

The sequence of metabolic changes leading to ketoacidosis is depicted in Fig. 19.1. In the early stages of DKA, the profound insulin deficiency leads not only to hyperglycemia but also to a rise in plasma glucagon which in turn stimulates hepatic gluconeogenesis and lipolysis. Hyperglycemia and ketoacidosis then cause osmotic diuresis, vomiting, hyperventilation, and vasodilatation, leading to hypotension which stimulates the release of catecholamines and cortisol, in turn leading to a vicious cycle of worsening metabolic decompensation provocative of further metabolic hormone release. Simultaneously, insulin deficiency reduces insulin-stimulated glucose disposal in peripheral tissues, such as muscle and adipose tissue, thereby fuelling the rise in glucose.

The combination of severe insulin deficiency and excess catabolic hormones promotes the breakdown of adipose tissue triglyceride (lipolysis), leading to the release of large quantities of long chain non-esterified fatty acids (NEFAs) into the circulation. These are the principal substrate for ketogenesis in the liver. Insulin deficiency and high catabolic hormone levels also promote ketogenesis. Because ketone bodies are strong organic acids that dissociate fully at physiologic pH, the increased levels rapidly outstrip the buffering capacity of the body fluids and tissues, leading to metabolic acidosis.

Hyperglycemia and acidosis both contribute to fluid and electrolyte depletion. Hyperglycemia causes an osmotic diuresis and this is compounded by ketonuria, leading to substantial loss of water and electrolytes (dehydration). Insulin deficiency and glucagon excess exacerbate sodium loss in the kidney. Metabolic acidosis leads to exchange of intracellular potassium ions for extracellular hydrogen ions, the potassium then being lost in excreted body fluids. The body attempts to compensate for the excessive metabolic acids by hyperventilation.

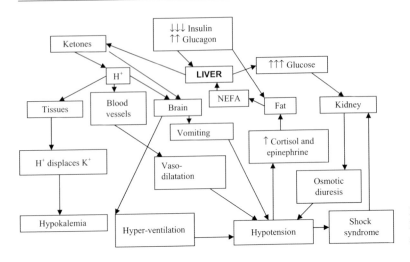

Fig. 19.1 Pathogenesis of diabetic ketoacidosis. NEFAs, non-essential fatty acids.

Further loss of electrolytes occurs because of acidosis-induced vomiting. The loss of body water in ketoacidotic adults is often 5 L or more. When dehydration progresses to the point of hypovolemic shock, reducing renal blood flow inhibits elimination of glucose and ketone bodies, so fuelling rises in their plasma concentrations. Phosphate and magnesium deficiency commonly accompany ketoacidosis but whether they are of clinical significance is uncertain.

Thus the patient with ketoacidosis has:
• Profound insulin deficiency
• High levels of catabolic hormones (glucagon, cortisol, epinephrine)
• Severe hyperglycemia
• Significant acidosis
• Dehydration
• Potassium depletion.

These are the key metabolic derangements that underpin the clinical presentation, natural history, and treatment rationale.

PREGNANCY AS A RISK FACTOR FOR DIABETIC KETOACIDOSIS

"Facilitated anabolism" and "accelerated starvation"

The metabolic characteristics of pregnancy may predispose to the development of ketoacidosis. One important influence is human placental lactogen (hPL), a single chain peptide hormone synthesized by the trophoblast and released into the maternal blood. This hormone has the principal action of increasing the supply of glucose to the fetus by decreasing maternal stores of fatty acids. It does this by increasing maternal secretion of insulin. hPL also induces a reduction in maternal insulin sensitivity. Thus during pregnancy, maternal postprandial glucose concentration is greater than that in the non-pregnant state. This in turn increases the gradient in glucose concentration between mother and fetus, enhancing glucose transfer from the former to the latter. In the fasting state, enhanced insulin resistance at the level of the fat cells promotes the release of non-essential fatty acids (NEFAs) for use as a maternal alternative fuel, thereby sparing maternal glucose for fetal utilization. These processes of "facilitated anabolism"[6] and "accelerated starvation"[7] make women with pregestational diabetes more susceptible to diabetic ketoacidosis which, when initiated, can develop quickly and sometimes at relatively low levels of hyperglycemia.[1]

Continuous subcutaneous insulin infusion (or "pump" treatment)

The use of continuous SC insulin infusion (CSII) is popular in pregnancy and because of the very small insulin reservoir, this may also represent a risk factor, although the increase in ketoacidosis found in early studies of CSII has been less evident in recent publications[8,9] (see chapter 10). In addition Type 1 diabetes, for which DKA is a well-recognized presenting syndrome, is more likely to present during pregnancy because of the prevailing metabolic milieu.

High-dose glucocorticoids

Glucocorticoids are commonly used in high doses to induce fetal surfactant during pregnancies where there is a high risk of impending preterm delivery. In women with diabetes during pregnancy, high-dose glucocorticoids inevitably induce severe hyperglycemia[10] unless prompt compensatory management is coadministered.[11] This is therefore a situation in which very careful monitoring for the potential development of ketoacidosis is mandatory (see chapter 21).

Tocolytics

Similarly, beta-agonist medications, such as ritodrine and terbutaline, may sometimes be used to try and halt the onset of preterm labour. These drugs also can induce severe hyperglycemia in the context of diabetes during pregnancy and similar vigilance must be exercised to that recommended during the use of glucocorticoids. The combined use of glucocorticoids and beta-agonists is especially hazardous (see chapter 21).

RISKS TO MOTHER AND FETUS OF DIABETIC KETOACIDOSIS

Mother

DKA continues overall to carry an appreciable mortality (around 5% in Western countries), although fatal outcome tends to be concentrated at the extremes of age. Pregnant women who develop DKA may die from the same causes as their non-pregnant counterparts, and there are certain aspects of pregnancy that may render them more vulnerable.

The five major causes of death directly attributable to ketoacidosis (as opposed to a precipitating illness) are:
- Hypovolemic shock
- Aspiration pneumonia
- Cerebral edema
- Hypokalemia induced cardiac dysrhythmias
- Pulmonary embolism.

Hypovolemic shock

This is due to loss of fluid from osmotic diuresis and vomiting, possibly compounded by acidosis-induced hyperventilation and vasodilatation. It will respond to fluid replacement. Rarely acute tubular necrosis may lead to the need for temporary renal replacement therapy.

Aspiration pneumonia

This is a risk predominantly in those patients with ketoacidosis who have impairment of consciousness. Hyperglycemia inhibits gastric emptying and is a major contributory factor in the severity of DKA-associated vomiting. Pregnancy itself, of course, may be associated with decreased gastric emptying and a propensity to vomiting, and therefore may compound this component of the syndrome.

Cerebral edema

Cerebral edema occurs predominately in the young and the old, and especially in females. Thus, pregnant teenagers with Type 1 diabetes who develop DKA are at particularly high risk. The pathogenesis is thought to involve delayed normalization of the intracerebral defenses against dehydration (generation of intraneuronal osmotically active molecules that counterbalance the extra- to intra-cellular osmotic gradient). Over-rapid rehydration during treatment for DKA may contribute to the chance of cerebral edema. Accordingly, it is believed that the risk can be mitigated by avoiding over-rapid rehydration. So, once an adequate circulating volume has been re-established, the reduction in plasma osmolality should proceed gradually, giving the physiologic defenses time to readjust. Typically such patients appear initially to improve as their circulating volume is restored, and then they exhibit a secondary decline in cerebral function as cerebral edema develops.

Hypokalemia

Hypokalemia is an important risk factor for cardiac dysrhythmia, particularly if its onset is rapid. All patients with DKA have total body potassium depletion but because of potassium–hydrogen ion exchange and impaired renal function, the plasma potassium may be normal or even high at presentation. Hypokalemia generally occurs when potassium replacement is not started sufficiently early or in sufficient quantity to replace intracellular potassium, as it normalizes rapidly during metabolic management.

Pulmonary embolism

Patients with ketoacidosis are at increased risk of thromboembolism; the greater the hyperosmolality (hemoconcentration) the greater the risk. Pregnant women are already at increased risk of thromboembolism and therefore this is another component of the ketoacidosis syndrome which is potentially compounded by pregnancy. Prophylaxis with heparin is indicated.

Fetus

Fetal distress and intrauterine death may be associated with ketoacidosis.[12] Furthermore, there is some evidence that ketonemia during pregnancy has an adverse impact on the behavioral and intellectual development of the fetus.[13] DKA is therefore a very high-risk complication for fetal health.

The causes of fetal loss are thought to be:
- Reduced uteroplacental blood flow (osmotic diuresis/maternal acidosis)
- Maternal acidosis leading to fetal acidosis and electrolyte imbalance
- Maternal hypokalemia leading to fetal hypokalemia with myocardial suppression, and fetal arrthymia
- Maternal hypophosphatemia leading to reduced 2,3-diphosphoglycerate (2,3-DPG)
- Fetal hyperinsulinemia leading to increased fetal oxygen requirement.

CLINICAL MANAGEMENT

Clinical presentation

DKA usually evolves rapidly, i.e. in less than 24 hours. Typically the osmotic diuresis causes severe polyuria and polydipsia. As the degree and duration of hyperglycemia and dehydration progress, lethargy, confusion, and coma may supervene. Acidosis drives the development of vomiting, abdominal pain, and hyperventilation. There may be coexistent symptoms of intercurrent infections, such as productive cough and pleurisy in pneumonia, dysuria and loin pain in pyelonephritis, and fever and rigors in either.

The clinical signs are related to acidosis (hyperventilation, peripheral vasodilatation), hypovolemia (tachycardia, hypotension), and hyperglycemia (succussion splash due to delayed gastric emptying, coma due to cerebral dehydration). There may also be signs of intercurrent precipitating illnesses, such as pneumonia or pyelonephritis. Fever is rare even in the presence of infection because of peripheral vasodilatation, and indeed hypothermia is a potential complication.

The patient will usually report a recent history, including polyuria and polydipsia (and polyphagia?), possibly accompanied by rapid weight loss and generalized weakness. However, history taking may be compromised by discomfort due to abdominal pain, vomiting, drowsiness, confusion or even coma. Difficulty in diagnosis may be encountered in that polyuria, nausea, and abdominal cramping may be normal findings during pregnancy.

Assessment

Physiologic assessment

Hypotension and tachycardia, the cardinal signs of hypvolemia due to dehydration, will be prominent in severe cases; less severe presentations may exhibit only postural hypotension. Metabolic acidosis stimulates the medullary respiratory centre. The resulting breathing pattern is of rapid and deep respirations, sometimes called "air hunger" (Kussmaul respiration). Those who are able to detect it may smell acetone in the breath.

Conscious level must be carefully charted because, as indicated above, any secondary decline in conscious level during treatment must always suggest the possibility of cerebral edema.

Despite hypovolemia, which would ordinarily induce peripheral vasoconstriction, patients will usually be vasodilated because of the acidosis. This may in certain circumstances lead to hypothermia or to the masking of pyrexia. Pregnancy itself is a state of physiologic vasodilatation. Generalized abdominal discomfort and gastric splash are not unusual.

Bedside biochemical measures can usually confirm the diagnosis before laboratory blood results are available. Thus, in the context of the clinical features described above, bedside tests indicating hyperglycemia and heavy (+++) ketonuria or ketonemia are essentially confirmatory of ketoacidosis.

Laboratory assessment

DKA is characterized by the triad of hyperglycemia, ketonemia, and anion gap metabolic acidosis.

Hyperglycemia

The serum glucose concentration is usually greater than 25 mmol/L (456 mg/dL). Because of fasting insulin resistance during pregnancy, ketoacids form at lower maternal glucose concentrations than in the non-pregnant state. Therefore, DKA may develop at glucose concentrations less than 25 mmol/L (456 mg/dL)[14].

Ketonemia

Three ketone bodies are produced in DKA: two ketoacids (β-hydroxybutyric acid and acetoacetic acid) and one neutral ketone (acetone). Testing for ketones can be carried out on urine or serum with nitroprusside-based reagent sticks. Nitroprusside reacts with acetoacetate and acetone but not with β–hydroxybutyrate, so that very occasionally a negative nitroprusside reaction is obtained in the presence of severe ketosis. A bedside capillary measure of β-hydroxybutyrate is routinely employed in some centers and has the advantage of providing an easily obtainable numerical index of successful management.[15]

Metabolic acidosis

The anion gap metabolic acidosis is due to the production and accumulation of β-hydroxybutyric acid and acetoacetic acid. Compensatory hyperventilation leads to loss of CO_2 and reduction of serum bicarbonate concentration, thus attenuating the fall in arterial pH. Typically in ketoacidosis, pH is between 6.9 and 7.3. Physiologically the serum anion gap provides an estimate of unmeasured anions in the serum, such as albumin. In metabolic acidosis it is increased by the presence of the pathologic anions, i.e. in DKA ketoacids. The anion gap is calculated by subtracting the major measured anions, chloride and bicarbonate, from the major measured cation sodium. Physiologically the gap is less that 15 mmol/L (<273 mg/dL). Patients with DKA usually have an anion gap of greater than 20 mmol//L (20 mEq/L). The normal anion gap of about 10–15 mmol/L (10–15 mEq/L) is accounted for by phosphate, sulfate and lactate ions, and ionized proteins. In the context of hyperglycemia and detectable ketones, none of the other causes of anion gap acidosis is likely (alcoholic ketoacidosis, lactic acidosis, advanced endstage chronic renal failure or poisoning [with salicylates, ethylene glycol or methanol]).

Other laboratory measurements
Sodium

Serum sodium concentration in ketoacidosis is variable. Osmotic water movement out of the cells, driven by hyperglycemia, leads to dilution and a reduction in sodium concentration, whereas glycosuria-induced osmotic diuresis results in water loss in excess of sodium and an increase in the sodium level. Occasionally the measured sodium concentration may be misleadingly low as a result of the phenomenon of pseudohyponatremia, in which DKA-associated hyperlipidemia is so severe that the serum is milky and contains less water and therefore less sodium.

Potassium

On presentation patients with DKA have an average potassium deficit of 3–5 mmol/kg. This is due to a combination of the cellular transmembrane exchange of potassium for hydrogen ions, the renal potassium losses accompanying the glucose-induced osmotic diuresis, and gastrointestinal losses due to vomiting. However, initially, because of displacement of intracellular potassium, dehydration-related hemoconcentration, and hypovolemic renal impairment, potassium levels in the serum are commonly normal, disguising the underlying whole body deficiency.

Urea and creatinine

When available, the initial laboratory tests typically show elevated urea and creatinine in keeping with acute renal impairment. In the past, plasma creatinine concentrations may have been falsely elevated in ketoacidosis due to assay interference by acetoacetate but this is now unusual.

Blood count

The majority of patients with ketoacidosis have a leukocytosis but this does not necessarily imply associated infection. Hemoglobin may initially be high due to dehydration-related hemoconcentration.

Other laboratory measurements

A variety of enzymes, including amylase, transaminases and creatinine kinase, may be raised non-specifically. Significant hyperlipidemia, hypophosphatemia, and hypomagnesemia may also occur.

Other tests

If there is a suggestive history or clinical signs, chest X-ray may be appropriate to confirm pneumonia, urine culture to look for urinary infection or blood culture to diagnose septicemia.

TREATMENT

Two protocols for the management of DKA from different UK centers are given by way of illustration (Tables 19.1 and 19.2). Each of the protocols is broadly similar and they generally concur with American Diabetes Association (ADA) recommendations. The first used by the author involves the infusion of insulin at a dose dictated by the ambient glucose and total daily insulin dose preceding DKA. The second protocol employed by the Belfast group includes a preceding insulin bolus followed by an extended insulin regimen, and utilizes capillary ketone body measurements both in the management and as a point of titration for the hourly insulin infusion. General principles of management are similar and need to be followed rigorously.

Table 19.1 Protocol 1: Management of diabetic ketoacidosis.

CONFIRM DIAGNOSIS

DKA is characterized by:

- Hyperglycemia (BG usually >25 mmol/L [>455 mg/dL] but may be lower, 15–25 mmol/L [273–455 mg/dL] in pregnancy
- Metabolic acidosis (bicarbonate <18 mmol/L [18 mM] or pH <7.30)
- Ketosis (urinary ketones +++, or raised plasma β-hydroxybutyrate)

INITIAL CLINICAL EVALUATION

Initial examination:

- Assess and record level of consciousness, e.g. use Glasgow coma score (GCS)
- Determine hemodynamic/volume status (BP, pulse)
- History and examination for possible precipitating illness
- NB High risk If GCS ≤ 8 or systolic BP ≤ 90 mmHg

Initial investigations:

- Serum glucose
- Arterial pH/venous bicarbonate
- Urinalysis for ketones
- Renal function (Na^+, K^+, urea, creatinine) and full blood count (Hb, WBC, platelets)
- Calculated osmolality (= 2 [Na^+ + K^+] + [urea] + [glucose])
- ECG (if K^+ >5 mmol/L [5 mEq/L])
- Other tests as indicated by the clinical presentation to identify precipitating factor (e.g. septic screen, chest X-ray)

MANAGEMENT

1. Fluids:
   - If systolic BP < 90 mmHg start IV plasma expander
   - Otherwise typical fluid regime:
     - 1 L normal saline (0.9%) over 1 h, followed by
     - 1 L normal saline (0.9%) over 2 h followed by
     - 1 L dextrose–saline (glucose 4.5%, saline 0.045%) every 4–5 h when BG <15 mmol/L (<270 mg/dL)
   - Aim for at least 2 L fluid over the first 3 h and 6 L over the first 24 h
2. Insulin: As per IV insulin sliding scale chart (below) – start with appropriate scale (if usual daily insulin dose is <40 U, start with scale A; 40–80 U start with scale B; 80–120 U start with scale C; >120 U start with scale D)

Rates of IV insulin infusion. Infusion rates A–D depend on total daily insulin dose preceding DKA (see text)

Sliding scale regime		Insulin infusion rate (U/h)			
		A	B	C	D
Plasma glucose (mmol/L [mg/dL])	0–3.9 [0–71]	0	0	0	0
	4–6.9 [72–125]	1	2	3	4
	7–8.9 [126–162]	2	4	6	8
	9–10.9 [163–198]	3	6	9	12
	11–12.9 [199–235]	4	8	12	16
	13+ [236+]	6	12	18	24

3. If GCS ≤ 8, pass a nasogastric tube to prevent aspiration/protect airway
4. Thromboprophylaxis (tinzaparin 4500 U SC once daily, enoxaparin 40 mg SC once daily or unfractionated heparin 5000–7500 U SC once or twice daily)
5. Treatment of identified precipitating factor (infection, etc)

Table 19.1 *Continued.*

MONITOR RESPONSE TO TREATMENT

1. Check bedside capillary glucose hourly
2. At 2 h after starting treatment check:
   - Venous bicarbonate /pH
   - Urea and electrolytes – potassium level leading to regulation of K^+ infusion:
     ○ If K^+ > 5.5 mmol/L (>5.5 mEq/L) do not infuse potassium
     ○ If K^+ 3.6–5.5 mmol/L (3.6–5.5 mEq/L) infuse 20 mmol/L (20 mM) potassium in each liter of saline or dextrose–saline
     ○ If K^+ < 3.6 mmol/L (<3.6 mEq/L) infuse 40 mmol/L (40 mEq/L) potassium in each liter of saline or dextrose–saline
   - Adjust IV insulin infusion according to sliding scale chart (see above)
   - Consider urinary catheter if no urine output
3. At 4, 12, and 24 h:
   - Venous bicarbonate (ABGs are unnecessary if bicarbonate is increasing)
   - U&E (potassium level) – replace potassium as above
4. If GCS deteriorates suspect cerebral edema:
   - Urgent CT/MR brain scan
   - Slow IV fluids and insulin
   - Consider mannitol

DISCONTINUATION OF INTRAVENOUS TREATMENT

- Continue IV insulin and fluids until acidosis has remitted (bicarbonate > 18 mmol/L [80 mM] urinary ketones ≤++) and the patient is eating and drinking. Thereafter, SC insulin regime may be commenced
- To prevent rebound hyperglycemia do not stop the IV insulin infusion until at least 60 min after the first SC injection of short- or rapid-acting insulin

BG, blood glucose; BP, blood pressure; Hb, haemoglobin; WBC, white blood cell; ECG, electrocardiogram; U&E, urea and electrolytes; ABG, arterial blood gas; IV, intravenous; SC, subcutaneous

Fluids

If the patient is in "frank shock" fluid replacement should commence with an IV plasma expander. This should be continued until systolic blood pressure is greater than 90 mmHg. Otherwise fluid replacement should consist of normal saline (0.9%). A serum Na greater than 150 mmol/L (150 mEq/L) should be followed by a more hypotonic solution. Most patients will require at least 6 L over the first 24 hours. After the first 3 hours the rate of infusion should be adjusted according to the clinical state of the patient. It must be kept in mind that once blood pressure is sustained at an adequate level, no further hypotensive damage will ensue. The enhanced risk of cerebral edema due to over-rapid fluid replacement has been previously discussed.

Insulin

Soluble insulin should be given as a continuous IV infusion of quick (short)-acting insulin. The first choice is regular insulin, the second either lispro or aspart. Insulin infusion charts such as those outlined in the protocols

can be used to guide the rate of IV insulin administration. In the first protocol, the initial rate of infusion is chosen according to the record of preceding insulin requirements (or scale A if these are not known), and subsequent adjustments made on the basis of hourly blood glucose tests (Protocol 1; Table 19.1). In the second protocol, the insulin infusion is preceded by an insulin bolus, followed by administration of 5 U of insulin/h (Protocol 2; Table 19.2). In the latter protocol, involving hourly measurement of ketone bodies, using capillary β-hydroxybutyrate (ketometer) was shown to be clinically effective and to accelerate resolution of the ketoacidosis when the hourly insulin infusion was continued until the ketometer reading was less than 0.5 mmol/L (0.5 mEq/L) (Protocol 2).[15,16] The ADA recommends an IV bolus of regular insulin at 0.1 U/kg body weight, followed by a continuous infusion of regular insulin at a dose of 0.1 U/kg/h.[17]

With these protocols, a steady fall in blood glucose of around 5 mmol/L (90 mg/dL)/h into the physiologic range should be anticipated. The ADA recommends that if the rate of fall is less at 4 hours after initiation of treatment, the rate of infusion should be doubled every hour

Table 19.2 Protocol 2: Management of diabetic ketoacidosis.[15,16]

Initial blood investigations:
- Plasma glucose, urea and electrolytes
- Venous "Astrup" (pH, standard bicarbonate)
- Plasma osmolality
- Capillary blood β-hydroxybutyrate (ketometer)

Intravenous infusion: 0.9% isotonic normal saline:
- 2000 mL in first 1½ h
- 1000 mL in next 2 h
- 2000 mL in next 8 h
- 500 mL every 4 h

If Na > 155 mmol/L (>155 mEq/L) consider 0.45% (half isotonic) saline

Insulin:
- 20 U soluble insulin IM initially
- 5 U each hour thereafter, either IM or by (the standard strength of insulin is 100 U/mL) continuous IV infusion (via syringe pump)

Potassium
- 15 mmol (15 mEq)/h from time of first insulin
- If K^+ falls to <4 mmol/L (<4 mEq/L) , increase to 30 mmol/h
- If K^+ falls to <3 mmol/L (<3 mEq/L), increase to 40 mmol/h (and *stop insulin* until corrected)
- If K^+ is >6 mmol/L, (>6 mEq/L) stop potassium

Sodium bicarbonate:

If pH < 7.0, consider 75 mmol (75 mEq) $NaHCO_3$ (500 mL 1.4% sodium bicarbonate) + 20 mmol K^+ in 30 min via piggy-back or Y connector to maintain infusion. Always use 1.4% $NaHCO_3$ Isotonic which is 145 mmol/L (145 mEq/L)

If patient is unconscious or semiconscious; nasogastric tube must be passed to prevent aspiration of vomitus

Other investigations once initial therapy is underway:

Hemoglobin, white cell count, throat swab, urine culture, blood culture, sputum culture (if available), ECG, coagulation screen, blood group and cross-match if hypotensive

Observations and monitoring:
- BP hourly, temperature 2 hourly
- Hourly capillary blood for glucose strip and β-hydroxybutyrate strip monitoring (ketometer)
- Repeat laboratory plasma glucose, electrolytes, "Astrup" (and others if indicated) at 2, 5, and 8 h (and 8 hourly until full recovery)

When capillary blood glucose <10 mmol/L (180 mg/dL):
- Continue insulin at 5 U/h until ketometer reads <0.5 mmol/L
- Continue fluid replacement with normal saline (+KCl) as necessary
- Begin 10% dextrose infusion to prevent hypoglycemia
- Usually commence 10% dextrose at 80 ml/h and adjust hourly

Piggy-back into normal saline infusion (use same access line as for normal saline)

When capillary β-hydroxybutyrate is normal, <0.5 mmol/L (<5 mg/dL) (i.e. ketometer reading <"50"):
- Stop hourly insulin or insulin infusion pump
- Begin 500 mL 5% dextrose with 8 U soluble insulin added to bag over 6 h
- Maintain capillary blood glucose close to 6 mmol/L (108 mg/dL) (give extra SC boluses of insulin 2–4 hourly as necessary)
- If additional fluid required at this stage (i.e. >500 mL/6 h) continue normal saline

Return to regular insulin regime:
- When clinical improvement permits, recommence oral feeding and regular SC insulin
- Keep 5% dextrose/insulin infusion going until patient has tolerated first meal
- Continue oral potassium for 5 days (50 mmoL [50 mEq/L] K^+ = 4 g KCl; four tablets of Sando K daily, or 50 mL Kay-Cee-L daily)

ECG, electrocardiogram; SC, subcutaneous

until a steady glucose decline is achieved. Insulin may be decreased to 1–2 U/h once acidosis is corrected.

Continuous IV insulin infusion should be continued until the metabolic state is stable and the patient is eating and drinking normally. At this point, SC insulin should be resumed and if all SC insulin has been stopped, there should be at least a 1-hour overlap between recommencement of SC insulin and discontinuation of the IV insulin infusion, because insulin has a very short half-life (<6 minutes) and it often takes 30–60 minutes before SC insulin starts to act fully. The total insulin required during the previous 24 hours can be used as a guide to initial requirements. Resistance to insulin action is common during the period immediately after resolution of the acute metabolic disturbance, and so careful monitoring of the glucose with frequent tactical adjustments using soluble insulin may be required for up to 2 weeks.

Potassium

Potassium should be checked at baseline and thereafter at regular intervals. The propensity for potassium to fall with insulin treatment should be anticipated with adequate replacement according to the protocol. If the plasma potassium level is greater than 5–6 mmol/L (>5–6 mEq/L) no supplementary potassium should be infused until the next measurement. If the plasma potassium is greater than 6 mmol/L (>6 mEq/L) an electrocardiogram (ECG) should be checked for hyperkalemic changes. If the potassium falls below 3–3.5 mmol/L (3–3.5 mEq/L) the potassium infusion should be increased and the ECG monitored for signs of impending dysrhythmia. Oral potassium may be needed for several days following resolution of DKA.

Airway protection

If there is any impairment of consciousness, a nasogastric tube should be passed and the stomach drained. Further appropriate action should be taken, i.e. position and airway protection, to minimize the risk of aspiration.

Bicarbonate

Bicarbonate is contraindicated in most patients. It is usually dangerous to administer bicarbonate because it can exacerbate tissue hypoxia, contribute to central nervous system acidosis, promote hypokalemia, and cause local tissue necrosis if the infusion fluid extrava-

sates. In the rare event that severe acidosis with a pH less than 6.9 is causing impaired tissue perfusion due to reduced cardiac contractility or if distressing hyperventilation or left ventricular failure are present, then consideration can be given to the cautious infusion of 75 mmol (75 mEq) sodium bicarbonate (500 ml 1.4% sodium bicarbonate). A concentration of 1.4% of $NaHCO_3$ isotonic should always be used, which is 145 mmol/L (145 mEq/L).

Thromboprophylaxis

As explained earlier, all pregnant women with ketoacidosis are at increased risk for thromboembolism. Tinzaparin 4500 U SC once daily, enoxaparin 40 mg SC once daily or unfractionated heparin 5000–7500 U SC once or twice daily are the usual prophylactic treatments. The dose may have to be revised downwards if weight is less than 50 kg or upward if weight is greater than 100 kg. Treatment should be continued until the patient is fully mobile.

Cerebral edema

Cerebral edema is a rare but potentially fatal complication of DKA. Should cerebral edema ensue, the declining level of consciousness (often a relapse following an improvement) will often progress rapidly to coma and then to cardiorespiratory arrest due to the herniation of the base of the brain through the foramen magnum (coning). If cerebral edema is suspected, the diagnosis should be confirmed by computed tomography (CT) or magnetic resonance (MR) scanning of the brain. Unsurprisingly there are no clinical trials of the treatment for this complication, but most authorities agree that the rate of IV fluid infusion should be slowed, hypotonic fluids should be avoided, the rate of insulin delivery (fall in glucose) should be slowed, and IV mannitol to raise cerebral spinal fluid (CSF) osmolality should be considered.

Antibiotics

Antibiotics should not routinely be administered in ketoacidosis. They should be given only if there is reasonable clinical suspicion of intercurrent infection and according to local guidelines, e.g. for pyelonephritis or community acquired pneumonia.

The typical course of management for the first 24 hours is illustrated in the two protocols.

Fetal assessment

Once treatment has commenced and the maternal condition begins to improve, it will be necessary to determine whether the fetus is still alive by the use of ultrasound. There is little point in undertaking more detailed assessment, such as cardiotocography (CTG), until the mother is in a condition where, if the gestation were appropriate, delivery could be undertaken. This is because if CTG is performed while the mother is still in DKA, it will almost certainly show a pathologic pattern and yet no action can be undertaken because of the maternal condition. Only if the abnormal tracing persists after correction of the acidosis should an expedited delivery be considered.

PREVENTION

DKA in pregnancy should not occur. It is preventable. Frequent blood glucose monitoring must be used to guide progressive increases of insulin dosing to match the escalating physiologic insulin requirements of pregnancy. If steroids or tocolytics are used, supplementary insulin must be prescribed according to even more intensive blood glucose monitoring. If self-monitored blood glucose exceeds 15 mmol/L (273 mg/dL), the mother must always check for ketones. In the event of self-detected hyperglycemia and ketonuria, prompt action by the mother using supplementary insulin guided by more intensive monitoring according to carefully specified "sick-day rules" (e.g. Table 19.3) will prevent progression to DKA even if serious infection is the precipitant. Twenty-four hour telephone access to the diabetes care team should also be available.

Table 19.3 "Sick-day rules".

ILLNESS AND DIABETES

When you are ill your blood glucose will rise even if you do not eat. Controlling your blood glucose is more difficult and you should contact your Diabetes Centre for help and advice.

What should you do?

- Never stop taking your insulin
- Monitor your blood glucose frequently
- Check for ketones in your urine frequently – If you have more than a "small" level of ketones (as indicated by the chart on the bottle), contact the your Diabetes Centre immediately
- If you have repeated vomiting and/or "large" levels of ketones in your urine, go to hospital as soon as possible
- Increase the amount of fluid that you drink
- If you don't feel like eating, replace solid foods with a still sweet drink, such as fruit juice. Milky drinks, ordinary fruit yoghurt and ice cream also provide carbohydrates

IF IN DOUBT CONTACT YOUR DIABETES CENTRE (24 h contact numbers should be provided on any literature)

REFERENCES

1 Ramin KD. Diabetic ketoacidosis in pregnancy. *Obstet Gynecol Clin North Am* 1999;**26**:481–8.
2 Cullen MT, Reece EA, Homko CJ, Sivan E. The changing presentations of diabetic ketoacidosis during pregnancy. *Am J Perinatol* 1996;**13**:449–51.
3 Kreisberg RA. Diabetic ketoacidosis: New concepts and trends in pathogenesis and treatment. *Ann Intern Med* 1978;**88**:681.
4 Kitabchi AE, Umpierrez GE, Murphy MB. Diabetic ketoacidosis and hyperglycemic hyperosmolar state. In: DeFronzo RA, Ferrannini E, Keen H, Zimmet P (eds). *International Textbook of Diabetes Mellitus*, 3rd edn. Chichester: John Wiley & Sons, 2004:1101.
5 Krentz AJ, Nattrass M. Acute metabolic complications of diabetes: diabetic ketoacidosis, hyperosmolar non-ketotic hyperglycaemia and lactic acidosis. In: Pickup JC, Williams G (eds). *Textbook of Diabetes*, 3rd edn. Oxford: Blackwell Science, 2003:32.
6 Freinkel N. Banting Lecture. Of pregnancy and progeny. *Diabetes* 1980;**29**:1023–35.
7 Metzger BE, Freinkel M. Accelerated starvation in pregnancy: implications for dietary treatment of obesity and gestational diabetes mellitus. *Biol Neonate* 1987;**51**:78–85.
8 Chen R, Ben-Haroush A, Weissman-Brenner A, Melamed N, Hod M, Yogev Y. Level of glycemic control and pregnancy outcome in type 1 diabetes: a comparison between multiple daily insulin injections and continuous subcutaneous insulin infusions. *Am J Obstet Gynecol* 2007;**197**:404.e1–5.
9 Mukhopadhyay A, Farrell T, Fraser RB, Ola B. Continuous subcutaneous insulin infusion vs intensive conventional insulin therapy in pregnant diabetic women: a systematic review and metaanalysis of randomized, controlled trials. *Am J Obstet Gynecol* 2007;**197**:447–56.
10 Bouhanick B, Biquard F, Hadjadj S, Roques MA. Does treatment with antenatal glucocorticoids for the risk of premature delivery contribute to ketoacidosis in pregnant women with diabetes who receive continuous subcutaneous insulin infusion (CSII)? *Arch Intern Med* 2000;**160**:242–3.
11 Kaushal K, Gibson JM, Railton A, Hounsome B, New JP, Young RJ. A protocol for improved glycaemic control following corticosteroid therapy in diabetic pregnancies. *Diabet Med* 2003;**20**:73–5.

12 Girling J, Dornhorst A. Pregnancy and diabetes mellitus. In: *Textbook of Diabetes*, 3rd edn. Pickup JC, Williams G (eds). Oxford: Blackwell Science, 2003:65.

13 Rizzo T, Metzger BE, Burns WJ, Burns K. Correlations between antepartum maternal metabolism and child intelligence. *N Engl J Med* 1991;**325**:911–6.

14 Oliver R, Jagadeesan P, Howard RJ, Nikookam K. Euglycaemic diabetic ketoacidosis in pregnancy: an unusual presentation. *J Obstet Gynaecol* 2007;**27**:308.

15 McBride MO, Smye M, Nesbitt GS, Hadden DR. Bedside blood ketone body monitoring. *Diabetic Med* 1991;**8**: 688–90.

16 Wiggam MI, O'Kane MJ, Harper R, *et al.* Treatment of diabetic ketoacidosis using normalization of blood β-hydroxybutyrate concentration as the endpoint of emergency management. A randomized controlled study. *Diabetes Care* 1997;**20**;1347–52.

17 American Diabetes Association. Hyperglycemic crises in adult patients with diabetes. A consensus statement from the American Diabetes Association. *Diabetes Care* 2006;**29**: 2739–48.

Section 5

Delivery and postdelivery care

20 Obstetric management of labor, delivery, and the postnatal period

Michael Maresh

St Mary's Hospital for Women, Manchester, UK

PRACTICE POINTS

- Women with any form of diabetes should be assessed for vaginal delivery and individualized decisions made following discussion between the woman and her clinicians, taking into consideration both maternal and fetal factors.
- Women with pregestational diabetes should be offered elective delivery at 38–39 weeks assuming no other maternal or fetal factors have caused significant concern previously.
- Women with insulin-requiring gestational diabetes should be considered for elective intervention at 38–39 weeks as this is associated with a reduction in shoulder dystocia and birthweight, but no significant increase in cesarean rates.
- Women suspected clinically or on ultrasound to have a fetus with macrosomia should be considered for earlier induction at 37–38 weeks or for cesarean delivery.
- Women with gestational diabetes not requiring insulin therapy do not need specific intervention prior to term unless other factors are present.
- Routine delivery by cesarean if macrosomia is suspected will increase the already high cesarean rates with minimal benefit as ultrasound-estimated weights are not that reliable, shoulder dystocia is unpredictable; brachial plexus injury still may occur and cesarean morbidity is significant.
- In labor, specific care must be taken with regard to monitoring fetal condition, maintaining maternal normoglycemia and watching for signs of potential disproportion.

CASE HISTORY

A 32-year-old woman with Type 1 diabetes was pregnant for the second time. Her first pregnancy had been relatively uncomplicated and she had been induced at 38 weeks of gestation. Her daughter was born vaginally with the aid of forceps and weighed 3.82 kg. In her second pregnancy diabetes control was suboptimal and there was concern about excessive fetal growth both clinically and on ultrasound scanning. A decision was made to induce labor at 37+ weeks, but the day prior to the planned induction she presented in labor with ruptured membranes. Continuous fetal heart rate monitoring showed a normal pattern and the amniotic fluid remained clear. She progressed rapidly to 8 cm of cervical dilation, but no further dilation occurred over the next 3 hours, with the head remaining above the level of the ischial spines. The senior resident obstetrician commenced an oxytocin infusion and 2 hours later her cervix was fully dilated with the head below the level of the ischial spines and she was pushing involuntarily. However, after 60 minutes she remained undelivered and the senior resident performed a forceps delivery, but then encountered severe shoulder dystocia. Eventually delivery was achieved by extraction of the posterior arm and then the posterior shoulder. Her son was born in poor condition weighing 4.63 kg. His Apgar scores were 2 at 1 minute and 6 at 5 minutes and after resuscitation he was transferred to the special care baby unit. He had considerable bruising and was found to have a fractured humerus and clavicle, but he made a complete recovery. The woman elected to be sterilized later that year.

- What factors influence the decision on the timing of delivery?
- What factors influence the decision on the mode of delivery?
- If induction of labor is necessary, what is the optimum method?
- How is fetal condition assessed in labor?
- How is progress assessed in labor and when should oxytocin be used?
- How may shoulder dystocia be avoided and what is the optimal management when it occurs?

A Practical Manual of Diabetes in Pregnancy, 1st Edition.
Edited by David R. McCance, Michael Maresh and David A. Sacks.
© 2010 Blackwell Publishing

- Are there any specific anesthetic issues which need consideration?
- Does there need to be any specific postnatal management?

BACKGROUND

Obstetric intervention in pregnant women with pregestational diabetes prior to spontaneous labor has been standard practice for decades. The objectives were, and still are, to avoid the fetus dying *in utero* and to avoid the hazards of obstructed labor or shoulder dystocia associated with fetal macrosomia. In an effort to achieve these goals, cesarean section rates for women with pregestational diabetes in most parts of the world are more than 50%. Iatrogenic prematurity has resulted in high rates of admission to neonatal intensive care in Type 1 diabetes. While it may be the objective of the health professional to obtain a normal outcome (spontaneous labor, normal delivery, and no neonatal care admission) in women with pregestational diabetes, this is achieved in only a minority of cases. By contrast, such a goal should be achievable in the majority of women with gestational diabetes not requiring insulin. Although there are general guidelines to follow, an individualized approach to the timing and mode of delivery is essential. This is particularly so in Type 1 diabetes where many factors need consideration, including glycemic control, diabetes complications, past obstetric history, fetal growth, and the availability of healthcare resources in labor. The management of labor should follow standard practice as for the woman without diabetes. Particular attention is needed with regard to fetal monitoring and signs of delay in labor.

TIMING OF DELIVERY

The decision of when during pregnancy to deliver a woman who has diabetes reflects the obstetrician's opinion of the gestational age at which the risk of possible excessive fetal growth, plus the risk of unexpected fetal demise, is balanced by the risks of induction of labor and/or cesarean section. Data from the 2002–2003 UK survey[1] showed that 35.8% of women with pregestational diabetes delivered at under 37 weeks of gestation compared to 7.4% in the general population. While an increased incidence of spontaneous preterm birth compared to the general population was anticipated from previous studies, 26.4% of the total births were delivered iatrogenically preterm. Wide variation in practice exists within the UK, suggesting that the attitude of health professionals plays

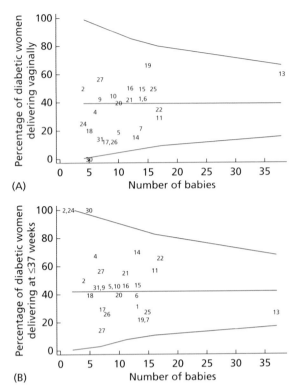

Fig. 20.1 Funnel plot showing variations in (A) vaginal delivery rates and (B) preterm delivery rates in women with established pregestational diabetes across 25 units in the North West of England. The 99% confidence intervals are marked. Some of the smaller units lie outside these limits.[2] The numbers within the plots are the codes for the individual units.

a major role in determining the timing and route of delivery for diabetic women. A method of demonstrating the significance of this variation across a region in the UK using a funnel plot has been described (Fig. 20.1A).[2]

Large studies are needed to address the risks and benefits of delivery prior to 40 weeks. The few relevant studies have either been composed entirely or predominantly of women with gestational diabetes. A US study[3] randomized 187 women with insulin-requiring gestational diabetes and 13 with pregestational diabetes to either intervention at 38 weeks or expectant management. As anticipated, intervention was associated with a lower rate of babies weighing at or above the 90th centile for gestational age (10% *vs* 23%; p = 0.02) and a trend towards a reduction in shoulder dystocia (0% *vs* 3%; not significant). Similarly, a case-controlled study in insulin-requiring gestational diabetes from Israel (n = 260)[4] showed a reduced prevalence of shoulder dystocia in women delivering at 38–39 weeks compared to those delivering at or beyond 40 weeks (1.4% *vs* 10.2%; p < 0.05). Neither study showed an increase in cesarean section rate with induction of labor prior to term. While it might be expected that induction by 38–39 weeks will reduce the risk of stillbirth or early neonatal death of normally formed babies, there is no evidence as yet to support this.

Type 1 and Type 2 diabetes

The current UK guidelines advise that diabetic women should be offered elective delivery after 38 completed weeks,[5] assuming no other significant factors have developed before this time. Current US guidelines recommend that if diabetes is well-controlled, the pregnancy may be allowed to go to, but not beyond, term.[6] In practice, the clinician is often faced with a decision as to whether or not to deliver even earlier and there may also be contraindications to such intervention. In making a decision about the timing of delivery, it is necessary to individualize care, taking into account a number of maternal and fetal factors, including:

- Poor maternal glycemic control – as episodes of maternal hyperglycemia may cause fetal acidemia, the fetus may be at risk of unexpected death *in utero*
- Progression of maternal diabetic complications – maternal renal impairment, hypertension, neuropathy or retinopathy may all cause significant concerns about maternal health (see chapters 15–17)
- Fetal macrosomia – as assessed by serial ultrasound (see chapter 12)
- Fetal growth restriction or compromise – as assessed by ultrasound and other methods of fetal surveillance (see chapter 12)
- Maternal preference, particularly if there is a poor obstetric history.

Neonatal facilities should not influence the decision, as if premature delivery is indicated and facilities are not available locally, then *in-utero* maternal transfer to a maternity unit with these facilities should occur.

In the UK 2002–2003 survey[1] of pregestational diabetes, there was a 39% induction rate (general population rate 21%). The main reasons stated for induction were routine (48%), general obstetric complications (14%), presumed fetal compromise (9%), anticipated large baby or polyhydramnios (9%), and diabetes complications (2%).

Gestational diabetes

Women with gestational diabetes range from those with undiagnosed Type 2 diabetes to those with mild impairment of glucose tolerance diagnosed for the first time during pregnancy which is corrected following appropriate dietary measures. Again care should be individualized at least to a degree. The studies mentioned above[3,4] relate primarily to insulin-requiring gestational diabetic women and accordingly there is a case for considering elective intervention in these women at 38–39 weeks, particularly if macrosomia is suspected, as these studies showed a reduced incidence of shoulder dystocia in the intervention groups. In addition, other maternal or fetal factors may indicate the need for either early or delayed intervention. However, for women who have been managed satisfactorily with diet alone and who have no specific other risk factors (e.g. macrosomia), treatment should be similar to the general obstetric population.

MODE OF DELIVERY

Incidence of cesarean section and vaginal delivery

Type 1 and Type 2 diabetes

Studies show an increased incidence of delivery by cesarean section compared to the general population. The figure from the UK survey of 3474 women in 2002–2003 was 67% compared to the overall population rate of 24%.[1] Although the data were not presented by type of diabetes, the rate tends to be lower in women with Type 2 diabetes, as these women are often older and multiparous, and may well have had their previous pregnancies at a time when they had normal or only impaired glucose tolerance. This wide variation in rates is illustrated by a funnel plot for the North West of England (Fig 20.1B).

Gestational diabetes

In gestational diabetes cesarean section rates tend to be higher than those of the background population. However, studies have shown that this may be attributable to other factors, such as maternal obesity, which is independently associated with fetal macrosomia[7] and probably to traditional obstetric practice.[8,9] The multiethnic international Hyperglycemia and Adverse Pregnancy Outcome (HAPO) study has provided additional data as women with abnormal glucose tolerance during pregnancy short of diabetes (defined by a 75-g oral glucose tolerance test [OGTT] at approximately 28 weeks of gestation) were managed with the caregiver and participant being blinded to the OGTT result.[10] Although the strength of the positive association between maternal glucose concentrations and primary cesarean section rate was attenuated after controlling for confounding variables, there still remained a significant relationship between hyperglycemia during pregnancy and cesarean section rates. In addition, labeling a woman with gestational diabetes may result in clinicians favoring cesarean delivery, thus negating any possible treatment-induced reduction of macrosomia being translated into a greater likelihood of vaginal delivery. In the randomized controlled Australian Carbohydrate Intolerance Study (ACHOIS) trial there was no difference in the cesarean rates between treated and untreated gestational diabetes groups despite the latter group having been double-blinded.[8] In the Canadian Tri-Cities case–control study, the cesarean delivery rate for women with treated gestational diabetes was 33.6% compared with 29.6% for those who were untreated, despite the treated group having reduced macrosomia.[9] The cesarean rate for controls was 20.2%, but multivariate analysis showed that compared to the untreated group, it was not the gestational diabetes which increased the risk.

Indications for cesarean or attempted vaginal delivery

The indications for cesarean section are often multiple, making analyses of the reasons difficult. However, apart from general obstetric complications, a number of factors can be considered individually:

Previous cesarean section

Existing data, mainly from studies in gestational diabetes, do not suggest that women with diabetes should be treated differently from those without diabetes and accordingly should be considered for vaginal birth after cesarean (VABC). None of the studies is able to address the issue of whether there is an increased risk of scar dehiscence in diabetes. One study reviewed only women with diet-controlled gestational diabetes.[11] Other studies suffer from problems with the control groups.[12,13] However, the Washington State study[13] included women with both pregestational and gestational diabetes and showed that fewer women with diabetes attempted VBAC (non-diabetic 64.4%; gestational 58.1%; established 51.0%) and that their success rates were significantly lower (non-diabetic 62.0%, gestational 45.8%, established 36%). These results might be anticipated as any

delay in progress in labor in a diabetic woman should raise concern as to the possibility of impending dystocia and the potential for scar rupture.

Routine practice

In some hospitals cesarean delivery in women with pregestational diabetes is almost the routine (Fig. 20.1A). If maternity units have anxieties about caring for diabetic women in labor, women should be offered the choice of transfer to a unit with more experience in the management of pregnant women who have diabetes. This raises the controversial issue as to whether care for such pregnancies should be centralized into a smaller number of larger centers staffed with personnel experienced in the management of diabetes in pregnancy. There are outcome data which tend to support the latter practice.[14,15]

Maternal diabetic complications

Some express the opinion that from a maternal health perspective a cesarean is safest for the mother whose diabetes is complicated by, for example, hypertension or severe retinal disease. There are no data on this and in the UK survey this was considered the primary indication in only 3%.[1] However, in women with vascular complications, there may be associated fetal growth restriction and a cesarean may be indicated for fetal reasons.

Concern about fetal condition

Antenatal fetal surveillance (see chapter 12) may suggest that a fetus is less likely to cope with the hypoxic stresses of labor. The 2008 UK National Institute for Health and Clinical Excellence (NICE) guidelines[5] concluded from a review of the evidence that the risk of stillbirth was a determining factor in the decision to perform a cesarean delivery, and this was the primary indication in 28% of cases in the 2002–2003 UK survey.[1] The survey showed that intrapartum stillbirths accounted for 10% of all stillbirths. The neonatal death rate for the infants of diabetic women was 9.3 per 1000, which was 2.6 times (95% CI 1.7–3.9) that of the general population.[1]

Excessive fetal weight

This was the other major factor considered in the UK NICE guidelines,[5] but in the 2002–2003 UK survey,[1] this was recorded as the primary indication for cesarean in only 4%. However, in 14% of women the indication for section was delay in progress in labor. In many of these women, the concern may have been about excessive fetal weight, with the possible sequelae of perinatal death or morbidity (see below). The UK survey showed that the birthweight distribution of the stillbirths was similar to that of the live births.[16]

Maternal stature, ethnic group, and corrected birthweight centiles may also assist decision-making. In the multiparous woman with a suspected large fetus, other relevant factors include the previous successful vaginal delivery of a baby of similar weight to that estimated for the current pregnancy or a comparison of antenatal ultrasound serial biometry of a previous fetus with those of the current pregnancy.

Shoulder dystocia and brachial plexus injury

The possibility of shoulder dystocia and subsequent brachial plexus injury undoubtedly influence the clinician's decision as to how best to deliver the baby of the diabetic mother. It is always uppermost in the mind of clinicians looking after a woman with diabetes in labor. In view of this, there has been much analysis of the role of cesarean delivery in this regard.

The current UK rate of shoulder dystocia in women with pregestational diabetes is 7.9%.[1] A large US regional study reported population rates of 3%,[17] while a large study from Boston, US revealed an incidence of 1.2%.[18] Brachial plexus injury was reported in 4.5 per 1000 UK births to mothers with pregestational diabetes,[1] which was estimated to be 10 times greater than the general population rate of 0.42 per 1000.[19] The difference between rates in women with or without diabetes is less marked in the Boston study, but the diabetic group included women with gestational diabetes.[18] In the UK study of pregestational diabetes, 25% of the babies with brachial plexus injury were delivered by cesarean section.[1] The mechanism for the injury in the latter cases is unclear, but excessive head traction may still be applied at cesarean delivery. Similarly, only two-thirds of the vaginal deliveries with brachial plexus injury were described as having been complicated by shoulder dystocia,[1] similar to that reported in the general population.[17–19]

Pregestational maternal diabetes and infant birthweight appear to be independent risk factors for brachial plexus injury[16] with an odds ratio of 9.6 (95% CI 6.2–14.9) for infants weighing more than 4000 g compared to those weighing less. The odds ratio increased to 17.9 (95% CI 10.3–31.3) for birthweights above 4500 g and to 45.2 (95% CI 15.8–128.8) above a birthweight of 5000 g. In the HAPO study, the prevalence of shoulder dystocia was 1.2% (n = 311), but rates varied from 0.1% to 3.4% among centers.[10] In the latter study, there was a significant relationship between worsening glucose tolerance and shoulder dystocia even after controlling for con-

founding variables. However, in clinical practice, birthweight predictions may not be that helpful as typically 40–60% of cases of shoulder dystocia occur in babies weighing less than 4000 g.[20] For brachial plexus injury, similar percentages of cases have been reported to occur in babies weighing less than 4000 g, both in non-diabetic and diabetic (gestational and pregestational) women.[18]

Although there are limitations in the use of fetal weight estimated by ultrasound (chapter 12), in a study of women predominantly with gestational diabetes, it was used at 37–38 weeks of gestation to aid delivery decision-making.[21] Elective cesarean section was performed when the ultrasound fetal weight estimation was more than 4250 g and labor induced when the weight estimation was on or greater than the 90th centile but less than 4250 g. Compared to the period before weight estimations were performed, there was a significant reduction in the incidence of shoulder dystocia from 2.4% to 1.1% (OR 2.2). The rate of shoulder dystocia in the macrosomic group (defined as ≥4000 g) delivered vaginally was 7.4%, but there was a significant 15% rise in the rate of cesarean section from 21.7% prior to the introduction of weight estimations to 25.1% thereafter. Analysis of available data has suggested that using a predicted weight threshold of 4500 g, an additional 443 cesarean sections would be required to prevent one permanent brachial plexus injury.[22] Apart from the economic aspects, the benefit of reducing shoulder dystocia must be carefully weighed against the short- and long-term morbidities of cesarean section, not least of which is hysterectomy. In the UK the risk of having a hysterectomy at the time of cesarean is 1 in 220 for a woman who has previously had two or more cesareans.[23]

PRETERM LABOR AND DELIVERY

The prevalence of delivery before 34 weeks among women in the UK with pregestational diabetes was 9.4% (328 of 3474) and before 37 weeks was 35.8%.[1] While the spontaneous preterm delivery rate was 9.4% (general obstetric population 4.7%), of all the preterm deliveries 73% were iatrogenic. Great variation in the incidence of preterm delivery may be seen when comparing different hospitals, which undoubtedly is a reflection of individual hospital policy (Fig. 20.1A).[2] A detailed Danish prospective study of pregnancies complicated by Type 1 diabetes attempted to analyse the causes of preterm delivery.[24] Having excluded women with significant hypertensive or renal problems, 16 (23%) women were found to have delivered before 36 weeks, mostly for obstetric reasons such as spontaneous labor with or without preceding ruptured membranes or bleeding. The strongest predictor of preterm delivery was a higher hemoglobin A1c (HbA1c) concentration throughout pregnancy compared with the women who went to term. This coupled with a mean birthweight of 3.02 kg at a mean gestation of 32.6 weeks is in accord with suboptimal diabetic control, macrosomia, and probably polyhydramnios being associated with spontaneous preterm delivery.

Predicting whether a woman who presents prematurely with contractions is actually going to deliver is often difficult. For the women without diabetes, there is rarely a contraindication to administering steroids to aid fetal lung maturity. However, in the diabetic woman, such therapy must be given with caution as it can precipitate diabetic ketoacidosis. Frequent monitoring of blood glucose and additional insulin are required (see chapter 21), and this applies also to the women with gestational diabetes. Tocolysis may be used, particularly to delay delivery and thus allow the effects of steroids to be beneficial. However, if tocolytics are used, beta-sympathomimetics are best avoided as they are likely to further worsen diabetic control. Other drugs such as calcium channel antagonists (e.g. nifedipine) or magnesium sulfate are preferable as they do not interfere with diabetic control.

If preterm labor supervenes, then management should be as for the non-diabetic woman with premature labor. There is no specific indication for a cesarean section. Continuous electronic monitoring should be utilized once labor is established. Shoulder dystocia may still occur preterm (e.g. 35–36 weeks) as a macrosomic fetus could weigh 4 kg at this gestation, and accordingly careful attention should be made with regard to progress in established labor (see below).

PLANNED CESAREAN DELIVERY – PRACTICAL ISSUES

As always prior to elective intervention, the accuracy of the expected date of delivery must be checked. If ultrasound biometry from the first trimester or at least before 24 weeks is not available, then this is one of the few indications for consideration of amniocentesis to ascertain fetal lung maturity (see chapter 12).

It should be feasible to manage women with diabetes in exactly the same way as women without diabetes other than with regard to their insulin regime (see chapter 21). As many of these women will be obese or have other diabetic complications, a preoperative anesthetic review

is advised. Regional anesthesia is preferred to general anaesthesia, as with non-diabetic women. Additional reasons for favoring regional anesthesia include the possibility of hypoglycemia developing whilst under general anesthesia and the risk of aspiration of stomach contents, as the diabetic woman may have decreased gastric emptying associated with a degree of autonomic neuropathy. Possible hemodynamic effects and hypotension, which may be associated with regional anesthesia, should not cause significant problems.

Difficulty with delivery of the shoulders is sometimes experienced and excessive head traction may be avoided by extracting the shoulders digitally; excessive head traction is likely to be the cause of some cases of brachial plexus injury following cesarean.

Prophylactic antibiotics are recommended for planned as well as emergency cesarean sections in view of increased infection risk. Thromboprophylaxis, even in the absence of other risk factors, is also advisable in all cases. The issue of tubal ligation should be raised beforehand with all women having their second or subsequent baby. Postoperative care should be as for any woman after a cesarean apart from with regard to her diabetes treatment (see chapter 21).

INDUCTION OF LABOR – PRACTICAL ISSUES

In view of the general recommendation to consider elective delivery by 38–39 weeks in women with pregestational and insulin-requiring gestational diabetes (see above), induction of labor is widely utilized. Prostaglandins are normally required first to ripen the cervix and initiate labor, and this can then be followed by artificial membrane rupture when the cervix is beginning to dilate. Usually oxytocin is required as well and is considered further below. Management should be conducted as for women without diabetes, apart from a few specific points. Induction should take place on the delivery suite or in an alternative well-staffed environment where careful monitoring of fetal condition can be performed using cardiotocography (CTG) and there can be regular monitoring of maternal blood glucose. During the initial phase with prostaglandins, if the woman is not in significant pain and labor has not commenced, she should be permitted to continue to eat and receive short- or ultrashort-acting insulin to cover this, coupled with routine pre- and postprandial glucose measurements. When labor is established, it is customary to monitor capillary blood glucose hourly; insulin regimes are discussed in chapter 21. She should also be reviewed by an anaesthesiologist (anesthetist), as there remains a relatively high risk of a cesarean being required in labor. In the UK 2002–2003 survey, of the 1975 women with pregestational diabetes who went into spontaneous labor or were induced, 43% had a cesarean.[1]

SPECIFIC OBSTETRIC ISSUES IN THE FIRST STAGE OF LABOR

Progress in labor and use of oxytocin

The major concern is that of unexpected disproportion between fetus and mother, and possible traumatic delivery. Careful monitoring of progress in labor is required, which may be facilitated by the use of a partograph or Friedman curve. While difficulties with delivery may occur after a relatively rapid first stage of labor, slow progress in the active phase of labor (i.e. ≥ 5 cm cervical dilation) requires careful review by an experienced obstetrician. In the woman having her first labor, stimulation of the uterus with oxytocin may be considered if the contractions have never been very frequent or strong. However, after good progress in labor followed by cessation of cervical dilatation, oxytocin must be used with caution. Intrauterine pressure catheters, whilst not widely used, may be helpful in this situation by quantifying the uterine response to oxytocin. In the woman who has had a previous vaginal delivery, delay in the active phase of labor is normally an indication for cesarean delivery and oxytocin is almost always contraindicated (Fig. 20.2).

Total length of labor

As labor is often induced it may be of considerable duration. There is no need to impose arbitrary time limits as long as progress is being made and both fetal and maternal condition is satisfactory. With regard to the mother, it should be feasible to maintain normal glycemic and metabolic control by careful attention to intravenous fluid regimes despite a prolonged labor (see chapter 21).

Monitoring fetal condition in labor

The fetus of the diabetic mother is probably at higher risk of developing intrapartum asphyxia than the fetus of the woman without diabetes, hence the recommendation for continuous electronic fetal monitoring in labor.[25] This increased risk may at least in part relate to the direct association between maternal hyperglycemia and fetal acidemia.[26] An example of the effect of maternal hyperg-

lycemia on the CTG of a woman in early labor is shown in Fig. 20.3. The presence of maternal disorders such as pre-eclampsia, the incidence of which is increased with established diabetes, and which is associated with fetal growth restriction, further makes the need for careful fetal monitoring essential. In early labor, CTG monitoring may be performed intermittently if there is maternal normoglycemia (between 4 and 7 mmol/L [72–126 mg/dL]); once labor is established it should be performed continuously.[25] If the CTG shows a suspicious or pathologic pattern, the first step should be to check that the maternal glucose is normal. If hyperglycemia is present, then this should be corrected by supplementary intravenous insulin (see chapter 21) and the CTG pattern may well improve as a result (Fig. 20.3). If the mother is normoglycemic, or obtaining normoglycemia fails to correct the CTG abnormality, then other methods of assessing fetal condition should be utilized. A fetal blood sample may be taken if cervical dilatation permits. In the US, fetal blood sampling is not routine practice and other tests such as scalp stimulation are utilized. A systematic review of intrapartum stimulation tests in general pregnant populations has been undertaken.[27] Scalp stimulation tests appear to be a moderately good predictive test for fetal acidemia. Interpretation and action on the basis of such tests in the presence of maternal normoglycemia should be the same as for the non-diabetic woman.

Analgesia in labor

As maternal stress may result in hyperglycemia, adequate analgesia in labor may be beneficial for glycemic control. There are no contraindications to the use of opioids or epidurals for analgesia. Indeed, given the increased risk of cesarean delivery with maternal diabetes, the presence of an epidural is usually sufficient for anesthesia (with an appropriate dosage regime) if a cesarean is required.

SPECIFIC OBSTETRIC ISSUES IN THE SECOND STAGE OF LABOR

The main issues in the second stage are similar to those in the first stage, namely concerns about fetal condition and delay. A pathologic CTG in the second stage should be managed in the same way as for the non-diabetic mother, apart from the need for greater caution in the consideration of an instrumental delivery. Delivery of a woman with diabetes should not be conducted by relatively inexperienced staff, unless the latter are closely supervised. In view of the increased risk of shoulder

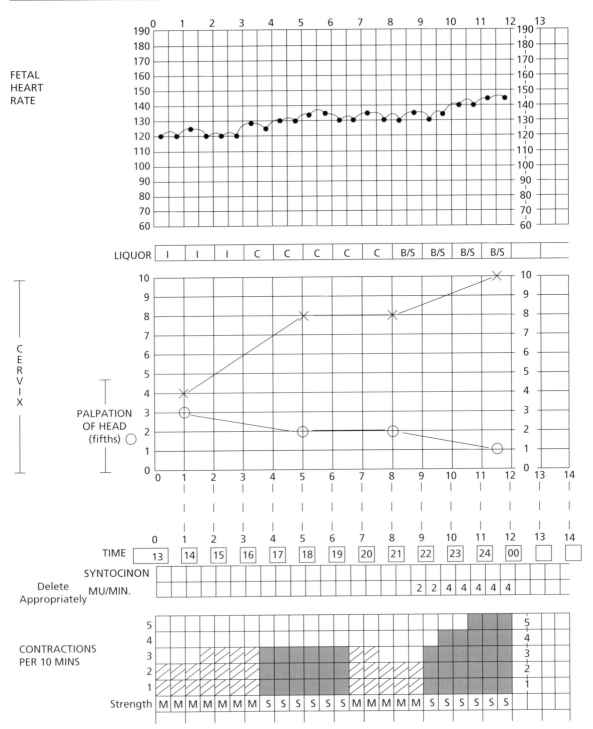

Fig. 20.2 Partogram of a woman in spontaneous labor who has had one previous normal delivery. After slightly slow progress in cervical dilation up to 8 cm there was cessation of progress. Contraction frequency declined slightly and an oxytocin infusion was commenced. Full dilatation was achieved, but delivery was complicated by severe shoulder dystocia. Time is shown on the horizontal axis in hours. Liquor – I – intact membranes, C – clear liquor, B/S – blood stained; X – cervical dilatation/cm; O – descent of the head abdominally in fifths.

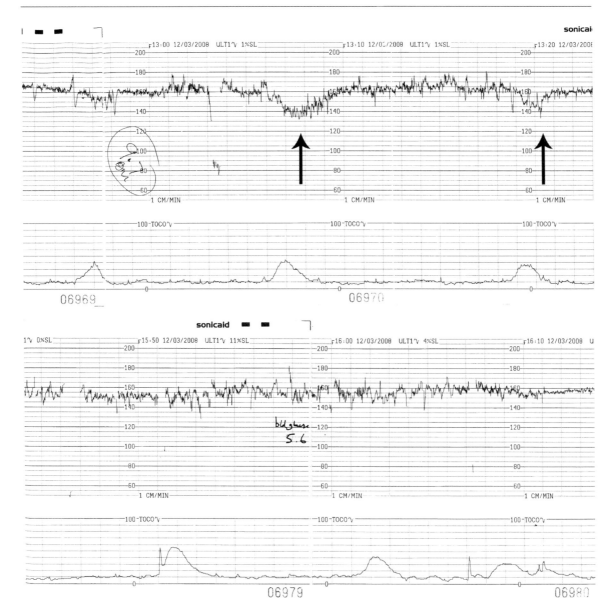

Fig. 20.3 Cardiotocograph (CTG) of a woman in early labor. This demonstrates the association between maternal hyperglycemia (blood glucose 9.7 mmol/L [175 mg/dL]– annotated on the CTG) and a pathologic fetal heart rate pattern (tachycardia and two decelerations which are marked with arrows) (top trace). With subsequent correction of the hyperglycemia (5.6 mmol/L [101 mg/dL] – annotated on the CTG), the fetal heart rate pattern became normal (normal rate and no decelerations) (bottom trace).

dystocia in all deliveries of diabetic women, whether birth is spontaneous or by low forceps or vacuum delivery, the attendants must be prepared for potential shoulder dystocia. Any early signs of shoulder dystocia should be acted upon using standard maneuvres, such as McRoberts position and suprapubic pressure. If operative deliv-

ery (other than low forceps/vacuum) is required, then an experienced obstetrician needs to make an assessment in the operating theater with good anesthesia. Unless there has been significant descent and rotation of the head during the time required to move the woman into the operating theater and to obtain effective anesthesia, then serious consideration should be given to recourse to a cesarean delivery. A relatively difficult delivery of the fetal head may well be followed by an extreme case of shoulder dystocia, followed, in turn, by brachial plexus injury, neonatal asphyxial brain damage, or both. About 10% of cases of documented shoulder dystocia in pregestational diabetes were followed by brachial plexus injury.[1]

There is wide variation in the rates of reported full recovery from such injury, but in the UK study of 276 cases only 52% had made a complete recovery by 6 months, with a partial recovery in 46% and no recovery in 2%.[19]

SPECIFIC ISSUES POSTNATALLY

Attempts must be made to manage the mother postnatally in a similar way to the non-diabetic mother, particularly with regard to the encouragement to breastfeed. There are some specific issues which require medical input.
- Reduction of insulin and blood glucose control is discussed in detail in chapter 21.
- Women with Type 2 diabetes may revert to oral hypoglycemic agents, such as metformin and glyburide (glibenclamide), even if they are breastfeeding (see chapter 11).
- There may be a need to revise antihypertensive regimes, including the recommencement of angiotensin-converting enzyme (ACE) inhibitors.
- With many women having a cesarean section, attention must be paid to the increased risks of wound infection associated with diabetes.
- Thromboprophylaxis for at least 5 days postnatally is recommended.
- Discussion should be commenced prior to discharge about contraception and possible family size limitations (see chapter 23).

FOLLOW-UP ARRANGEMENTS

Type 1 and Type 2 diabetes

On discharge from hospital, all women must have arrangements made for a follow-up review, typically at 6 weeks, but it may need to be earlier if required from a diabetic perspective. This may be either by the team that has looked after the woman in pregnancy or with the specialist diabetes team that normally supervises care, whether this is in the primary or secondary healthcare

sector. Women with Type 2 diabetes are at particular risk of missing out on optimum care, as demonstrated by the finding that in the year prior to pregnancy their care was less comprehensive than that for those with Type 1 diabetes.[28] For women who have developed significant retinopathy requiring ophthalmic specialist involvement, it is essential that ongoing follow-up is arranged (see chapter 17). As the ophthalmic team manages these women outside of the diabetic obstetric clinic, there is a risk that this communication will not occur and so an appointment with the ophthalmic team should be made prior to the woman's discharge from hospital.

Gestational diabetes

All women with abnormal glucose tolerance diagnosed during pregnancy should have arrangements made for an assessment of their glucose tolerance about 6 weeks post-delivery. It is controversial as to whether a full GTT is required or whether a fasting value is sufficient. Until this issue is resolved, it would seem prudent to advise blood glucose estimation in both the fasting state and also 2 hours after a 75-g glucose load. Those women with greater degrees of glucose intolerance during pregnancy may well have undiagnosed diabetes and it is vital that these women are followed up appropriately. For those who have persisting impaired glucose tolerance, lifestyle advice, including weight loss and daily exercise, as well as annual glucose testing (either fasting or a full GTT), are required. For those who revert to normal glucose tolerance, similar advice still needs to be given because of the long-term risks (see chapter 24).

CONCLUSIONS

While the evidence base is limited, a consensus view is that women with Type 1 and Type 2 diabetes should be offered elective delivery at 38–39 weeks, assuming no other maternal or fetal factors have caused significant concern previously. This should lower the risk of shoulder dystocia and probably of fetal death *in utero*.

Women with insulin-requiring gestational diabetes should be considered for elective intervention at 38–39 weeks as this is associated with a reduction in shoulder dystocia and birthweight, but no significant increase in cesarean rates. Women suspected clinically or on ultrasound to have a fetus with macrosomia should be considered for earlier induction at 37–38 weeks or for cesarean delivery. Women with gestational diabetes not requiring insulin therapy do not need specific intervention prior to term unless other factors are present.

All women with any form of diabetes should be assessed for vaginal delivery and individualized decisions made following discussion between the woman and her clinicians, taking into consideration both maternal and fetal factors. The practice of routine cesarean section for women with diabetes is inappropriate and centers which adopt such a policy should offer women the choice of delivering at another centre which does not have this policy. Women who have diabetes and who have had a previous cesarean section should be counseled in the same way as women without diabetes and advised to aim for a vaginal delivery unless there are other relevant factors.

Diabetic vascular complications alone are not an indication for cesarean delivery, although they may be associated with other maternal or fetal complications which make a cesarean the preferred option. Routine delivery by cesarean if macrosomia is suspected will result in a further increase in the already high cesarean rates with minimal benefit, as ultrasound-estimated weights are not that reliable and shoulder dystocia is unpredictable.

Cesarean section is not without its morbidity, particularly for those women who wish for a large family, and cases of brachial plexus injury still occur following cesarean delivery.

In labor specific care must be taken with regard to monitoring fetal condition, maintaining maternal normoglycemia, and watching for signs of potential disproportion.

Post-delivery attempts must be made to manage the mother in a similar way to those without diabetes, particularly with regard to the encouragement of breastfeeding. Diabetes management is covered in chapter 21. Follow-up arrangements must be made for all women (Type 1 and Type 2, and gestational diabetes) to advise on future management.

FUTURE DIRECTIONS

Research on the management of labor and delivery is sparse, and largely based on studies in gestational diabetes. The major issue, apart from the management of diabetes, is preventing asphyxial damage in labor and traumatic delivery without unnecessary recourse to routine cesarean section. This is closely linked to better antenatal prediction of shoulder dystocia and research on whether measurement of markers (such as erythropoietin, see chapter 12) can help predict the fetus at risk of developing asphyxia in labor. Whether centralization of care results in a higher rate of normal outcomes (nonpreterm, vaginal delivery, and a healthy baby) remains to be answered.

REFERENCES

1 Confidential Enquiry into Maternal and Child Health. *Pregnancy in Women with Type 1 and Type 2 Diabetes in 2002-03, England, Wales and Northern Ireland.* London: CEMACH, 2005. www.cemach.org.uk

2 Young RJ, Holmes EM, Casson IF, Maresh M. The North West Diabetic Pregnancy Audit: a practical system for multi-centre diabetic pregnancy audit. *Diabet Med* 2008;**25**:496–500.

3 Kjos SL, Henry OA, Montoro M, Buchanan TA, Mestman JH. Insulin-requiring diabetes in pregnancy: a randomised trial of active induction of labor and expectant management. *Am J Obstet Gynecol* 1993;**169**:611–15.

4 Lurie S, Insler V, Hagay ZJ. Induction of labor at 38 to 39 weeks of gestation reduces the incidence of shoulder dystocia in gestational diabetic patients class A2. *Am J Perinatol* 1996;**13**:293–6.

5 National Collaborating Centre for Women's and Children's Health. *Diabetes in Pregnancy: Management of Diabetes and its Complications from Preconception to the Postnatal Period.* London: RCOG, 2008.

6 ACOG Practice Bulletin. Clinical Management Guidelines for Obstetrician – Gynecolgists. Number 60, March 2005. Pregestational diabetes mellitus. *Obstet Gynecol* 2005;**105**:675–85.

7 Ehrenberg HM, Durnweld CP, Catalano P, Mercer BM. The influence of obesity and diabetes on the risk of cesarean delivery. *Am J Obstet Gynecol* 2004;**191**:969–74.

8 Crowther CA, Hiller JE, Moss JR, McPhee AJ, Jeffries WS, Robinson JS. Effect of treatment of gestational diabetes mellitus on pregnancy outcomes. *N Engl J Med* 2005;**352**:2477–86.

9 Naylor CD, Sermer M, Chen E, Sykora K. Cesarean delivery in relation to birth weight and gestational glucose tolerance. Pathophysiology or practice style? *JAMA* 1996;**275**:1165–70.

10 The HAPO Study Cooperative Research Group. Hyperglycemia and adverse pregnancy outcomes. *N Engl J Med* 2008;**358**:1991–2002.

11 Marchiano D, Elkousy M, Stevens E, *et al.* Diet controlled gestational diabetes mellitus does not influence the success rates for vaginal birth after cesarean delivery. *Am J Obstet Gynecol* 2004;**190**:790–6.

12 Coleman TL, Randall H, Graves W, *et al.* Vaginal birth after cesarean among women with gestational diabetes. *Am J Obstet Gynecol* 2001;**184**:1104–7.

13 Holt VL, Mueller BA. Attempt and success rates for vaginal birth after cesarean section in relation to complications of the previous pregnancy. *Paediatr Perinatal Epidemiol* 1997;**11** (Suppl 1):63–72.

14 Hadden DR, Alexander A, McCance DR, Traub AI. Obstetric and diabetic care for pregnancy in diabetic women: 10 years outcome analysis, 1985–1995. *Diabet Med* 2001;**18**:546–53.

15 Maresh M, Dawson A, Abdul-Azis, *et al*. Pregnancy outcome with Type I diabetes in seven tertiary centres in the United Kingdom. *J Obstet Gynaecol* 2000;**20** (Suppl 1):S63.

16 Macintosh M, Fleming K, Bailey J, *et al*. Perinatal mortality and congenital anomalies in babies of women with type 1 or type 2 diabetes in England, Wales, and Northern Ireland: population based study. *BMJ* 2006;**333**:177–80.

17 Nesbitt TS, Gilbert WM, Herrchen B. Shoulder dystocia and associated risk factors with macrosomic infants born in California. *Am J Obs Gynecol* 1998;**179**:476–80.

18 Ecker JL, Greenberg JA, Norwitz ER, Nadel AS, Repke JT. Birth weight as a predictor of brachial plexus injury. *Obstet Gynecol* 1997;**89**:643–7.

19 Evans-Jones G, Kay SPJ, Weindling AM, *et al*. Congenital brachial palsy: incidence, causes, and outcome in the United Kingdom and Republic of Ireland. *Arch Dis Child Fetal Neonatal Ed* 2003;**88**:F185–9.

20 Gherman RB, Chauhan S, Ouzounian JG, Lerner H, Gonik B, Goodwin TM. Shoulder dystocia: The unpreventable obstetric emergency with empiric management guidelines. *Am J Obstet Gynecol* 2006;**198**:657–72.

21 Conway DL, Langer O. Elective delivery of infants with macrosomia in diabetic women: reduced shoulder dystocia versus increased caesarean deliveries. *Am J Obstet Gynecol* 1998;**178**:922–5.

22 Rouse DJ, Owen J. Prophylactic cesarean delivery for fetal macrosomia diagnosed by means of ultrasonography – A Faustian bargain? *Am J Obstet Gynecol* 1999;**181**:332–8.

23 Knight M, Kurinczuk JJ, Spark P, Brocklehurst P. Cesarean delivery and peripartum hysterectomy. *Obstet Gynecol* 2008;**111**:97–105.

24 Lauszus FF, Fuglsang J, Flyvbjerg A, Klebe JG. Preterm delivery in normoalbuminuric, diabetic women without pre-eclampsia: The role of metabolic control. *Eur J Obstet Gynecol* 2006;**124**:144–9.

25 Clinical Effectiveness Support Unit. The Royal College of Obstetricians and Gynaecologists. The Use of Electronic Fetal Monitoring. London: RCOG Press, 2001. www.rcog.org.uk

26 Salvesen DR, Brudnell MJ, Proudler AJ, Crook D, Nicolaides KH. Fetal pancreatic beta-cell function in pregnancies complicated by maternal diabetes mellitus: relationship to fetal acidemia and macrosomia. *Am J Obstet Gynecol* 1993;**168**:1363–9.

27 Skupski DW, Rosenberg CR, Eglinton GS. Intrapartum fetal stimulation tests: a meta-analysis. *Obstet Gynecol* 2002;**99**:129–34.

28 Confidential Enquiry into Maternal and Child Health. *Diabetes in Pregnancy. Are We Providing the Best Care? Findings of a National Enquiry. England, Wales and Northern Ireland.* London: CEMACH, 2007. www.cemach.org.uk

21 Diabetic management in labor, delivery, and post delivery

Ciara McLaughlin & David R. McCance

Regional Centre for Endocrinology and Diabetes, Royal Victoria Hospital, Belfast, Northern Ireland, UK

PRACTICE POINTS

- Diabetic management during labor and delivery should be according to a standard protocol in centers with neonatal intensive care facilities.
- Maintenance of maternal euglycemia is essential to prevent neonatal hypoglycemia.
- Unless the neonate is symptomatic, blood glucose testing should be deferred until after the first feed to prevent unnecessary treatment or admission to neonatal intensive care.
- Post delivery, all mothers with diabetes should be encouraged to breastfeed and should be supported appropriately.
- Whether or not maternal use of oral hypoglycemic agents poses a risk to the breastfed infant of a diabetic woman is unresolved.

CASE HISTORY

A 32-year-old woman with a 15-year history of Type 1 diabetes presented to her family doctor at 13 weeks of gestation in her second pregnancy. At her last hospital review 6 months previously, no diabetic complications were noted. The current pregnancy was unplanned. Her hemoglobin A1c (HbA1c) at booking was significantly raised at 8.6%. Apart from insulin therapy (soluble preprandial insulin and isophane at bedtime) she was taking no other medication. She was referred urgently to the local joint diabetes antenatal clinic. Despite continuing advice, her attendance at the clinic was erratic, her home capillary glucose readings were frequently above target, and her HbA1c did not fall below 7%. Her labor was induced at 38 weeks of gestation. During labor, hourly maternal capillary blood glucose levels were maintained

A Practical Manual of Diabetes in Pregnancy, 1st Edition.
Edited by David R. McCance, Michael Maresh and David A. Sacks.
© 2010 Blackwell Publishing

between 5.2 and 7.1 mmol/L using an intravenous (IV) insulin/dextrose regime. She delivered a baby boy weighing 4500 g per vaginum. Four hours following delivery the baby appeared irritable and was slow to feed. Laboratory plasma glucose was 1.9 mmol/L (34 mg/dL) and the baby was admitted to neonatal intensive care for IV dextrose infusion. Subsequently the baby required tube feeding for 24 hours until normal feeding was established. The baby was exclusively bottle fed. When the mother was able to tolerate food her insulin requirements were adjusted to doses approximating the prepregnancy insulin regime.

- What is the relevance of intrapartum glycemic control to neonatal hypoglycemia?
- What is the target maternal glucose level during labor?
- How should this be achieved?
- What are the issues regarding maternal insulin requirements postpartum?
- What advice should be given to the mother regarding breastfeeding and diabetes?
- What are the differences in management between women with Type 1 diabetes, Type 2 diabetes, and gestational diabetes?

BACKGROUND

Diabetic pregnancy continues to present a substantial risk for both mother and baby.[1-4] Much of this risk occurs at the time of labor and delivery. This book has highlighted the critical role of optimal diabetes control and obstetric care prior to and during pregnancy in order to reduce and eliminate some of these adverse outcomes. Equally important is the management of diabetes in labor, delivery, and post delivery, and this should interface seamlessly with antenatal diabetes care. Poor or inappropriate diabetes management at this time can have major implications for the well-being of the mother and neonate. The focus of the physician caring for the diabetic woman during labor is to maintain normal maternal blood glucose levels in order to prevent maternal ketoacidosis, to avoid fetal acidemia with unnecessary intervention, and to reduce the risk of neonatal hypoglycemia with its subsequent separation of mother and baby.[2] After delivery, regular diabetic supervision is required to ensure the stability of maternal glycemia in the face of changing insulin requirements. The postpartum period also provides a unique opportunity to influence behavior that may have significant implications for the long-term health of both mother and child.

PATHOPHYSIOLOGY

In the normal pregnancy without diabetes, despite an increase in insulin resistance, blood glucose levels remain between 4.0 mmol/L and 4.5 mmol/L (72–81 mg/dL). This corresponds to a doubling of insulin secretion by beta cells in the pancreas. Glucose passes from mother to fetus via facilitated diffusion, whereas insulin (unless antibody bound) does not cross the placenta at physiologic concentrations. In pregnancy complicated by Type 1 diabetes, the physiologic change in pancreatic beta cell function usually observed in normal pregnancy is impaired. The dose of insulin required tends to increase as the pregnancy progresses. This results from the physiologic increase in insulin resistance caused by maternal diabetogenic hormones, including increased free cortisol levels and the secretion of several pregnancy-related hormones, such as human placental lactogen. Under the Pedersen hypothesis,[1] it is envisaged that maternal hyperglycemia promotes abnormal stimulation of the fetal pancreatic beta cells, resulting in marked fetal hyperinsulinemia. This mechanism can potentially explain many of the fetal complications seen during labor and delivery.

Type 2 and gestational diabetes are associated with both increased insulin resistance and abnormalities of insulin secretion (see chapter 2). During pregnancy, there is an increase in insulin resistance that facilitates growth and diversion of glucose to the fetus. In pregnancy complicated by Type 2 diabetes, the ability to increase insulin production via hypertrophy and hyperplasia of pancreatic beta cells is impaired.

LOCATION OF DELIVERY

It is recommended that pregnancy, labor, and delivery of women with pregestational and gestational diabetes should be supervised in centers with tertiary maternal and neonatal care, particularly in the US, where the levels of obstetric and neonatal care vary substantially from one hospital to the next. As there is a substantial risk of neonatal hypoglycemia and other complications, close monitoring and supervision are required. Although traditionally, many infants were admitted to a specialist neonatal unit, this is probably unnecessary in the majority of cases and should be reserved for standard peridelivery problems and/or for those babies suffering from significant neonatal hypoglycemia.[2,4]

PRETERM LABOR

Use of tocolytic agents and antenatal steroids

Preterm labor can be particularly hazardous for the infant of the diabetic mother. Beta-sympathomimetic agents, which may be used to suppress uterine contractions, are capable of causing rapid and extreme elevations in maternal glucose concentrations and possibly ketoacidosis. Corticosteroids, used to accelerate fetal lung maturation, may also result in significant and prolonged maternal hyperglycemia. During treatment with these drugs, regular diabetes supervision is essential. Maternal glucose should be carefully monitored, hourly if necessary, and 2–4 hourly once maternal glucose levels are stable. Even women with gestational diabetes may have their diabetes control worsened significantly; they must also have regular monitoring of their glucose levels and insulin may be required.

Various glucose/insulin algorithms involving increased insulin dosage have been described, and this requirement should be anticipated. We have successfully used an algorithm comprising additional doses of subcutaneous insulin during steroid treatment (intramuscular administration of betamethasone 12 mg repeated after 12 hours), aiming to maintain preprandial glucose levels below 6 mmol/L (<108 mg/dL) without excessive hypoglycemia.[5] This algorithm which is administered as an inpatient involves:

1 Day 1 (the day on which the first dose of betamethasone is given): the night time dose of insulin is increased by 30%
2 Day 2: all insulin doses are increased by 50%
3 Day 3: all insulin doses are increased by 50%
4 Day 4: all insulin doses are increased by 30%
5 Day 5: all insulin doses are increased by 20%
6 Days 6 and 7: the insulin dose is gradually reduced to presteroid levels.

A broadly similar, although less aggressive, approach has been employed in Scandanavia.[6] Another group[7] reported its experience of a supplementary intravenous sliding scale (in addition to the woman's usual subcutaneous insulin regime) to indicate the required dosage of insulin infusion in six women receiving antenatal steroids. The additional infusion was commenced immediately before the first steroid injection and continued until 12 hours after the second injection. Patients moved up to a higher level of insulin administration as dictated by glucose levels. Using this method, 75% of all glucose measurements were within 4–10 mmol/L (72–180 mg/dL).

The UK Confidential Enquiry into Maternal and Child Health (CEMACH)[2,3] highlighted that only 293 of 328 women giving birth before 34 weeks received a full course of antenatal steroids; the most common reason for non-administration was birth of the baby before the full course could be given.

Summary of recommendations

- When tocolysis is indicated in women with diabetes, an alternative to betamimetics should be used to avoid hyperglycemia and ketoacidosis.
- The use of antenatal steroids for fetal lung maturation with diabetes is associated with a significant worsening of glycemic control and this must be anticipated.
- Women with insulin-treated diabetes who are receiving steroids for fetal lung maturation should be closely monitored and receive supplementary insulin according to an agreed protocol.
- Further appraisal of the optimal methods to achieve euglycemia in this context is needed.

EVIDENCE IN SUPPORT OF THE NEED FOR GOOD GLUCOSE CONTROL DURING LABOR

Neonatal hypoglycemia

This is a relatively common complication following birth among infants of mothers with diabetes, with prevalence rates ranging from 10% to 60%.[8–10] It is well recognized that blood glucose in the neonate tends to fall early after birth, reaching a nadir between 1 and 2 hours. This is an almost universal finding and is unlikely to be of pathologic significance. Subsequently, even in the absence of nutritional intake, blood glucose rises significantly by 3 hours of age. The diagnosis of hypoglycemia therefore

requires the persistence of neonatal hypoglycemia beyond the first few hours of birth as these babies have failed to mount an appropriate lipolytic and ketogenic response. The aim is to minimize the incidence and severity of hypoglycemia (<2.6 mmol/L [<47 mg/dL]) by early feeding and careful monitoring. This level is not necessarily used to diagnose the condition, but does indicate the level at which further intervention may be required. This is based on a study which showed that adverse neurodevelopmental outcomes were associated with repeated values below this level.[11] The presumptive mechanism is thought to be neonatal hyperinsulinism resulting from hyperglycemia during labor, although a persisting autonomous fetal insulin secretion may also occur earlier in pregnancy in poorly controlled maternal diabetes.[12]

The results of a series of observational studies, summarized in Table 21.1,[13–18] are in general agreement that neonatal hypoglycemia is closely related to maternal hyperglycemia in labor and during delivery. In addition, in a retrospective study involving 107 women with Type 1 diabetes, Taylor et al[10] showed that neonatal hypoglycemia correlated with maternal hyperglycemia in labor, but not with HbA1c during pregnancy.

Fetal acidemia

It has also long been recognized that maternal hyperglycemia is associated with an increased risk of fetal acidemia. Two observational studies in women with Type 1 diabetes considered the effect of intrapartum blood glucose control on fetal distress. In one study of 149 subjects,[19] perinatal asphyxia was reported in 27% (n = 40). The maximum maternal blood glucose during labor was higher in babies with perinatal asphyxia than in those without (9.5 ± 3.7 vs 7.0 ± 3.0 mmol/L [171 ± 67 vs 126 ± 54 mg/dL]; p < 0.0001). In the other study of 65 subjects,[17] mean blood glucose during labor in women using continuous subcutaneous insulin infusion (CSII) (n = 28) was 4.8 ± 0.6 mmol/L (86 ± 11 mg/dL) (range 3.8–5.8 mmol/L) compared with 7.2 ± 1.1 mmol/L (130 ± 20 mg/dL) (range 5.6–8.3 mmol/L) (p < 0.025) among those using a constant IV insulin infusion (n = 37). Acute fetal distress occurred in 27% of the IV infusion group versus 14.3% of the CSII group (p < 0.001); cesarean section occurred in 38% versus 25% (p < 0.05), respectively.

These data suggest that maintenance of maternal blood glucose between 4 and 7 mmol/L (72–126 mg/dL) during labor and delivery reduces the incidence of both neonatal hypoglycemia and "fetal distress".[4]

Table 21.1 Observational studies which have examined the relation between intrapartum capillary blood glucose (CBG) and neonatal hypoglycaemia (NH).

Authors (year)	Subjects	Methods/definitions	Findings
Andersen et al[13] (1985)	53 Type 1	Plasma glucose measured at birth and 2 h later; NH (<1.7 mmol/L [<31 mg/dL])	Maternal BG at birth correlated positively with neonatal BG at birth (r = 0.82; p <0.001) and negatively with neonatal BG at 2 h (r = –0.46; p < 0.001); If maternal BG at birth was >7.1 mmol/L (>128 mg/dL) (11/30) 37% rate of NH vs 0% if maternal BG < 7.1 mmol/L (<128 mg/dL)
Miodovnik et al[14] (1987)	122 Type 1	IV glucose ± insulin infused to maintain CBG 3.9–5.6 mmol/L (70–101 mg/dl); NH (< 1.7 mmol/L [< 31 mg/dl])	47% babies whose mothers had CBG > 5 mmol/L (>90 mg/dL) developed NH compared to 14% with CBG < 5 mmol/L (<90 mg/dL)
Curet et al[15] (1997)	233 insulin-requiring (77 Type 1, 156 Type 2)	Day of delivery – 10% glucose/fructose infusion; IV insulin at 1–4 U/h to maintain BG 3.3–5.0 mmol/L (59–90 mg/dL); NH (< 1.7 mmol/L [< 31 mg/dL])	Incidence of NH was 16.5%. Mean intrapartum BG level was significantly lower in mothers of babies without hypoglycemia (p < 0.05)
Lean et al[16] (1990)	29 insulin-treated	See Protocol 2 (Table 21.3)	NH occurred in 11 babies; neonatal BG correlated negatively with maternal BG at delivery (r_s = –0.58, p < 0.01)
Feldberg et al[17] (1988)	65 Type 1	Comparison of CSII (n = 28) with constant IV insulin infusion (n = 37)	8 cases of NH in constant IV insulin group; no cases in CSII group (p < 0.05)
Balsells et al[18] (2000)	54 insulin-treated	IV glucose (8.3 g/h); IV insulin infusion via syringe pump	5 babies developed NH; maternal BG in last 2 h of birth was associated with NH

RECOMMENDATIONS FOR THE MANAGEMENT OF GLYCEMIC CONTROL DURING LABOR AND DELIVERY

The main objective of glycemic control during labor is to avoid maternal hyperglycemia in order to minimize the risks of neonatal hypoglycemia and fetal acidemia as discussed above.

With elective cesarean delivery

- The physician (see below) responsible for care during labor should be informed of the admission.
- Women should ideally be first on the operating list.

- The mother should fast from 22.00 h the previous evening (except for sips of water).
- The woman is allowed to take her long-acting insulin the preceding evening as usual, but does not take her usual insulin on the morning of delivery.
- A glucose/insulin infusion is begun 1–2 hours before surgery.
- Close liaison is required with the anesthesiologist (anesthetist).
- Maternal capillary blood glucose should be monitored hourly.
- The aim is to maintain blood glucose levels between 4 and 7 mmol/L (72–126 mg/dL) according to protocol.
- The dose of insulin is adjusted in response to maternal capillary glucose.

In the UK, the physician is usually a diabetologist or internist specializing in diabetes, while the obstetrician manages the obstetric care and a neonatologist is present at delivery. In the US, it is more customary for the obstetrician in consultation with the perinatologist, the perinatologist exclusively, or the obstetrician in consultation with both the perinatologist and endocrinologist (diabetologist), to manage all aspects of the patient's care during pregnancy, labor, and delivery

With induction of labor

- For standard induction with prostaglandins, women should continue to eat normally and to have their normal doses of insulin until in established labor.
- Once labor is established, a regime of IV dextrose/insulin is commenced.
- Maternal capillary blood glucose should be monitored hourly.
- The aim is to maintain blood glucose levels between 4 and 7 mmol/L (72–126 mg/dL) according to protocol.
- The dose of insulin is adjusted in response to maternal capillary glucose.

With spontaneous labor

- The capillary glucose should be measured on admission and thereafter hourly.
- If the capillary glucose is between 4 and 7 mmol/L (72–126 mg/dl) and delivery is imminent, hourly glucose measurement should be continued.
- If capillary glucose is greater than 7 mmol/L (>126 mg/dL) or delivery is not imminent, an IV dextrose/insulin infusion should be commenced as per protocol.
- The subsequent steps are as for induction of labor (see above).

For mothers with gestational diabetes controlled on diet alone, maternal capillary blood glucose should be monitored every 1–2 hours once labor is established with the aim of keeping levels below 7 mmol/L (<126 mg/dL). If this is not achieved, an insulin/dextrose infusion may be required. Women with gestational diabetes who required insulin during the course of their pregnancy should be treated as detailed for women who required insulin during pregnancy.

Women with Type 1 diabetes who use a CSII in pregnancy should have an agreed plan documented as to how blood glucose is to be achieved during labor and delivery. It is usually feasible to continue using CSII in labor and good results have been achieved. For example, in the study of Feldberg et al[17] (see below), the insulin dosage was extended from pregnancy into labor and ranged between 0.5 and 1.2 U/h. However, delivery unit staff may have anxieties about this approach due to unfamiliarity, thus necessitating the close involvement of medical personnel trained to adjust the CSII pump. Similarly, with cesarean section, anesthesiologists (anesthetists) may prefer to revert to an intravenous insulin regime.

MATERNAL BLOOD GLUCOSE CONTROL DURING LABOR AND DELIVERY

There is no consensus over how best to achieve optimal maternal glucose control during labor and delivery. Perhaps the critical point is that the method of insulin delivery with which the physician and nursing staff are most familiar is the one which should be used. The first stage of labor is associated with a decrease in the need for insulin and a constant glucose requirement.[20] Most of the data are observational and many regimes have arisen through personal experience. Details of three protocols are outlined by way of illustration. In Belfast, for many years we have successfully used an intravenous glucose/insulin infusion supplemented by additional insulin doses (Protocol 1; Table 21.2).[21] Alternatively, some centers use a constant glucose infusion with insulin being infused separately by an infusion pump. The latter type of protocol was assessed during labor in 25 women with insulin-treated diabetes (Protocol 2; Table 21.3)[16]. Blood glucose was maintained at 6.0 ± 1.8 mmol/L (108 ± 32 mg/dL) for a mean of 6 hours before delivery. Neonatal hypoglycemia (plasma glucose <2.0 mmol/L [36 mg/dL]) occurred in 11 (44%) babies. A further protocol was evaluated in terms of its ability to achieve normoglycemia during labor and delivery among 229 pregnancies in 174 women with Type 1 diabetes (Protocol 3; Table 21.4).[22] Maternal glycemia during labor was 6.1 ± 1.6 mmol/L (110 ± 29 mg/dL) with a 13% incidence of neonatal hypoglycemia.

Feldberg et al[17] in a small non-randomized trial of subjects with Type 1 diabetes, showed a significant decrease in neonatal hypoglycemia using CSII (maintained throughout gestation and delivery) (n = 28) compared with those using an IV regime (n = 39). Neonatal hypoglycemia occurred in 8% of infants in the IV insulin regime group and not at all in the CSII group; however, the subjects may have been self-selecting, leading to some bias. A randomized controlled trial[23] examined the influence of rotating glucose-containing and glucose-free IV

Table 21.2 Protocol 1. (adapted from [21])

At onset of established labor or before cesarean section:

Maternal capillary blood glucose (mmol/L [mg/dL])	5% dextrose infusion (mL)	Insulin (short acting) added to each 500 mL (U)	Time for 500 mL infusion (h)	Drops per minute
< 2.0 [36]	500	0	2	84
2.0–3.9 [36–70]	500	0	6	28
4.0–7.9 [72–142]	500	6	6	28
8.0–11.9 [144–214]	500	12	6	28
12.0–15.9 [216–287]	500	16	6	28
>16 [288l]	Contact diabetes staff			

- Postpartum the 5% dextrose glucose/insulin infusion is maintained until the subject is eating; supplementary doses of insulin are halved.
- Approximately half of the normal subcutaneous prepregnancy dose is given, adjusted to amount of food intake, and rapidly titrated to capillary blood glucose levels.
- Mother's blood glucose target is relaxed to range 6–8 mmol/L (108–144 mg/dL) before meals.

Table 21.3 Protocol 2.[16]

At onset of established labor or at breakfast time before induction/cesarean section:
- Nil by mouth until after delivery
- Start IV dextrose 10% containing KCl 1 g (13 mmoL) in 500 mL, 100 mL/h via IMED pump
- Hourly blood glucose estimation by glucose meter
- Set up insulin infusion by IV pump, mounted onto the IV line, initially at 2 U/h when blood glucose > 7 mmol/L (>126 mg/dL) (50 U human soluble insulin in 50 mL of 0.9% saline, 2 ml/h)
- Adjust insulin infusion rate to maintain blood glucose at 4.0–7.0 mmol/L (72–126 mg/dL) according to glucose meter:
  - If <4 mmol/L (<72 mg/dL), and not rising: decrease insulin by 1 U/h to a minimum of 0.5 U/h
  - If >7.0 mmol/L (>126 mg/dL), and not falling: increase insulin by 0.5 U/h

After delivery of the placenta:
- Halve the rate of insulin infusion, to a minimum of 0.5 U/h
- Adjust as before to maintain blood glucose at 4.0–7.0 mmol/L (72–126 mg/dL)
- Refer to medical records or contact diabetic clinic team for advice about subcutaneous insulin dose before next main meal (usually about 50% of total daily insulin during late pregnancy)
- Stop IV fluids and insulin 30 min after subcutaneous insulin

Table 21.4 Protocol 3.[22]

Commence protocol on morning of delivery or following admission in spontaneous labor:
- 10% dextrose solution IV at 80 mL/h
- Short-acting insulin IV using an infusion pump, starting at 1 U/h
- Capillary blood glucose (CBG) measured hourly until delivery
- Target CBG values are 3.4–7.8 mmol/L (61–140 mg/dL) and the insulin infusion is adapted as follows:
  - Maintain at 1 U/h if CBG 3.4–7.8 mmol/L (61–140 mg/dL)
  - Increase to 1.5 U/h if CBG 7.8–10.0 mmol/l (140–180 mg/dL)
  - Increase to 2 U/h if CBG 10.0–12.2 mmol/L (180–220 mg/dL)
  - Increase to 3 U/h if CBG above12.2 mmol/L (220 mg/dL)
- In the case of hypoglycemia (CBG ≤ 3.3 mmol/lL [≤59 mg/dL]), stop the insulin infusion for 30 min and if the CBG remains low give 30% dextrose IV

fluids *versus* an insulin infusion on intrapartum maternal glycemic control in women with insulin-requiring diabetes. There was no difference in mean maternal capillary blood glucose levels in the two groups (5.77±0.48 mmol/L [104 ± 9 mg/dL] *vs* 5.73 ± 0.99 mmol/L [103 ± 18 mg/dL],

respectively; p = 0.89). Neonatal hypoglycemia (blood glucose < 0.6 mmol/L [<11 mg/dL] within the first 24 hours) was 6.7 *versus* 19% in the two groups, respectively, but this and various other outcome measures were not significantly different between the two groups. In subjects without diabetes, Singhi[24] reported that rates of neonatal hypoglycemia were three times higher in mothers who had received intrapartum glucose therapy compared with those who had not, although a later randomized comparison did not confirm these findings.[25]

MATERNAL GLUCOSE CONTROL POSTPARTUM

As soon as the cord is cut, the rate of the insulin infusion should be approximately halved as insulin sensitivity returns to normal within minutes of the shutdown of the utero-placental circulation. Regular capillary blood glucose readings and intravenous fluids are continued until the mother is able to eat normally. For those with Type 1 diabetes, insulin requirements tend to fall substantially after delivery. As a general rule, it is usually reasonable for the women to resume her usual insulin regime in doses approximating those used prepregnancy. Regular diabetes supervision, however, is required at this time to review the insulin needs, which will also vary depending on whether or not the mother has chosen to breastfeed. In the latter situation, lower doses of insulin may be required (see below).

For mothers with Type 2 diabetes, again insulin requirements fall to near prepregnancy levels. Insulin should be withdrawn with regular monitoring of capillary blood glucose. At this point, the mother will usually return to the method by which her diabetes was controlled prior to conception, although this may vary depending on whether or not she intends to breastfeed. Those mothers who were previously on oral hypoglycemic agents can resume these agents postpartum if they do not intend to breastfeed. If breastfeeding is desired, the question of whether or not to prescribe oral hypoglycemic agents is controversial and will depend on individual circumstances and assessment of the risks and benefits (see chapter 11). If blood glucose levels, after careful monitoring, are not satisfactory with dietary measures alone, insulin should be reinstituted for a period. The mother may be able to return to oral hypoglycemic therapy once breastfeeding has ceased.

For those patients with gestational diabetes, insulin can usually be discontinued following delivery. Capillary glucose monitoring should continue for several days to ensure a return of both fasting and postprandial values to the normal range. If these are satisfactory, blood testing can cease and the patient is booked for formal assessment of glucose tolerance and review approximately 6 weeks after delivery.

BREASTFEEDING

Dietetic advice at this stage is essential. The recommendation is that postpartum calorie requirements are increased from 25 kcal/kg/day for non-breastfeeding women to 27 kcal/kg/day for those women who wish to breastfeed (based on postpartum weight). The optimal insulin program must be individualized but is guided by home blood glucose monitoring results. Because maternal hypoglycemia is most likely to occur within an hour of breastfeeding, this is an important time to measure blood glucose. In most cases, hypoglycemia can be avoided by eating a small snack before breastfeeding rather than making excessive adjustment of insulin dosage. During lactation, nocturnal insulin requirements fall due to glucose siphoning into the breast milk; thus most of the insulin requirement is during the day to cover the increased caloric needs of breastfeeding.[20] As high maternal glucose levels elevate milk glucose, the aim should be to keep maternal glycemia as normal as possible.

Unfortunately, the intention-to-breastfeed rate in women with diabetes is lower than the initial breastfeeding rate in the general population,[2] and even for those intending to breastfeed, there are a number of barriers to this happening successfully. A recent CEMACH survey reported a lack of early close contact and early feeding on the delivery unit, as well as high rates of infant formula being given as the first feed as relevant factors.[2] The CEMACH survey also found that one-third of all admissions to a neonatal unit (NICU) were due to a standard unit policy of admitting well babies of mothers with diabetes. Half of these admissions were felt to be avoidable.[2] This prolonged separation of mother and child due to NICU admission, along with the fact that often infant formula is given to all babies admitted to the NICU, even if the mother had expressed an earlier wish to breastfeed, may contribute to reduced rates of breastfeeding.

There are of course other perceived benefits of breastfeeding for both mother and child, which, in the absence of contraindications, have lead to it being strongly recommended for all mothers with diabetes whether pregestational or gestational.

A study by Kjos et al[26] looked at the effect of lactation on glucose metabolism in 809 primarily Latino women. These women were assessed using an oral glucose tolerance test between 4 and 12 weeks postpartum. The postpartum glucose results were significantly lower in the breastfeeding group. Those who did not breastfeed developed postpartum diabetes at a two-fold higher rate than those women who did. These results persisted when controlled for relevant risk factors.

A significant amount of epidemiologic research has examined the relationship between breastfeeding and chronic disease.[27] Several studies have suggested that breastfeeding has a protective effect against obesity in childhood and adulthood.[28–30] A meta-analysis of 17 studies by Harder et al[31] found that the duration of breastfeeding was inversely associated with the risk of being overweight with a dose-dependent relationship. In a longitudinal cohort study among 720 Pima Indians aged 10–39 years who had been breastfed exclusively in the first 2 months of life, there was a 59% reduction in the rate of Type 2 diabetes compared with those who were exclusively bottle fed.[32] Plagemann et al[33] suggested that early neonatal ingestion of breast milk from women with diabetes (compared with those ingesting donor milk) may increase the risk of becoming overweight. In another study, however, no association was found between either neonatal breast milk intake or duration of breastfeeding on childhood risk of being overweight or having impaired glucose tolerance when these children were studied in infancy.[34] A link between breastfeeding and lower rates of Type 1 diabetes has also been established.[35]

Some of these studies involve populations with high rates of Type 2 diabetes and obesity that limit their generalization to all populations. Further research is required in this important area given the increasing incidence of gestational and Type 2 diabetes within women of reproductive age.

Three authoritative bodies recommend a 6-month period of exclusive breastfeeding with continued breastfeeding for a total period of 12 months.[36–38]

Oral hypoglycemic agents and breastfeeding

With the rise of gestational and Type 2 diabetes among women of child-bearing age, and the likely increase in the use of oral hypoglycemic agents for the management of gestational diabetes following recently published data,[39,40] the question of the safety of these drugs during breastfeeding has become more important. Many women with Type 2 diabetes will be taking oral hypoglycemic agents prior to pregnancy. Currently, the majority of these are switched to insulin during pregnancy, but this may also change in the future as has been discussed elsewhere in this book. At present the wisdom of prescribing oral hypoglycemic drugs to breastfeeding mothers remains uncertain. The small number of studies that have looked at the passage of oral hypoglycemic agents into breast milk are reviewed in chapter 11. If a mother is keen to breastfeed, she should be encouraged to do so, and the physician must weigh up the risks and benefits of each individual case, including her willingness to continue

with, or the availability of, insulin therapy. Recently published UK guidelines support the ingestion of glibenclamide and metformin in breastfeeding mothers.[4]

SUMMARY AND FUTURE DIRECTIONS

Women with pregestational and gestational diabetes should be delivered in centers capable of providing tertiary maternal and neonatal care according to standard protocols. The literature is concordant that the risks of neonatal hypoglycemia and fetal distress are minimized by optimal maternal glucose control in labor and during delivery. There is a lack of consensus on how best to define and achieve optimal maternal glycemic control, and randomized trials comparing CSII with more traditional glucose/insulin infusions may be of use in this regard. With the rising tide of gestational and Type 2 diabetes, the issues surrounding lactation have become more pertinent. Further study is needed to examine the safety of oral hypoglycemic drugs in breastfeeding women.

REFERENCES

1 Pedersen J. The Pregnant Diabetic and her Newborn – Problems and Management. Copenhagan: Munksgaard, 1977.
2 Confidential Enquiry into Maternal and Child Health. Diabetes in Pregnancy: Are We Providing the Best Care? Findings of a National Enquiry: England, Wales and Northern Ireland. London: CEMACH, 2007.
3 Confidential Enquiry into Maternal and Child Health. Pregnancy in Women with Type 1 and Type 2 Diabetes in 2002–2003, England, Wales and Northern Ireland. London: CEMACH, 2005. www.cemach.org.uk
4 National Institute for Clinical Excellence. Diabetes in Pregnancy: Management of Diabetes and its Complications from Pre-conception to the Postnatal Period. London: NICE, 2008. www.nice.org.uk/CG063
5 Kennedy A, Hadden DR, Ritchie CM, Gray O, McCance DR. Insulin algorithm for glycemic control following corticosteroid therapy in type 1 diabetic pregnancy. Irish J Med Sci 2003;172:40.
6 Mathiesen ER, Christensen AB, Hellmuth E, et al. Insulin dose during glucocorticoid treatment for fetal lung maturation in diabetic pregnancy: test of an algorithm. Acta Obstet Gynecol Scand 2002;81:835–9.
7 Kaushal K, Gibson J, Ralton A. A protocol for improved glycaemic control following corticosteroid therapy in diabetic pregnancies. Diabet Med 2003;20:73–5.
8 Berk MA, Mimouni F, Miodovnik M, et al. Macrosomia in infants of insulin dependent diabetic mothers. Pediatrics 1989;83:1029–34.

9 Evers IM, Valk H, Visser GHA. Risk of complications of pregnancy in women with type 1 diabetes: nationwide prospective study in the Netherlands. *BMJ* 2004;**328**:915–8.

10 Taylor R, Lee C, Kyne-Grebalski D, *et al.* Clinical outcomes of pregnancy in women with type 1 diabetes. *Obstet Gynecol* 2002;**99**:537–41.

11 Lucas A, Morley R, Cole TJ. Adverse neurodevelopmental outcome of moderate neonatal hypoglycaemia. *BMJ* 1988;**297**:1304–8.

12 Pedersen J. Weight and length at birth of infants of diabetic mothers. *Acta Endocrinol* 1954;**16**:330–42.

13 Andersen O, Hertel J, Schmolker L, *et al.* Influence of the maternal plasma glucose concentration at delivery on the risk of hypoglycaemia in infants of insulin-dependent diabetic mothers. *Acta Paediatr Scand* 1985;**74**:268–73.

14 Miodovnik M, Mimouni F, Tsang RC. Management of the insulin-dependent diabetic during labor and delivery. Influences on neonatal outcome. *Am J Perinatol* 1987;**4**:106–14.

15 Curet LB, Izquierdo LA, Gilson GJ, *et al.* Relative effects of antepartum and intrapartum maternal blood glucose levels on incidence of neonatal hypoglycaemia. *J Perinatol* 1997;**17**:113–5.

16 Lean ME, Pearson DW, Sutherland HW. Insulin management during labour and delivery in mothers with diabetes. *Diabet Med* 1990;**7**:162–4.

17 Feldberg D, Dicker D, Samuel N, *et al.* Intrapartum management of insulin-dependent diabetes mellitus (IDDM) gestants. A comparative study of constant intravenous insulin infusion and continuous subcutaneous insulin infusion pump (CSIIP). *Acta Obstet Gynecol Scand* 1988;**67**:338–8.

18 Balsells M, Corcoy R, Adelantado JM, *et al.* Gestational diabetes mellitus: Metabolic control during labour. *Diabetes Nutr Metab* 2000;**13**:257–62.

19 Mimouni F, Miodovnik M, Siddiqi TA, Khoury J, Tsang RC. Perinatal asphyxia in infants of diabetic mothers is associated with maternal vasulopathy and hyperglycaemia in labour. *J Paediatr* 1988;**113**(2):345–53.

20 Jovanovic L, Kitzmiller JL. Insulin therapy in pregnancy. In: Hod M, Jovanovic L, Di Renzo GC, de Leiva A, Langer O (eds). *Textbook of Diabetes and Pregnancy*, 2nd edn. London: Informa Healthcare; 2008:205.

21 Watt P, Hughes J, Moore A, Traub AI, Hadden DR. A protocol for diabetes in pregnancy. In: Dornhorst A, Hadden DR (eds). *Diabetes and Pregnancy: An International Approach to Diagnosis and Management*. Chichester: Wiley, 1996:253–64.

22 Lepercq J, Abbou H, Agostini C, *et al.* A standardised protocol to achieve normoglycaemia during labour and delivery in women with type 1 diabetes. *Diabet Metab* 2008;**34**:33–37.

23 Rosenberg VA, Eglinton GS, Rauch ER, *et al.* Intrapartum maternal glycaemic control in women with insulin requiring diabetes: a randomised clinical trial of rotating fluids versus insulin drip. *Am J Obstet Gynecol* 2006;**195**:1095–9.

24 Singhi S. Effect of maternal intrapartum glucose therapy on neonatal blood glucose levels and neurobehavioural status of hypoglycaemic term newborn infants. *J Perinat Med* 1988;**16**:217–24.

25 Nordstrom L, Arulkumaran S, Chau S, *et al.* Continuous maternal glucose infusion during labor: effects on maternal and fetal glucose and lactate levels. *Am J Perinatol* 1995;**12**:357–62.

26 Kjos SL, Henry O, Lee RM, Buchanan TA, Mishell DR. The effect of lactation on glucose and lipid metabolism in women with recent gestational diabetes. *Obstet Gynecol* 1993;**82**:451–5.

27 Davis MK. Breast feeding and chronic disease in childhood and adolescence. *Pediatr Clin North Am* 2001;**48**:125–41.

28 Von kries R, Koletzko B, Sauerwald T, *et al.* Breast feeding and obesity: cross-sectional study. *BMJ* 1999;**319**:147–50.

29 von Kries R, Koletzko B, Sauerwald T, *et al.* Does breast feeding protect against childhood obesity? *Adv Exp Med Biol* 2000;**478**:29–39.

30 Ravelli AC, van der Meulen JH, Osmond C, Barker DJ, Bleker OP. Infant feeding and adult glucose tolerance, lipid profile, blood pressure and obesity. *Arch Dis Child* 2000;**82**:248–52.

31 Harder T, Bergmann R, Kallischnigg G, Plagemann A. Duration of breastfeeding and risk of overweight: A meta-analysis. *Am J Epidemiol* 2005;**162**:397–403.

32 Pettitt DJ, Forman MR, Hanson RL, Knowler WC, Bennett PH. Breast feeding and incidence of non-insulin dependent diabetes mellitus in Pima Indians. *Lancet* 1997;**350**:166–8.

33 Plagemann A, Harder T, Franke, *et al.* Long-term impact of neonatal breast feeding on body weight and glucose tolerance in children of diabetic mothers. *Diabetes Care* 2002;**25**:16–22.

34 Rodekamp E, Harder T, Kohlhoff R, *et al.* Long-term impact of breast feeding on body weight and glucose tolerance in children of diabetic mothers: role of the late neonatal period and early infancy. *Diabetes Care* 2005;**28**:1457–62.

35 Dosch HM, Becker DJ. Infant feeding and autoimmune diabetes. *Adv Exp Med Biol* 2002;**503**:133–40.

36 Satcher DS. DHHS blueprint for action on breast feeding. *Public Health Rep* 2001;**116**:72–3.

37 American Academy of Pediatrics, Work Group on Breastfeeding. Breastfeeding and the use of human milk. *Pediatrics* 1997;**100**:1035–9.

38 American Dietetic Association. Position of the American Dietetic Association: promotion of breast feeding. *J Am Diet Assoc* 1997;**97**:662–6.

39 Langer O, Conway DL, Berkus MD, *et al.* A comparison of glyburide and insulin in women with gestational diabetes mellitus. *N Engl J Med* 2000;**343**:1134–8.

40 Rowan JA, Hague WM, Gao W, Battin MR, Moore MP for the MiG trial Investigators. Metformin versus insulin for the treatment of gestational diabetes. *N Engl J Med* 2008;**358**:2003–15.

22 Care of the neonate

Jane M. Hawdon

UCL EGA Institute for Women's Health, University College London Hospitals NHS Foundation Trust, London, UK

PRACTICE POINTS

- Neonatal mortality rates associated with pregestational diabetes are about twice those in the general population.
- Preterm delivery with its associated neonatal morbidity is five times as common with pregestational diabetes than in the general population and is often avoidable.
- Major congenital anomalies are between three and five times as common in pregnancies with pregestational diabetes than in the general population.
- Other recognized neonatal complications of diabetes in pregnancy include macrosomia, birth injury, hypoxic–ischemic encephalopathy, and hypoglycemia.
- The majority of babies born to mothers with diabetes do not have complications and do not require additional specialist care.
- Separation of babies and mothers and formula feeding should only occur if clinically indicated; such policies should not be "routine".

CASE HISTORY

Mrs AB had insulin-dependent diabetes since her teenage years. She planned her pregnancy and attended a pre-pregnancy clinic to discuss best possible control at this crucial time. She envied her closest friend who was planning a home birth for her own baby, but appreciated that even with good diabetic control there were risk factors for her baby which meant hospital birth was advisable. Early ultrasound scans showed normal growth and normal fetal anatomy.

Mrs AB had threatened preterm labor at 28 weeks. She was admitted to hospital and was given intramuscular betamethasone, to reduce the chances of respiratory distress syndrome if the baby were to be born preterm. Fortunately, contractions settled and the pregnancy continued to near term. A junior obstetrician advised Mrs

AB that she would need a cesarean section "because she has diabetes". She asked to speak to the consultant who, following review, considered there were no risk factors and that normal delivery could be anticipated. Mrs AB was relieved as she had read that there is an increased risk of breathing problems if babies are delivered by cesarean section.

Baby Tom was born at 38 weeks of gestation by normal delivery. His birthweight was 3.6 kg (91st centile). Tom was placed skin-to-skin on his mother's chest immediately after birth, and within 30 minutes had been to the breast and was noted to have a good latch and suck. At 4 hours of age he had a blood glucose level measured (using the machine in the neonatal unit laboratory). This was 1.5 mmol/L (27 mg/dL). The midwife considered Tom had normal tone, color, and vital signs, and encouraged his mother to feed him again. He fed well and she felt that he had taken some colostrum. He remained alert and with normal tone, and from his skin-to-skin position fed intermittently but each time with good latch and suck. At 8 hours of age, blood glucose level was 2.2 mmol/L (40 mg/dL) and the midwife again evaluated Tom's condition as normal. As his blood glucose level was increasing and his clinical condition was good, no additional feeds to breastfeeds were given. Tom continued to feed well and blood glucose levels remained above 2.0 mmol/L (>36 mg/dL). Blood glucose monitoring was discontinued after 24 hours and Tom went home the next day.

Tom's health visitor was initially concerned at his 6-week check that his weight had fallen to the 50th centile. However, she then recalled the history of diabetes in pregnancy and considered that Tom was showing "catch down" to his natural weight.

- Why advice against home birth?
- Why did Tom have minimal complications after birth?
- Why did Tom receive formula milk?
- Why did Tom's weight fall to a lower centile?

A Practical Manual of Diabetes in Pregnancy, 1st Edition.
Edited by David R. McCance, Michael Maresh and David A. Sacks.
© 2010 Blackwell Publishing

BACKGROUND

The impact of pregestational diabetes and gestational diabetes upon the mother during pregnancy is covered in other chapters. Adverse consequences for the fetus and the neonate arise either from the directly harmful metabolic environment, or the obstetric interventions required when maternal control is poor, or from inappropriate "routine" practices. Optimizing diabetic control minimizes risks to the mother and fetus, and reduces the risk of the postnatal complications described below. Whilst in many cases this is achieved and a healthy mother and baby result, it is important to be aware of the complications that can occur.

As the population of women with Type 2 diabetes becomes younger, particularly in some ethnic groups, the proportion of women with pregnancies complicated by pregestational Type 2 diabetes has risen to approximately one-third of pregnancies complicated by diabetes.[1,2] These women have perinatal mortality rates and rates of fetal macrosomia that are no different from those with Type 1 diabetes.[1] Finally, the fetus and neonate of the mother who develops gestational diabetes are at risk of some of the same adverse consequences if the gestational diabetes is not recognized and well managed.[3]

CARE OF THE HEALTHY INFANT AFTER PREGNANCY COMPLICATED BY DIABETES

For many women, especially those who access prenatal counseling and enhanced diabetes care and then continue to have good control during pregnancy, fetal and neonatal complications related to diabetes in pregnancy are unlikely. It is important to recognize that a baby at very low risk of complications should be managed according to normal standards for the healthy newborn baby.[4,5] In particular, it is important to avoid unnecessary separation of mother and baby, and to facilitate successful breastfeeding if this is the mother's chosen method of feeding. Failure to follow these principles and the resulting iatrogenic complications are also covered below.

NEONATAL COMPLICATIONS – ETIOLOGY AND MANAGEMENT

Despite the aspiration that improved maternal diabetes care will minimize perinatal morbidity and mortality, recent data suggest that despite some improvements over time, insufficient progress has been made.[1,2,6–11] Some

Table 22.1 Neonatal complications after diabetes in pregnancy.

Directly related to diabetes in pregnancy
- Congenital anomalies
- Intrauterine growth restriction
- Intrapartum hypoxia–ischemia
- Macrosomia, obstructed labor, birth injury
- Neonatal death
- Polycythemia/jaundice
- Hypoketonemic hypoglycemia
- Hypocalcemia, hypomagnesemia
- Hypertrophic cardiomyopathy

Complications of necessary, or unnecessary, obstetric interventions
- Complications of preterm delivery
- Complications of cesarean section – respiratory distress, impact on breastfeeding

Iatrogenic
- Inappropriate separation of mother and baby
- Inappropriate formula supplementation – impact on breastfeeding

Table 22.2 Neonatal outcomes in the UK.[1]

	IDM (%)	UK (%)	Rate ratio
Neonatal death	9.3 per 1000	3.6 per 1000	2.6
Preterm delivery	37	7.3	5
Congenital anomaly	5.5	2.1	2.6
Birthweight >90th centile	52	10	5.2
Shoulder dystocia	7.9	3	2.6
Erb palsy	4.5 per 1000	0.42 per 1000	11
Apgar <7 at 5 min	2.6	0.76	3.4
Admission to NNU	56	10	5.6
Term admission to SC*	33	10	3.3

*Avoidable admission to SC, 67.1% of SC term admissions
IDM, baby of mother with pregestational diabetes; UK, rate for general UK population; NNU, any admission to a neonatal unit, all levels of care; SC, admission to a neonatal unit, special care only

neonatal complications arise from the effects of being born preterm or by cesarean section, and are not specific to diabetes, while others are secondary to intrauterine or intrapartum hypoxia–ischemia or the abnormal diabetic metabolic environment that the fetus may be exposed to during pregnancy. Finally, some neonatal problems are iatrogenic (Tables 22.1 and 22.2).

Perinatal mortality

Data from the UK for 2002–2003 indicate that the overall UK perinatal mortality rate (stillbirths and first-week neonatal deaths) with pregestational diabetes was 31.8 per 1000 compared with a national rate of 8.5 per 1000 (RR 3.8, 95% CI 3.0–4.7).[1] This was similar to the rates in cohort studies from The Netherlands (1999–2001),[6] Scotland (1998–1999),[10] English Northern region (1996–2004),[2] and North West England (1990–1994).[9] Higher rates of 37 per 1000 and 48 per 1000, respectively, were reported in older cohort studies from Scotland (1979–1995)[11] and the Northern region (1994).[8] For the cohort of babies from the Confidential Enquiry into Maternal and Child Health (CEMACH) undergoing a more detailed enquiry, the most common causes of death were related to congenital abnormality and intrapartum complications (Table 22.3).[7]

Severe fetal compromise resulting in intrauterine loss is covered in chapter 12. The stillbirth rate for women with Type 1 and Type 2 diabetes in the UK 2002–2003 cohort was 26.8 per 1000, compared with a national rate of 5.7 per 1000 (RR 4.7, 95% CI 3.7–6.0).[1] Similar rates have been reported in other UK and European studies.[6,9–11]

These are pregnancies at the extreme of the spectrum for adverse sequelae of diabetes in pregnancy; it follows that fetuses less severely affected will survive, but carry a burden of neonatal compromise. Indeed, in the UK CEMACH cohort, the neonatal death rate was 9.3 per 1000 for babies born to mothers with diabetes, compared with a national rate of 3.6 per 1000 (RR 2.6, 95% CI 1.7–3.9).[1] Neonatal mortality rates were very similar to this in the Dutch and Scottish cohort studies,[6,11] but were higher in the older studies from the UK Northern Region and North West England.[8,9]

Preterm delivery

In the UK CEMACH cohort (2002–2003), the rate of preterm delivery (<37 weeks of gestation) for babies born to mothers with pregestational diabetes was 35.8% compared to a rate of 7.4% in the general population.[1] The Netherlands cohort study has provided similar data.[6] The causes of preterm delivery are covered in chapter 20.

As with other maternal conditions that affect pregnancy, there is always a balance between continuing a pregnancy until term and reducing the time that both fetus and mother are exposed to a harmful environment. However, for women in the UK cohort, 19% had preterm delivery that was not spontaneous or explained by maternal or fetal compromise and thus could have been avoided.[1] This would have prevented some 235 admissions to neonatal care over the study period.

If preterm delivery is planned, this must be in a unit that can provide neonatal intensive care, which may require transfer of the mother to an appropriate unit, preferably within a perinatal network system as operates in the UK.

Now that it is widely recognized that mothers with diabetes should receive steroid injections if preterm delivery is anticipated, babies of diabetic mothers do not in general have worse respiratory distress than other babies of equivalent gestation. In the UK cohort, 70% of women who delivered live babies between 24 and 34 weeks of gestation received prophylactic antenatal steroids.[1] However, there have been concerns regarding potential worsening of maternal glycemic control and resulting perinatal and maternal morbidity if steroid therapy is given. In the UK cohort, for five of the 68 women who were not given steroids, the reason cited was "health professionals concerned about effect of steroids on maternal glycemic control".[7] The rationale for giving steroid therapy and subsequent maternal management are discussed elsewhere (chapter 21).

If a baby is born preterm, there is no evidence that the usual complications of prematurity are more severe than for a baby born at a similar gestational age to a mother who does not have diabetes. Preterm babies of diabetic mothers should be managed according to standard protocols. In particular, mothers should be encouraged to express and store breast milk. Additional problems specific to the baby of a diabetic mother may be present and need additional management (see below).

Table 22.3 Causes of perinatal mortality in the UK.[1]

Cause of death*	Number (%) in enquiry (n = 98)	Number (%) in general population (n = 5756)	p value for difference
Unexplained	58 (59)	2516 (44)	0.002
Congenital anomaly	18 (18)	1087 (19)	0.68
Intrapartum causes	10 (10)	429 (8)	0.30
Immaturity	4 (4)	1027 (18)	< 0.001
Infection	1 (1)	252 (4)	0.10

*Extended Wigglesworth classification

Effects of delivery by cesarean section

In the 2002–2003 UK cohort, the cesarean section rate for women who have diabetes was 67%[1] and in The Netherlands study 44.3%,[6] compared with the overall UK national rate of 22%. In the UK study, 9% of cesarean sections were not explained by maternal or fetal compromise and 4% were "routine for diabetes" or "maternal request".[1] As stated above, a number of these "routine" cesarean sections were at a preterm gestation. Even in pregnancies complicated by gestational diabetes (rather than pregestational diabetes), there appears to be a higher rate of cesarean section (see chapter 20).

Whilst the baby may be protected from hypoxic–ischemic brain injury by avoiding labor and vaginal delivery, the potential adverse impacts on the baby of unnecessary cesarean section are two-fold: delayed and disrupted breastfeeding and respiratory morbidity (transient tachypnea of the newborn or surfactant deficiency).[12,13] These in turn frequently result in avoidable admission to a neonatal unit and separation of mother and baby.

Effects of antenatal and intrapartum hypoxia–ischemia

Hypoxia–ischemia is the combined pathology of impaired oxygenation of the blood and reduced perfusion (secondary to the effect of hypoxia on cardiac function). This is potentially damaging to all organ systems, and particularly the brain. The mechanisms by which intrauterine loss and neonatal complications occur secondary to hypoxia–ischemia are not fully understood (see chapters 3 and 12). However, it is likely that macrosomia and obstructed labor may contribute to intrapartum hypoxia–ischemia and increase the risk of neonatal complications.

In the UK enquiry, 10% of perinatal deaths were related to intrapartum causes.[7] These represent the end of a spectrum; many babies affected by intrapartum hypoxia–ischemia will be born alive and require expert resuscitation. This is one of the reasons why delivery of babies of diabetic mothers must occur in units where advanced neonatal life support is available. If a neonate has unexpected and severe complications of hypoxia–ischemia, he/she will require transfer to a neonatal unit which provides intensive care, if this is not available in the hospital of birth. As total body cooling becomes an established treatment for hypoxic–ischemic encephalop-

athy, then time is of the essence in commencement of this treatment at a specialist center.[14]

Relative cellular hypoxia causes increased erythropoietin secretion and in turn increased fetal red cell production.[15] The resulting neonatal polycythemia may then cause excessive neonatal jaundice (as the red cell burden is lyzed) and occasionally hyperviscosity syndrome. Renal vein thrombosis or thrombosis in other vessels is rare, but occurs more frequently in babies whose mothers have diabetes compared to those whose mothers do not.

Clinicians caring for these babies must be alert to these complications and test for them if there are abnormal clinical signs, such as irritability, lethargy, and poor feeding. The effects of polycythemia and hypoglycemia may be additive in terms of reduction of glucose delivery to the brain, and polycythemia associated with clinical signs, such as irritability or lethargy, must be treated with partial exchange transfusion, according to standard neonatal guidance.

Congenital anomalies

It has long been recognized that there is a higher incidence of congenital anomalies in pregnancies complicated by diabetes than in the general population.[16] The most recent UK data demonstrated that 4–6% of fetuses of diabetic mothers had one or more major congenital anomalies.[1,10] The reported incidence was higher in The Netherlands and in the older UK cohort studies from the North East and North West of England.[6,8,9]

The most common anomalies are congenital heart disease (the incidence in the CEMACH cohort 1.7% was three times that in the general population) and anomalies of limb, musculoskeletal system or connective tissue (incidence 0.7%).[1] Neural tube defects, although numerically rare, are 3.4 times more common than in the general population.[1] The possible etiologies of these anomalies and strategies for their prevention are covered in chapters 8 and 14.

The most important predelivery issues for the obstetrician and neonatologist are to ensure that there has been adequate counseling of parents, involving the specialist team who will care for the baby postnatally, and to ensure that delivery takes place at an appropriate center (dependent on the nature of the anomaly) to enable early access to specialist care. Routine postnatal echocardiography to screen for congenital heart anomalies is not indicated, unless an abnormality has been suspected on antenatal scanning or the baby presents with clinical signs of congenital heart disease.[5]

Macrosomia – obstructed labor, birth injury, and organomegaly

Macrosomia and large for gestational age are not interchangeable terms. Macrosomia describes a baby who is heavier than his/her genetically deteremined birthweight, has the clinical appearance of a baby who has had somatic growth in excess over head growth, and may be present in a baby of "normal" birthweight. Macrosomia and organomegaly attributed to fetal hyperinsulinemia are well-recognized characteristics of pregnancies complicated by diabetes, but evidence is inconsistent regarding the potential impact on these morbidities of improved diabetic control and duration of diabetes.[1,3,11,17] The rate of macrosomia (birthweight above 90th centile) was 52% in the recent UK cohort.[1]

The clinical significance of macrosomia pertains to the the risk of complications presented by delivery of a large infant, such as shoulder dystocia, obstructed labor, perinatal hypoxia–ischemia, and birth injury (e.g. brachial plexus injury and fractured clavicle or humerus). Recent UK cohort data provide rates for some of these: shoulder dystocia 7.9% (over twice the rate in the general population), Erb palsy 4.5 per 1000 births (10 times the rate in the general population), and fractures (usually of the clavicle and humerus) 7 per 1000 births.[1] In the context of the high rate of preterm delivery and cesarean section in this cohort, the complication rate is likely to be even higher with more normal deliveries at term.

Management of these complications is covered in standard neonatal texts. Some, such as fractures, cause no long-term morbidity, but significant long-term neurodevelopmental morbidity may be associated with hypoxia–ischemia secondary to obstructed labor and Erb palsy.

Finally, parents and health professionals must be prepared for "catch down" in postnatal growth of macrosomic babies, especially when breastfed. This is a normal and healthy adaptation, and provided the baby appears to be feeding well and is healthy, there should be no concern if there is an initial period of slow weight gain such that weight trajectory crosses down the centile lines. Rather, to over feed the baby and have him/her remain overweight has long-term health consequences, e.g. later risk of cardiovascular disease and diabetes.[9] This is a further reason to promote and support breastfeeding, which protects against long-term metabolic disturbances.[18,19]

Hypertrophic cardiomyopathy

Hypertrophic cardiomyopathy, characterized by hypertrophied septal muscle which obstructs the left ventricular outflow tract, may be sufficiently severe to cause fetal or neonatal death.[15] In less severe cases, the presentation is usually within the first weeks of postnatal life with cardiorespiratory distress and congestive heart failure. The majority of infants need supportive care only, as resolution of the signs can be expected in 2–4 weeks. The septal hypertrophy regresses within 2–12 months. Routine postnatal echocardiography is not required unless there are clinical signs.[5]

Intrauterine growth restriction

Intrauterine fetal growth restriction, often associated with severe diabetic vasculopathy, may lead to further problems after birth. The small for gestational age infant of the diabetic mother appears to be at even greater risk of adverse outcome, especially neurodevelopmental sequelae.[20] Often this is compounded by a requirement for preterm delivery. Delivery must be planned at an appropriate unit as specialist neonatal care is likely to be required.

Impaired postnatal metabolic adaptation

With the cessation of placental nutrition at birth, the healthy newborn baby undergoes metabolic adaptation to ensure energy provision to vital organs and subsequently to sustain growth and further development. The key fuels are glucose and ketone bodies (the latter being the product of beta oxidation of fatty acids). The infant of the diabetic mother is at risk of transient hyperinsulinism, which in turn causes a high rate of glucose uptake and conversion to fat, reduced hepatic glucose production, and reduced lipolysis and thus reduced ketone body production[15,21] (Fig. 22.1). At the extreme end of the spectrum, this will result in hypoketonemic hypoglycemia with markedly reduced fuel availability for the brain and other vital organs.

The ultimate concern is that of brain injury and long-term neurodevelopmental sequelae. Reviews of a number of published studies have suggested an association between the occurrence of neonatal hypoglycemia and adverse neurodevelopmental outcome, but none has been able to exclude other potentially confounding complications of maternal diabetes, which may also influence outcome.[15,21] Whilst it is clear that untreated

Maternal hyperglycemia and amino acids

↓

Excess transport across placenta

↓

Fetal hyperinsulinism

↓

Neonatal hyperinsulism

↓

Hypoketonemic hypoglycemia

Fig. 22.1 Impaired neonatal metabolic adaptation.

Table 22.4 Issues in the management of neonatal hypoglycemia.

- Poor maternal blood glucose control, especially prior to delivery, increases risk
- CEMACH survey – accurate blood glucose monitoring method in only one-quarter of cases
- Formula supplementation is likely to suppress metabolic adaptation
- Formula feeding may increase risk of later obesity and metabolic disturbance
- Unnecessary separation of mother and baby must be avoided

hypoglycemia that is sufficiently severe and prolonged to cause clinical signs may cause brain injury, there is no evidence that brain injury occurs in the absence of clinical signs ("asymptomatic hypoglycemia"). Clinical signs suggestive of (but not specific to) hypoglycemia are:
- Abnormal tone
- Abnormal level of consciousness
- Poor oral feeding
- Fits which may be atypical, e.g. presenting as apnea.

The purpose of clinical monitoring (see below) is to detect hypoglycemia at an early stage when it becomes clinically significant and to institute appropriate management.[3,5,22]

Fortunately, although cohort studies report that many babies have low blood glucose levels leading to admission to a neonatal unit, in practice today in the UK very few babies develop clinically significant hypoglycemia associated with clinical signs (see above). Reasons for this are likely to include standards of maternal diabetic control during labor (see chapter 21), such that significant postnatal hyperinsulinism is uncommon, the transient nature of hyperinsulinism, the ability of the neonate to produce and utilize ketone bodies, and early preventive management (see below).

There are no clinical studies of sufficient rigor to provide evidence for the circumstances in which neonatal hypoglycemia may cause brain injury, and thus it is not possible to provide evidence-based guidelines for the prevention and management of clinically significant neonatal hypoglycemia following maternal diabetes. Therefore, recommendations in this chapter, in referenced texts written by clinical experts, in the UK CEMACH survey, and in the UK National Institutes for Health and Clinical Evidence (NICE) guidelines remain empirical, urging clinicians to individualize management for each baby and emphasizing the importance of careful clinical evaluation[5,15,21–25] (Table 22.4).

Clinical monitoring

Unless the baby has clinical complications sufficiently severe to require admission to a neonatal unit, mother and baby should remain together. This may be on a postnatal ward, provided there is sufficient midwifery or nursing resource to allow regular clinical monitoring of mother and baby as required. Some hospitals elect to look after these babies and mothers on transitional care units, where enhanced midwifery or nurse staffing is available.

Those caring for the baby must regularly monitor the baby for feeding behavior and abnormal neurological signs, and must document their findings. Unless there are risk factors for other complications (e.g. infection) and as long as the baby appears well, it is not necessary to monitor vital signs (temperature, pulse, respiration rate) or to screen for other potential complications, e.g. polycythaemia.[5] If at any stage there are abnormal clinical signs, the blood glucose level must be measured and an urgent pediatric review arranged.

It is generally accepted that infants of diabetic mothers should have regular blood glucose monitoring, and the timing for this and the thresholds for intervention are discussed below and in Table 22.6. Given that clinically significant hyperinsulinism and hypoglycemia appear to be rare in the UK, this is likely to be an over-cautious policy applied to prevent babies "slipping through the net". It could be argued that provided there is regular clinical monitoring by experienced staff, such that worrying signs are detected early and blood glucose level checked at that time, routine blood glucose monitoring of clinically healthy babies is not required. However, in practice in the UK, initial blood glucose monitoring is almost always undertaken and is recommended in the most recent national UK guidance.[5]

Blood glucose monitoring must be by an accurate, laboratory-based method. No reagent strip with meter measurement has been demonstrated to be sufficiently accurate to diagnose or exclude neonatal hypoglycemia.[23] Some neonatal units have an accurate and quality assured analyzer situated in the unit laboratory to allow rapid but accurate blood glucose monitoring. This is the recommended standard.[5,3,7,21,22,23,26] However, recent data indicate that only around 25% of babies have blood glucose monitoring using accurate methods.[1]

Blood glucose monitoring should be commenced at around 3–4 hours of age. To commence it sooner than this is not informative as babies experience a physiologic transitional fall in blood glucose level in the first hours after birth, often even in healthy babies to levels below 2.0 mmol/L (<36 mg/dL). Therefore, in an otherwise healthy baby, a low blood glucose level in the first 3–4 hours does not help to differentiate a baby who has significant but transient hyperinsulinism from a baby who is not affected by hyperinsulinism.

Blood glucose monitoring should be prefeed in order to detect a nadir in blood glucose level. In a baby with no clinical signs, a postfeed glucose level is not helpful and exposes the baby to excessive heel stabs.

If hyperinsulinism occurs, it will usually present in the first 1–2 days postnatally and will be transient, lasting a maximum of a few days. Therefore, if a baby is clinically stable and has shown no evidence of clinically significant hypoglycemia, blood glucose monitoring may be discontinued when laboratory measured glucose levels are persistently above 2.0 mmol/L (>36 mg/dL), and in these circumstances discharge to community care from 24 hours of age is appropriate if all else is well[5] (Table 22.5).

Clearly babies who are preterm or unwell and admitted to neonatal units will undergo blood glucose monitoring as part of their clinical care.

Feeding

Breastfeeding is the method of choice for all babies (barring notable rare exceptions, e.g. maternal HIV infection). However, in the UK cohort, only 53% of mothers with diabetes intended to breastfeed, and at 28 days only 27% of term babies were breastfed.[1]

Mothers should be encouraged antenatally to consider breastfeeding their baby and should receive sufficient information regarding the benefits to make their choice. Immediately after delivery, a healthy baby should be placed skin-to-skin with mother and an early breastfeed offered, with assistance to ensure that the baby achieves an effective latch. Breastfeeds should be offered every 3–4

Table 22.5 Practical aspects of neonatal blood glucose monitoring.

- Use an accurate laboratory-based method
- Start at 3–4 hours after birth
- Measurements advised approximately 4 hourly
- Intervention if clinical signs (regardless of blood glucose level) or two consecutive glucose levels < 2.0 mmol/L (<36 mg/dL)
- Stop monitoring when two consecutive levels > 2.0 mmol/L

hours (or more frequently if the baby demands), again with support if necessary.

Formula supplements to breastfeeds are required only if there are clinical indications, including intervention for hypoglycemia (see operational thresholds below). Formula supplements often result in reduced frequency of and hunger for breastfeeding, thus reducing breast milk supply and suppressing normal neonatal metabolic adaptation.[13] Therefore, if formula supplementation is required, this must be of the volume required and no more. If a mother elects to formula feed, requirements are not usually in excess of 100 ml/kg/day, but volumes should be adjusted according to clinical monitoring. Finally, the potential long-term metabolic risks of overfeeding and obesity in infancy must be considered.

If a mother and baby are separated, or if the baby requires formula supplements to breastfeeding, the mother should be encouraged to express breast milk, which allows lactation to be sustained and provides breast milk which can be given to the baby.

Operational thresholds for management

There is no doubt that a low blood glucose level associated with clinical signs (see above) must be treated. In the absence of abnormal clinical signs, recommendations for blood glucose thresholds at which to intervene must be pragmatic, and must balance the risks of developing clinically significant hypoglycemia against the risks of disrupting breastfeeding and separating mother and baby. The most recent UK guidance advises that, in the absence of clinical signs, two consecutive blood glucose levels below 2.0 mmol/L (<36 mg/dL) at least 3–4 hours after delivery require intervention to aim to raise the blood glucose level.[5]

Management of clinically significant hypoglycemia

Management of a low blood glucose level associated with abnormal clinical signs (see above) is a medical emergency necessitating full clinical evaluation and transfer to a neonatal unit. If clinical signs are not severe (e.g. alert baby but poor suck), it is reasonable to assess the effect of tube feeds at an appropriate interval. However, if blood glucose levels do not increase with tube feeds or the baby has serious clinical signs (e.g. reduced level of consciousness or fits), intravenous glucose must be given without delay, starting at 5 mg/kg/min (equivalent to 3 ml/kg/h of 10% dextrose) but being aware of the possible need to increase this as necessary if indicated by frequent blood glucose monitoring.[27] Intramuscular glucagon (200 µg/kg) is useful if there are clinical signs and a delay in achieving intravenous access, in that glycogen will be broken down to release glucose, but the effect will be transient, lasting less than 1 hour.

Hypocalcemia and hypomagnesemia

Transient neonatal hypocalcemia has been reported following diabetes in pregnancy, and both its incidence and severity appear to be related to the degree of maternal diabetes control.[15] It is usually associated with hyperphosphatemia and occasionally with hypomagnesemia. The aetiology is not entirely clear, but neonatal hypoparathyroidism has been demonstrated and may in part be secondary to maternal magnesium loss. Published studies and clinical experience indicate that hypocalcemia and hypomagnesemia are rarely of clinical significance, unless the baby has other complications, e.g. perinatal hypoxia–ischemia. Therefore, there is no indication to screen for them in the healthy baby. If associated with clinical signs, the deficits must be corrected, as recommended in standard neonatal textbooks.

Iatrogenic complications

It will be seen from the discussion above that the timing and method of delivery often impact upon neonatal morbidity. Occasionally decisions are made on fetal grounds, but more often are related to maternal complications. However, in a number of cases there are no clear maternal or fetal reasons for preterm delivery or delivery by cesarean section. Each places neonatal well-being at risk.

Even if there are no significant maternal or fetal complications and the pregnancy goes to term or near term, the evidence would suggest that the baby is still exposed to potential iatrogenic harm (Table 22.6). The UK CEMACH enquiry demonstrated frequent failings in medical and midwifery care which impacted upon the

Table 22.6 Potentially avoidable adverse outcomes for the baby.[1,7,22]

- 16% of preterm deliveries – no clear indication for induction or cesarean section
- 30% of preterm babies – no maternal steroids administered
- 5% of babies delivered with no intensive care/high-dependency care facility
- 25% of admitted term babies – reason given was "routine"
- 9% of babies who received formula – reason given was "routine"

baby's postnatal course and in particular establishment of feeding.[1,7,22] These included:
- "Routine" admission of babies to neonatal units
- "Routine" supplementation or replacement of breastfeeds with formula
- Delayed "skin-to-skin" contact and first feed
- Poor management of temperature control
- Testing of blood glucose with subsequent response to this too soon after delivery.

In addition to the harmful effects of these practices for mother and baby, they represent an avoidable use of neonatal unit resource.

LONG-TERM OUTCOMES

Studies of potential long-term neurodevelopmental sequelae in infants born to mothers with poorly controlled diabetes in pregnancy are inconsistent.[15,21] However, studies of infants born to mothers with well-controlled diabetes in pregnancy show a favorable neurodevelopmental outcome.[15] This is discussed in detail in chapter 25. Finally, the risk of insulin-dependent diabetes developing by the age of 20 years in the offspring of diabetic women is at least seven times that for non-diabetic mothers (lower than the risk if it is the father who has diabetes).[15]

MINIMIZING RISK

The findings from the UK national 2002–2003 survey and many other published studies have reinforced the recommendations for good practice, as these are associated with a reduction in postnatal complications and iatrogenic harm[1,7,22] (Table 22.7).

In addition, all hospitals must have written protocols for the prevention and management of potential neonatal complications, including hypoglycemia, and for admission to the neonatal unit.

Table 22.7 Key points for good practice to prevent neonatal complications.

- Antenatal counseling by experienced clinicians if complications are expected
- Written policies and guidelines for delivery and postnatal management
- Avoid unnecessary preterm delivery and/or cesarean section
- Give maternal steroids if preterm delivery anticipated
- Plan delivery where appropriate neonatal expertise is available
- Encourage breastfeeding as method of choice, do not give formula to a breastfed baby unless clinically indicated
- Offer early feed and skin-to-skin contact
- Commence blood glucose monitoring, using accurate method, at 3–4 hours after birth
- Do not treat for hypoglycemia unless two consecutive blood glucose levels are < 2.0 mmol/L (<36 mg/dL) or there are clinical signs of hypoglycemia
- Do not screen for other potential complications unless there are clinical signs
- Keep mother and baby together unless there is a clinical indication for admission of baby to a neonatal unit
- Advise mother and primary care health professionals of the normal pattern of "catch-down" growth in a macrosomic baby

The baby must be delivered in a unit where the appropriate expertise is present, the minimum standard being a hospital where advanced neonatal life support skills are immediately available. However, many babies in addition will require, often unexpectedly, care on a neonatal intensive care unit. Of equal importance is the need to avoid iatrogenic harm, such as unnecessary preterm delivery or cesarean section and unnecessary separation of baby and mother. These all require planning and cooperative working within the multidisciplinary team.

REFERENCES

1 Confidential Enquiry into Maternal and Child Health. *Pregnancy in Women with Type 1 and Type 2 Diabetes in 2002–2003*. London: CEMACH, 2005.

2 Bell R, Bailey K, Creswell T, *et al*. Trends in prevalence and outcomes of pregnancy in women with pre-existing type I and type II diabetes. *BJOG* 2008;**115**:445–52.

3 HAPO Study Cooperative Research Group, Metzger BE, Lowe LP, *et al*. Hyperglycemia and adverse pregnancy outcomes. *N Engl J Med* 2008;**358**:1991–2002.

4 National Collaborating Centre for Primary Care. *Postnatal Care: Routine Postnatal Care of Women and Their Babies.*

London: NICE, 2006. http://www.nice.org.uk/Guidance/CG37

5 National Institute for Health and Clinical Excellence. *Diabetes in Pregnancy*. London: NICE, 2008. http://www.nice.org.uk/Guidance/CG63

6 Evers IM, de Valk HW, Visser GH. Risk of complications of pregnancy in women with type 1 diabetes: nationwide prospective study in the Netherlands. *BMJ* 2004;**328**:915–18.

7 Confidential Enquiry into Maternal and Child Health. *Diabetes in Pregnancy: Are We Providing the Best Care? Findings of a National Enquiry*. London: CEMACH, 2007.

8 Hawthorne G, Robson S, Ryall EA, Sen D, Roberts SH, Ward Platt MP. Prospective population based survey of outcome of pregnancy in diabetic women: results of the Northern Diabetic pregnancy Audit, 1994. *BMJ* 1997;**315**:279–81.

9 Casson IF, Clarke CA, Howard CV, *et al*. Outcomes of pregnancy in insulin dependent diabetic women: results of a five year population cohort study. *BMJ* 1997;**315**:275–8.

10 Penney GC, Mair G, Pearson DW. Outcomes of pregnancies in women with type 1 diabetes in Scotland: a national population based study. *BJOG* 2003;**110**:315–18.

11 Silva Idos S, Higgins C, Swerdlow AJ, *et al*. Birthweight and other pregnancy outcomes in a cohort of women with pregestational insulin-treated diabetes mellitus, Scotland, 1979–1995. *Diabet Med* 2005;**22**:440–7.

12 Evans KC, Evans RG, Royal R, Esterman AJ, James SL. Effect of cesarean section on breast milk transfer to the normal term newborn over the first week of life. *Arch Dis Child Fetal Neonatal Ed* 2003;**88**:F380–2.

13 Hansen AK, Wisborg K, Uldbjerg N, Henriksen TB. Risk of respiratory morbidity in term infants delivered by elective cesarean section: cohort study. *BMJ* 2008;**336**:85–7.

14 Jacobs S, Hunt R, Tarnow-Mordi WO, Inder TE, Davis PG. Cooling for newborns with hypoxic ischaemic encephalopathy. *Cochrane Database Syst Rev* 2007, Issue **4**: CD003311.

15 Hawdon JM. The infant of a diabetic mother. In: Rennie J (ed) *Roberton's Textbook of Neonatology*, 4th edn. Edinburgh: Churchill Livingstone, 2005.

16 Molsted-Pedersen L, Tygstrup I, Pedersen J. Congenital malformations in newborn infants of diabetic women. *Lancet* 1964;**i**:1124–6.

17 Mello G, Parretti E, Mecacci F, *et al*. What degree of maternal metabolic control in women with type 2 diabetes is associated with normal body size and proportions in full term infants? *Diabetes Care* 2000;**23**:1494–8.

18 Owen CG, Martin RM, Whincup PH, Smith GD, Cook DG. Does breastfeeding influence risk of Type 2 diabetes in later life? A quantitative analysis of published evidence. *Am J Clin Nutr* 2006;**84**:1043–54.

19 Owen CG, Whincup PH, Kaye SJ, *et al*. Does initial breastfeeding lead to lower blood cholesterol in adult life? A quantitative review of the evidence. *Am J Clin Nutr* 2008;**88**:305–14.

20 Petersen MB, Pedersen SA, Greisen G, Pedersen JF, Molsted-Pedersen L. Early growth delay in diabetic pregnancy: relation to psychomotor development at age 4. *BMJ* 1998; **296**:598–600.

21 Hawdon JM. Hypoglycemia and brain injury – when neonatal metabolic adaptation fails. In: Levene MI, Chervenak FA (eds). *Fetal and Neonatal Neurology and Neurosurgery*, 4th edn. Edinburgh: Churchill Livingstone, 2009.

22 Confidential Enquiry into Maternal and Child Health. *Diabetes in Pregnancy: Caring for the Baby after Birth. Findings of a National Enquiry*. London: CEMACH, 2007.

23 Cornblath M, Hawdon JM, Williams AF, *et al.* Controversies regarding definition of neonatal hypoglycemia: Suggested operational thresholds. *Pediatrics* 2000;**105**: 1141–5.

24 Rozance PJ, Hay WW. Hypoglycemia in newborn infants: Features associated with adverse outcomes. *Biol Neonate* 2006;**90**:74–86.

25 Williams AF. Neonatal hypoglycemia: Clinical and legal aspects. *Semin Fetal Neonatal Med* 2005;**10**:363–8.

26 Deshpande S, Ward Platt MP. The investigation and management of neonatal hypoglycemia. *Semin Fetal Neonatal Med* 2005;**10**:351–61.

27 Hawdon JM. Disorders of blood glucose homeostasis in the neonate. In: Rennie J (ed) *Roberton's Textbook of Neonatology*, 4th edn. Edinburgh: Churchill Livingstone, 2005.

23 Contraception for the woman with diabetes

Penina Segall-Gutierrez[1] & Siri L. Kjos[2]

[1] Department of Obstetrics and Gynecology, Keck School of Medicine, University of Southern California, Los Angeles, CA, USA

[2] Department of Obstetrics & Gynecology, Harbor UCLA Medical Center, Los Angeles, CA, USA

PRACTICE POINTS

- The use of *effective* methods of contraception, until euglycemia is achieved and the woman is ready to conceive, will minimize the risks of unintended pregnancy and adverse pregnancy outcomes, and should be discussed with each sexually active woman with diabetes, regardless of her pregnancy intentions.
- Intrauterine devices are an excellent contraceptive option in women with diabetes, as they are metabolically neutral and have a failure rate similar to sterilization.
- Diabetic women who do not wish to or cannot use intrauterine contraception, have a variety of hormonal contraceptive options, and in most cases a suitable hormonal method can be identified. Combination hormone contraceptive methods may be used in diabetic women without micro- and macro-vascular disease and have minimal metabolic effects, and progestin-only methods are acceptable for most women who are not candidates for estrogen-containing methods.
- Barrier methods and methods of natural family planning, while metabolically safe, are not recommended as a first-line agent for women with diabetes because of their high failure rate.
- All women should be informed about emergency contraception, which is safe to use in diabetic women.
- For diabetic women without euglycemia, counseling in routine pregnancy options should include an accurate estimate of the risk for congenital malformations.

CASE HISTORY

Maria is a 43-year-old mother of four children with a 21-year history of Type 2 diabetes and an 8-year history of hypertension. She has recently started metformin as

A Practical Manual of Diabetes in Pregnancy, 1st Edition.
Edited by David R. McCance, Michael Maresh and David A. Sacks.
© 2010 Blackwell Publishing

prescribed by her physician. She has a body mass index (BMI) of 36 kg/m^2, blood pressure of 142/88 mmHg, and a fasting blood glucose of 7.6 mmol/L (137 mg/dL). She presents for a visit 4 weeks postpartum. She is both breast and bottle feeding. She used condoms before her first three pregnancies and the progestin-only pill between her third and fourth pregnancies, although she admits to somewhat variable compliance. She thinks she would like to resume using one of these methods, and that her family is probably complete. You counsel her regarding her contraceptive options, emphasizing efficacy, including sterilization and intrauterine devices, but also the possibility of her resuming the progestin-only contraceptive method or using condoms.

- Why is effective contraception so important in relation to diabetes in pregnancy?
- When should women be advised to start contraception after delivery?
- What are the types of contraceptives available?
- What are the advantages and disadvantages of each of these methods?
- What are the issues with contraception and breastfeeding?

BACKGROUND

The association of hyperglycemia during embryogenesis with an increased dose–response risk of both major and minor congenital malformations[1] is now clearly established and underscores the importance of offering women with pregestational diabetes, and those with a history of gestational diabetes mellitus (GDM), a safe and reliable contraceptive method both in the planning stage and as soon as possible after delivery. All women with diabetes should receive preconception counseling and achieve euglycemia prior to attempting conception. Using an effective method of contraception during this period is crucial. During pregnancy, postpartum contraceptive options and breastfeeding need to be discussed to achieve seamless contraception that begins after delivery. Exclusive breastfeeding during the first 6 months postpartum does provide pregnancy prevention and decreases the risk for obesity and metabolic syndrome in the offspring. However, by the time of the traditional 6-week postpartum visit, over 25% of women who intend to breastfeed may have abandoned breastfeeding, and only 35% are exclusively breastfeeding.[2]. Within six weeks of delivery, up to 5% of non-breastfeeding women will ovulate, putting them at risk for subsequent pregnancy.[3] Accordingly, it is important that discussions about contraception are held prior to postpartum hospital discharge and that plans are finalized at the 3–6-week postpartum visit.

Contraceptive choices depend on whether and when a woman desires to become pregnant. For women who do not desire pregnancy in the near future, long-acting reversible contraceptive (LARC) methods, e.g. intrauterine contraceptives and hormonal implants, are the most efficacious because they are not coitus dependent and do not require vigilance on the part of the patient. Continuation rates, efficacy rates, and World Health Organization (WHO) recommendations of the various methods are detailed in Table 23.1.[4,5] Studies examining contraceptive use in diabetic or prediabetic women have generally been retrospective and limited to short-term use.[6] Thus, many of the recommendations have been necessarily extrapolated from epidemiologic studies and clinical trials in non-diabetic women, and WHO classification of categories of contraceptive risk.[4] Most of the data available are a combination of level C evidence, expert opinion, and practitioner experience. While more contraceptive trials in diabetic women are needed, data from existing studies support the use of most contraceptive methods. Additionally, morbidity and mortality risks of pregnancy far outweigh those for using the most effective forms of contraception. Many women, including those with diabetes, have misconceptions about family planning methods. Eliciting concerns from the patient and providing evidence-based education may improve uptake of effective contraceptive methods and adherence.

This chapter will review contraception in women with Type 1, and Type 2 diabetes, and previous GDM. A simple question-based approach to individualized counseling is used, considering diabetic complications, comorbidities, metabolic effects, and lifestyle demands.

HOW MANY MORE CHILDREN WOULD YOU LIKE TO HAVE?

If the woman is convinced that her family is complete, two permanent options are available: vasectomy or female tubal sterilization. These methods require the patient to be counseled as to the permanent nature of the procedure and are generally not recommended for nulliparous women.

Vasectomy

The safest method for the woman with diabetes is for her male partner to have a vasectomy, which can be performed as an outpatient procedure. By interrupting the vas deferens, the passage of sperm is prevented from entering the female reproductive tract. The perfect use failure rate in the first year is reported as 0.1%, but studies reveal a failure rate of 0.0–0.74% at 1 year with a cumulative failure rate of 1.1% at 5 years.[5] The higher failure rate is usually considered secondary to the failure to use an alternate method of contraception until two consecutive sperm samples reveal no motile sperm. The use of this method does require a cooperative partner.

Female sterilization

If a cesarean delivery is planned, tubal sterilization can occur at that time. However, if the cesarean is unplanned, then even if counseling had taken place during pregnancy, there is the risk of a hurried decision which must be balanced against the risks of a subsequent sterilization operation. The most effective methods are postpartum partial salpingectomy and interval laparoscopic sterilization, both with a 10-year cumulative failure rate of 0.75%.[7] While sterilization is safe and effective, diabetes is an independent risk factor (adjusted OR 4.5) for one or more postoperative complications.[8]

A newer method of female sterilization has been developed that can be performed hysteroscopically in an outpatient setting without anesthesia, by inserting devices into the fallopian tubes that cause severe local inflammation. A hysterosalpingogram is advised at 3 months to document success. Data about this method in diabetic women are limited.

Table 23.1 Contraceptive failure and continuation rates at 1 year and 2004 World Health Organization (WHO) recommendations for hormonal and long-acting reversible contraceptive use in women with diabetes mellitus and associated conditions with 2008 updates. (Adapted from World Health Organization[4] and Trussel[5].)

	Combination estrogen and progestin methods (patch, pill, ring)	Progestin only oral contraception	Depo-medroxyprogesterone acetate injection	Etonorgestrel implant	Copper intrauterine device	Levonorgestrel releasing intrauterine device
Failure rate at 1 year (number of pregnancies in 1000 sexually active women using these methods)						
Perfect use	3	3	3	5	6	2
Typical use	80	80	30	5	8	2
Continuation rate at 1 year (%)	68	68	56	84	78	80
Recommendations for use (WHO score 1–4*)						
Diabetes						
Type 1 or 2 diabetes – without vascular disease; with or without insulin therapy	2	2	2	2	1	2
Type 1 or 2 diabetes – with neuropathy, retinopathy, nephropathy, other vascular disease, or diabetes >20 years duration	3 or 4	2	3	2	1	2
Multiple risk factors (i.e. diabetes mellitus + smoking, age >40, hypertension)	3 or 4	2	3	2	1	2
History of gestational diabetes mellitus	1	1	1	1	1	1
Breastfeeding						
<6 weeks postpartum	4	3	3	3	<48h = 1 48h to <4 weeks = 3 ≥4 weeks = 1	<48h = 3 48h to <4 weeks = 3 ≥4 weeks = 1
6 weeks–6 months, primarily breastfeeding	3	1	1	1		1
>6 months	2	1	1	1	1	1
Postpartum (not breastfeeding, if different from breastfeeding)	3	1	1	1		<48h = 1
<21 days				1		
≥21 days	1	1	1	1		
Post abortion	1	1	1	1	1	1
First trimester						
Second trimester	1	1	1	1	2	2

Table 23.1 *Continued*

	Combination estrogen and progestin methods (patch, pill, ring)	Progestin only oral contraception	Depo-medroxyprogesterone acetate injection	Etonorgestrel implant	Copper intrauterine device	Levonorgestrel releasing intrauterine device
Parity						
Nulliparous	1	1	1	1	2	2
Parous	1	1	1	1	1	1
Obesity (BMI $\geq$ 30mg/kg^2)	2	1	1 (2 if age <18 years)	1	1	1
Depressive disorders	1	1	1	1	1	1
Hyper- or hypo-thyroidism	1	1	1	1	1	1
Blood pressure						
History of hypertension, adequately controlled, or systolic 140–159 mmHg or diastolic 90–99 mmHg	3	1	2	1	1	1
Systolic $\geq$160 mmHg or diastolic $\geq$100 mmHg, or vascular disease	4	2	3	1	1	2
History of pregnancy-induced hypertension, now normal	2	1	1	1	1	1
Hyperlipidemia	2 or 3	2	2	2	1	2
Ischemic heart disease (history or current)	4	i2 c3	3	i2 c3	1	i2 c3
History of cerebrovascular accident	4	i2 c3	3	i2 c3	1	2

* 1, use the method without restriction; 2, use of the method generally outweigh the risks; 3, use of the method has theoretical or proven risks, but may be used if other methods not available or acceptable (usually requires monitoring); 4, use of the method represents an unacceptable health risk; c, continuation; I, initiation

ARE YOU INTERESTED IN USING A CONTRACEPTIVE METHOD THAT YOU DO NOT NEED TO THINK ABOUT ON A REGULAR BASIS?

Reversible long-acting methods of contraception (LARC) are recommended for use in women with diabetes and are also advocated worldwide by family planning leaders. Two main categories exist: intrauterine contraceptive devices (IUDs) and hormonal contraceptive implants. Their efficacy rivals that of permanent sterilization and they can be used by most women with diabetes, including during breastfeeding. Both are rapidly reversible. Because they require placement and removal by a healthcare professional, continuation rates are higher than for any other form of reversible contraception (see Table 23.1). This provides the healthcare provider with an opportunity to help patients achieve optimum glycemic control prior to removal for a desired pregnancy. While most diabetic women can safely use all LARC methods, various medical problems unrelated to diabetes, such as current breast cancer, may prohibit the use of hormonal LARC methods.

Intrauterine contraception

IUDs have little or no systemic or metabolic effects, and can be used in diabetic women with obesity, vascular disease, hypertension, retinopathy or hyperlipidemia. Most women with diabetes are excellent candidates for IUDs and patient selection follows the same guidelines as for non-diabetic women (e.g. no evidence of *current* pelvic inflammatory disease). Two types of IUDs are currently available, one which releases copper (Cu-IUD) and the other, a levonorgestrel-releasing intrauterine system (LNG-IUD). In an asymptomatic woman who does not have a mucopurulent cervicitis, cervical PCR for gonorrhea and chlamydia may be obtained at the time of insertion, but these results must be followed up for treatment in case of a positive culture. While IUDs are inserted using an aseptic technique, there is a slight risk for infection in the first 3 weeks after insertion. After this time, the risk of pelvic inflammatory disease is no longer increased compared to non-IUD users. Because the overall risk of infection is low in an asymptomatic woman, antibiotic prophylaxis is not routinely recommended.[9] IUDs may be placed in women with a remote history of pelvic inflammatory disease, nulliparous women, and after a non-septic spontaneous or elective abortion. If it is considered probable that the woman will return for insertion postpartum, then arrangements may be made for IUDs to be inserted 4–6 weeks after delivery. Alternatively, they may be inserted at cesarean delivery or within 48 hours after delivery, although this has been associated with an increased expulsion rate[10] when compared to the very low rate at 4–6 weeks post delivery.[11]

Follow-up studies reveal that mean weight gain after 5 years of use, at 2.4 kg in both hormonal and non-hormonal IUD users, is no different from what would be expected in the general population.[12] Although studies in diabetic women are limited, 12-month conception rates are comparable to the general population after discontinuation.[12] With regard to metabolic effects, in a 1-year randomized trial in diabetic women comparing the LNG-IUD with the Cu-IUD, no significant differences were found in fasting glucose levels, glycosylated hemoglobin or daily insulin requirements at 6 weeks, 6 months, or 12 months post insertion.[13]

Copper intrauterine device

The Cu-IUD is an excellent method of contraception for most women with diabetes. It is metabolically neutral with a 12-year cumulative pregnancy risk of 1.9%.[14] Prospective studies examining Cu-IUD use in women with Type 1 and Type 2 diabetes have found no increase in pelvic inflammatory disease or any decrease in efficacy.[15,16] The use of Cu-IUDs is associated with increased menstrual blood loss compared with controls and users of the LNG-IUD, making it a less desirable IUD for diabetic women with anemia of chronic disease or renal disease, heavy menstrual bleeding or on anticoagulation therapy.[17]

Levonorgestrel-releasing intrauterine device

In addition to its excellent efficacy, the LNG-IUD offers many non-contraceptive benefits, including protection from endometrial cancer, which is more common among obese women.[17] While it is protective against the development of anemia, there is often intermittent light vaginal bleeding in the first few months after insertion. Thereafter, menstrual blood loss is generally 70–90% less than before insertion. The levonorgestrel released into the uterine cavity reaches only 5% of the plasma levels observed with a 105-μg dose of oral levonorgestrel, resulting in minimal systemic effects. In a study of 48 women (mean age 44 years), there was a mean decrease in diastolic blood pressure with no significant change in systolic blood pressure, lipid profile, or liver function tests. However, at 1-year follow-up there was an increase in the mean fasting blood glucose concentration, although as the study was uncontrolled it is unclear if the IUD had an effect on this predestined metabolic decline.[18]

Progestin-releasing implants

The only progestin-releasing implant available in the US contains 68 mg of etonorgestrel (ENG-I). It consists of a single rod placed subdermally in the non-dominant arm by a trained inserter. It may be associated with irregular light bleeding and is effective for at least 3 years. Currently no studies address its use in diabetic women. In one study of women with polycystic ovarian syndrome

(PCOS) and insulin resistance, a group at high risk of developing Type 2 diabetes, there was a decline in insulin action as measured by the homeostasis model (HOMA) at 3–12 months from baseline, but no comparison was made with other contraceptive methods.[19] In healthy women, the implant was associated with an increase in insulin resistance.[20] While there were no significant changes in BMI, daily insulin requirement, mean HbA1c or retinal changes, Vicente *et al* showed a statistically significant decrease in high-density lipoprotein cholesterol (HDL), total serum cholesterol (TC), and triglyceride levels. The low-density lipoprotein (LDL) levels and HDL/TC ratio did not change, while albuminuria decreased.[21] However, the ENG-I is a better alternative to pregnancy in diabetic women who have difficulty complying with non-LARC contraceptive methods.

ARE YOU INTERESTED IN USING A CONTRACEPTIVE PILL AND ARE NOT IMMEDIATELY POSTPARTUM?

The combined oral contraceptive (COC) preparations available today contain low doses of estrogen and less androgenic progestins, and generally result in no or minimal effects on glucose tolerance and favorable changes in serum lipids. In diabetic women, these possible metabolic effects become important considerations when comorbidities, particularly hypertension or hyperlipidemia, are present. Evaluation of fasting serum lipids and blood pressure allows the selection of the best formulation with the least possible metabolic effect. As a rule, the lowest possible dose and potency formulation should be selected.

Estrogen has a mixed effect on serum lipids. While producing desirable effects on HDL and LDL cholesterol levels, estrogen can also increase serum triglyceride levels, which often are already elevated in women with Type 2 diabetes, and can also be related to poor glycemic control and thyroid disease. Estrogen is also associated with a dose-dependent increase in globulin production along with an increase in coagulation factors and angiotensin II levels, thereby increasing thromboembolic risk and producing a slight increase in mean arterial blood pressure.[22] With low-estrogen COCs (≤35 μg), the absolute increase in arterial thromboembolism is very low (1 in 12 000) and comparable to that among healthy COC users and non-users.[4,23] However, the risk for hemorrhagic stroke, ischemic stroke, and myocardial infarction is increased when cardiovascular risk factors (e.g. hyper-

tension, diabetes with vascular disease, smoking, migraine, or prior thrombotic disease) are present, when blood pressure is not measured prior to starting COC, or when higher doses of estrogen are used (≥50 μg).[4,24] Garg *et al* did not show progression to nephropathy or retinopathy in insulin-requiring diabetic COC users *versus* controls.[25] There are minimal data in women with microvascular disease using COCs and the WHO does not comment on this subcategory of patients. However, duration of diabetes for more than 20 years is a contraindication and Ahmed *et al* demonstrated an increased risk of developing macroalbuminuria in women with microalbuminuria prior to the routine use of angiotensin converting enzyme inhibitors or angiotensin receptor blockers.[26] Thus, it is reasonable to avoid COCs in diabetic women with microvascular disease.

Progestin formulations and doses vary widely in COCs. Most progestins are testosterone derivatives and have varying degrees of androgenic effects, e.g. decreasing sex-binding globulin, increasing insulin resistance, and adversely affecting serum lipids. Newer formulations of oral progestins (desogestrel, drospironone) or older lower dose/potency norethindrone formulations minimize androgenic side effects and therefore are generally preferable.[27] As their net effect is estrogen dominant, they may improve metabolic states in women with increased insulin resistance, unfavorable lipid profiles, and hirsutism, e.g. in women with previous GDM or with PCOS.

Short-term (<1 year) prospective studies in women with Type 1 diabetes have evaluated lower doses of older progestins, norethindrone (norethisterone ≤0.75 mg mean daily dose), triphasic levonorgestrel preparations, and newer progestins (gestodene, desogestrel). These studies showed no or minimal effect on glycemic parameters, serum lipids, and cardiovascular risk factors.

Many women with diabetes are also obese (BMI ≥ 30 kg/m²). While the WHO currently lists COC methods as being generally safe in women with obesity, one study found the risk of venous thromboembolism in COC users to be 1.4, 1.8, and 3.1 respectively among those with a BMIs of 25–30, 30–35, and greater than 35 kg/m² compared with COC users with a BMI of 20–25 kg/m².[2,28] Because no data exist in obese women with Type 2 diabetes, COCs are not a first-line method in women with marked obesity (BMI > 35 kg/m²).

Diabetic women with vascular complications, hypertension, and/or cardiovascular disease should not be prescribed estrogen-containing contraceptives due to the possible exacerbation of thromboembolic risk and hypertension. Diabetic women who smoke or have migraine, and probably those with a BMI greater than or equal to $35\,kg/m^2$ should also avoid them. Should the woman have a strong desire for estrogen-containing methods, e.g. because of severe acne, she should undergo regular monitoring of blood pressure and lipids. However, COCs can be prescribed in diabetic women without micro- or macro-vascular disease, but the formulations containing very low doses of estrogen ($\leq 20\,\mu g$) and less androgenic progestins should be selected.

Women with previous GDM share many of the risk factors of Type 2 diabetes, but short-term prospective studies have not demonstrated any adverse effect of low dose/potency COCs on glucose or lipid metabolism.[29–31] A long-term, controlled study found continued use of two COCs, one with monophasic norethindrone ($40\,\mu g$) and the other with triphasic levonorgestrel ($50–125\,\mu g$), did not contribute to the development of diabetes, with virtually identical 3-year cumulative incidence rates for those using oral contraceptives (25.4%) compared to non-hormonal methods (26.5%).[29]

The ACOG recommends that COCs should not be started before 6 weeks postpartum, after lactation is well established and the infant's nutritional status is well monitored.[32] While the possible effect of the quantity of breast milk on infant growth has not been determined, estrogen-containing methods are contraindicated during the first 6 weeks to avoid a further increased risk of postpartum thromboembolic events.[33]

Other combined hormonal methods

Recently, other routes of combined hormonal methods have become available, e.g. contraceptive vaginal rings and transdermal patches. Currently there are no data regarding their use in diabetic or prediabetic women. Data available in non-diabetic women suggest that they do not offer any metabolic advantages over COCs. Both methods are well tolerated by women with the benefit of less frequent application.[20,34] Pharmacokinetic comparison of the three regimes reveals the area under the curve for ethinyl estradiol is lower for the vaginal ring than for COCs or the transdermal patch, suggesting a theoretical advantage of this method.[35]

In summary, while COCs are not absolutely contraindicated in women with diabetes, their use should be limited to those subjects free from vascular complica-

tions. However, they are a safer alternative to unintended pregnancy and can generally be used if other options are not available or acceptable.

ARE YOU BREASTFEEDING AND LESS THAN 6 MONTHS POSTPARTUM, OR HAVE DIABETIC OR OTHER CONTRAINDICATIONS TO ESTROGEN AND WANT TO USE HORMONAL CONTRACEPTION?

While estrogen-containing contraception is contraindicated in women with diabetic micro- or macro-vascular disease, these women are candidates for progestin-only hormonal methods. These do not increase clotting factors or blood pressure. While they may decrease triglycerides, they may also decrease HDL cholesterol levels. All progestin-only formulations generally change the vaginal bleeding profile, from an initial increase in breakthrough bleeding to amenorrhea after more long-term use. These changes are rarely harmful, but are an important component of the anticipatory guidance given to the woman.

Progestin-only oral contraceptives

Oral progestins have been widely studied in healthy women. There have also been short-term studies in women with Type 1 diabetes. They have an established safety profile and may be rapidly discontinued if side effects occur.[36] They are taken continuously with no pill-free intervals and when taken carefully their efficacy is considered to be similar to COCs. However, as the effect of progestin-only oral contraceptives (PO-OCs or "mini-pills") on cervical mucus decreases after 22 hours, the need for emergency contraception arises when just one PO-OC is missed or is taken 3 hours late. These formulations are not associated with an increase in blood pressure or coagulation factors and thus, are an acceptable method for diabetic women with vascular disease, hypertension, cardiovascular, and thromboembolic risk factors.[4]

The level of steroid hormones transferred to breast milk is less than 1% of the maternal dose, which is comparable to endogenous hormone levels observed during ovulatory cycles. PO-OC preparations may be used during the first 6 weeks postpartum as they have no effect on breast milk volume or infant growth and weight.[33] In

Latina women with previous GDM, the use of PO-OCs in postpartum breastfeeding women was associated with an approximately three-fold increase in adjusted risk of developing Type 2 diabetes compared to COC use in non-breastfeeding women with prior GDM.[29] This risk increased with duration of use: use for longer than 8 months was associated with an almost five-fold increased risk. However, while both PO-OCs and depomedroxy-progesterone acetate (DMPA) (see below) have been associated with an increased risk of progression to overt diabetes in women with a history of GDM, the WHO considers both may be used without restriction in women with a history of GDM, but does not specifically address the issue of breastfeeding *and* GDM history with respect to contraceptive use (Table 23.1). Choosing an alternate method, such as an IUD, in breastfeeding women with prior GDM would be recommended.

Depomedroxypregesterone acetate

Few studies have compared metabolic effects of the various routes of progestin administration in either diabetic or non-diabetic women. In normal weight, non-diabetic women using DMPA, one controlled study found no difference in weight gain, energy intake or expenditure,[37] while the use of DMPA was associated with significant weight gain in high-risk Native American and obese women.[38,39] A recent observational study which compared DMPA with COC use in women with prior GDM for up to 9 years after delivery, found higher annual diabetes incidence rates in the DMPA users (19% *vs* 12%), but these were no longer apparent after correction for baseline cardiovascular and diabetes risk factors. The increased risk for progression to diabetes appears to be limited to subsets of women with prior GDM, who have elevated triglycerides levels greater than 1.7 mmol/L (>150 mg/dL) and had breastfed, each with a 2.3-fold increased adjusted risk.[40] In a separate analysis of women with prior GDM, longitudinal use of DMPA and COC had very slight changes in lipid profiles or blood pressure, but DMPA use was associated with a significant weight gain (~4 kg/year) compared to non-hormonal and COC use (≤1 kg/year).[41] In conclusion, DMPA is not a first choice method for diabetic or prediabetic women. However, in selected patients where daily compliance is problematic and other more effective methods cannot be used, a highly efficacious method such as DMPA may be preferable, with risks minimized by monitoring weight gain, glucose, and lipids.

WOULD YOU LIKE TO USE NATURAL OR NON-HORMONAL METHODS OF CONTRACEPTION?

Lactation amenorrhea method

Breastfeeding in diabetic women should be strongly encouraged. Studies have shown that breastfed infants of diabetic mothers have approximately half the risk during adolescence or early adulthood of developing obesity, diabetes or the metabolic syndrome. Yet in a recent survey only half of the diabetic women had received information about breastfeeding during pregnancy.[42] In non-breastfeeding women about 5% will ovulate within six weeks of delivery,[3] necessitating the need for contraception after 21 days. Exclusive breastfeeding when used as birth control is called the lactation amenorrhea method (LAM). To use LAM properly, women need to start exclusive breastfeeding immediately postpartum, breastfeed at least every 4 hours during the day and 6 hours during the night, and avoid milk supplementation and pumping. If the woman meets these criteria during the first 6 months postpartum with no return of menses, LAM provides 98% contraceptive efficacy.[5] Another method should be used if menses resume, 6 months have past since delivery or supplementary feeding is used. Women who rely on LAM should be advised about how to obtain emergency contraception (or given a prescription) in case they unexpectedly have to supplement feeding or menses resume.

Barrier methods

Barrier methods block fertilization by preventing access of the sperm into the uterus. Except for the diaphragm and cervical cap, they are obtainable without prescription, e.g. male and female condoms, contraceptive sponges, cervical shields, spermicidal jellies, and suppositories. Diaphragms and cervical caps should not be fitted or used until 6 weeks postpartum to allow for proper fitting. Barrier methods are metabolically neutral, and have no medical contraindications to their use. Their typical use failure rate is relatively high (from 15% for male condoms to 32% for the cervical cap with spermicide in parous women), as success is dependent on proper application with each coital act. Barrier method failure rates should be reduced by explanation of correct usage and providing back-up emergency contraception in advance of need. Condom use, in addition to pregnancy prevention, also decreases the transmission risk of human immunodeficiency virus (HIV) and other sexually-transmitted diseases. Women in non-monogamous relationships should be encouraged to use condoms irrespective of contraceptive benefits to reduce this risk.

Coitus interruptus or fertility awareness method

Approximately one in four women using coitus interruptus (withdrawal) or fertility awareness method (FAM, otherwise known as periodic abstinence) will become pregnant. Some women have religious beliefs that do not allow contraceptive methods other than FAM. While encouraging other more reliable methods, the risk of unintended pregnancy with FAM is still much lower than using no method, which has an 85% annual failure rate.

DO YOU KNOW ABOUT EMERGENCY CONTRACEPTION AND WHAT TO DO IF YOU FIND YOURSELF UNEXPECTEDLY PREGNANT?

All women should receive information about emergency contraception. A medical prescription may or may not be required, depending on state/country laws. If a prescription is required, it should be given as back-up to all diabetic women using non-LARC methods of contraception. Advance provision does not decrease usage of ongoing contraceptive methods or increase incidence of sexually-transmitted infections. Often referred to as the "morning after pill", it should be taken as soon as possible within 120 hours after recognized method failure, e.g. unprotected coitus, broken condom, or missed oral contraceptive pills.[43] The mechanism of action is via delay or inhibition of ovulation, and thus the shorter the time interval from coitus to administration of emergency contraception, the more effective the pregnancy protection. In diabetic women, the progestin-only regime, levonorgestrel (1.5 mg total dose), is recommended and has no contraindications to use. The "modified Yuzpe" regime (0.5 mg of levonorgestrel and 100 μg of ethinyl estradiol taken once and repeated in 24 hours), is less efficacious at preventing pregnancies than the levonorgestrel-only method (57% *vs* 85%), and is associated with significant gastrointestinal side effects.[41] After taking emergency contraception, a woman needs to start or restart a reliable contraceptive method. A pregnancy test should be administered if menses have not resumed within 4 weeks of starting a method.[44] Another and more effective method of emergency contraception is to insert a Cu-IUD (pregnancy rates between 0.0% and 0.2%) after unprotected coitus. It can be inserted up to the time of possible implantation (7 days after suspected ovulation).[45]

Despite efforts to improve contraceptive adherence and effectiveness, there will be contraceptive failures and unplanned pregnancies. It is advised to inform the patient of her positive pregnancy test result in a dispassionate manner, allowing the patient to express her feelings regarding the diagnosis of pregnancy. Women must be advised that pregnancy in Type 1 and Type 2 diabetes is associated with an increased risk of congenital malformations and that this risk is further increased if the diabetes is poorly controlled (see chapters 8 and 14). In patients who desire pregnancy continuation, strict glycemic control should be obtained as quickly as possible if not already present. In women with undesired pregnancies, potential poor pregnancy outcomes related to poor maternal glycemic control may influence the decision regarding pregnancy termination. Women should be counseled regarding the option of pregnancy termination regardless of their metabolic status. While there are no studies regarding surgical aspiration *versus* medical termination in women with diabetes, both are considered acceptable options.

CONCLUSIONS

In the selection of a contraceptive method, choices must be individualized to take account of the woman's preferences, her health, social situation, and expected compliance. It is the physician's duty to stress the importance of using *effective* methods of contraception until the woman is euglycemic and ready to conceive, which will minimize the risks of congenital anomalies.

IUDs are first-line LARCs in women with diabetes, as they are metabolically neutral and have a failure rate similar to sterilization. Data are limited regarding the etonorgestrel implant in diabetic women, which lasts for 3 years and also requires a visit to a physician's office for removal.

Diabetic women who do not wish to or cannot use intrauterine contraception have a variety of hormonal contraceptive options, and in most cases a suitable hormonal method can be identified.

Combination hormone contraceptive methods may be used in diabetic women without micro- and macro-vascular disease and have minimal metabolic effects. Women with hypertension, a history of myocardial infarction, stroke, diabetic complications, longstanding diabetes or who are less than 6 weeks postpartum, should not use any estrogen-containing contraceptives; progestin-only methods are acceptable alternatives. Barrier methods and methods of natural family planning, while metabolically safe, are not recommended as a first-line agent for women with diabetes because of their high failure rate. All women should be informed about emergency contraception which is safe to use in diabetic women.

For women who have completed child-bearing, vasectomy and/or female sterilization are options to consider. When faced with an unintended pregnancy, women must receive non-directive counseling in pregnancy options which must include additional guidance reflecting their risk for major congenital anomalies.

While contraceptive choice is ultimately up to the woman, the physician caring for women with diabetes should promote the use of effective methods, to permit planning and preparation for a healthy and successful pregnancy outcome and to avoid unintended, unplanned pregnancies, which expose the woman and her offspring to increased risks of medical complications and congenital anomalies.

CASE HISTORY

Maria is an excellent candidate for sterilization and this option should be explored. However, as she has some doubts about this, she should be counseled that should she conceive she is at increased risk of having a child with congenital anomalies secondary to suboptimal glycemic control. A subsequent pregnancy for Maria also has many risks due to her advanced age, hypertension, obesity, and longstanding diabetes. These factors would also contraindicate the use of any estrogen-containing contraceptive method. Maria has risk factors for anovulatory bleeding and endometrial cancer (obese, older age, and Type 2 diabetes) and would benefit from a progestin-containing method. She could use a PO-OC, but she should be given advice about back-up emergency contraception. She is an ideal candidate for a LARC method, such as the LNG-IUS, or alternatively either the Cu-IUD or progestin implant. While she could use DMPA, she must be counseled about possible weight gain associated with its use. In the end, Maria chose to use a LNG-IUS.

FUTURE DIRECTIONS FOR RESEARCH

The literature to date is largely confined to short-term studies in Type 1 diabetes. There is a need for research on long-term outcomes for almost all contraceptive methods in women with diabetes. In addition, with the increase in Type 2 diabetes, frequently in the context of other cardiovascular risk factors, more studies are needed to clarify whether contraceptive use in these subjects is associated with adverse outcomes. Finally, research into more effective ways of delivering contraceptive advice is required to reduce the number of unplanned pregnancies occurring when metabolic control is not ideal.

REFERENCES

1 Schaefer-Graf UM, Buchanan TA, Xiang A, Songster G, Montoro M, Kjos SL. Patterns of congenital anomalies and relationship to initial maternal fasting glucose levels in pregnancies complicated by type 2 and gestational diabetes. *Am J Obstet Gynecol* 2000;**182**:313–20.

2 Halderman LD, Nelson AL. Impact of early postpartum administration of progestin-only hormonal contraceptives compared with nonhormonal contraceptives on short-term breast-feeding patterns. *Am J Obstet Gynecol* 2002;**186**:1250–6; discussion 6–8.

3 Speroff L, Mishell DR Jr. The postpartum visit: it's time for a change in order to optimally initiate contraception. *Contraception* 2008;**78**:90–8.

4 World Health Organization. *Medical Eligibility Criteria for Contraceptive Use*, 2004 (updated 2008). www.who.int/reproductive-health/publications/mec/mec.pdf

5 Trussel J. Contraceptive efficacy. In: Hatcher RA (ed). *Contraceptive Technology*, 19th edn. New York: Ardent Media, 2007:747.

6 Visser J, Snel M, Van Vliet HA. Hormonal versus non-hormonal contraceptives in women with diabetes mellitus type 1 and 2. *Cochrane Database Syst Rev* 2006, Issue 4:CD003990.

7 Peterson HB, Xia Z, Hughes JM, Wilcox LS, Tylor LR, Trussell J. The risk of pregnancy after tubal sterilization: findings from the U.S. Collaborative Review of Sterilization. *Am J Obstet Gynecol* 1996;**174**:1161–8; discussion 8–70.

8 Jamieson DJ, Hillis SD, Duerr A, Marchbanks PA, Costello C, Peterson HB. Complications of interval laparoscopic tubal sterilization: findings from the U.S. Collaborative Review of Sterilization. *Obstet Gynecol* 2000;**96**:997–1002.

9 Farley TM, Rosenberg MJ, Rowe PJ, Chen JH, Meirik O. Intrauterine devices and pelvic inflammatory disease: an international perspective. *Lancet* 1992;**339**:785–8.

10 Grimes D, Schulz K, Van Vliet H, Stanwood N. Immediate post-partum insertion of intrauterine devices. *Cochrane Database Syst Rev* 2003, Issue 1:CD003036.

11 Chen JH, Wu SC, Shao WQ, *et al.* The comparative trial of TCu 380A IUD and progesterone-releasing vaginal ring used by lactating women. *Contraception* 1998;**57**:371–9.

12 French R, Van Vliet H, Cowan F, *et al.* Hormonally impregnated intrauterine systems (IUSs) versus other forms of reversible contraceptives as effective methods of preventing pregnancy. *Cochrane Database Syst Rev* 2004, Issue 3:CD001776.

13 Rogovskaya S, Rivera R, Grimes DA, *et al*. Effect of a levonorgestrel intrauterine system on women with type 1 diabetes: a randomized trial. *Obstet Gynecol* 2005;**105**: 811–5.

14 Long-term reversible contraception. Twelve years of experience with the TCu380A and TCu220C. *Contraception* 1997;**56**:341–52.

15 Kimmerle R, Weiss R, Berger M, Kurz KH. Effectiveness, safety, and acceptability of a copper intrauterine device (CU Safe 300) in type I diabetic women. *Diabetes Care* 1993;**16**:1227–30.

16 Kjos SL, Ballagh SA, La Cour M, Xiang A, Mishell DR Jr. The copper T380A intrauterine device in women with type II diabetes mellitus. *Obstet Gynecol* 1994;**84**:1006–9.

17 Varma R, Sinha D, Gupta JK. Non-contraceptive uses of levonorgestrel-releasing hormone system (LNG-IUS) – a systematic enquiry and overview. *Eur J Obstet Gynecol Reprod Biol* 2006;**125**:9–28.

18 Kayikcioglu F, Gunes M, Ozdegirmenci O, Haberal A. Effects of levonorgestrel-releasing intrauterine system on glucose and lipid metabolism: a 1-year follow-up study. *Contraception* 2006;**73**:528–31.

19 Meyer C, Talbot M, Teede H. Effect of Implanon on insulin resistance in women with polycystic ovary syndrome. *Aust N Z J Obstet Gynaecol* 2005;**45**:155–8.

20 Lopez LM, Grimes DA, Gallo MF, Schulz KF. Skin patch and vaginal ring versus combined oral contraceptives for contraception. *Cochrane Database Syst Rev* 2008, Issue 1:CD003552.

21 Vicente L, Mendonca D, Dingle M, Duarte R, Boavida JM. Etonogestrel implant in women with diabetes mellitus. *Eur J Contracept Reprod Health Care* 2008;**13**:387–95.

22 Dong W, Colhoun HM, Poulter NR. Blood pressure in women using oral contraceptives: results from the Health Survey for England 1994. *J Hypertens* 1997;**15**:1063–8.

23 Lidegaard O. Oral contraceptives, pregnancy and the risk of cerebral thromboembolism: the influence of diabetes, hypertension, migraine and previous thrombotic disease. *Br J Obstet Gynaecol* 1995;**102**:153–9.

24 Ischaemic stroke and combined oral contraceptives: results of an international, multicentre, case-control study. WHO Collaborative Study of Cardiovascular Disease and Steroid Hormone Contraception. *Lancet* 1996;**348**:498–505.

25 Garg SK, Chase HP, Marshall G, Hoops SL, Holmes DL, Jackson WE. Oral contraceptives and renal and retinal complications in young women with insulin-dependent diabetes mellitus. *JAMA* 1994;**271**:1099–102.

26 Ahmed SB, Hovind P, Parving H-H, *et al*. Oral contraceptives, angiotensin-dependent renal vasoconstriction, and risk of diabetic nephropathy. *Diabetes Care* 2005;**28**: 1988–94.

27 Proudler T, Felton C, Lees B, *et al*. The effects of different formulations of oral contraceptive agents on lipid and carbohydrate metabolism. *N Engl J Med* 1990;**323**:1375–81.

28 Nightingale AL, Lawrenson RA, Simpson EL, Williams TJ, MacRae KD, Farmer RD. The effects of age, body mass index, smoking and general health on the risk of venous thromboembolism in users of combined oral contraceptives. *Eur J Contracept Reprod Health Care* 2000;**5**:265–74.

29 Kjos SL, Peters RK, Xiang A, Thomas D, Schaefer U, Buchanan TA. Contraception and the risk of type 2 diabetes mellitus in Latina women with prior gestational diabetes mellitus. *JAMA* 1998;**280**:533–8.

30 Kjos SL, Shoupe D, Douyan S, *et al*. Effect of low-dose oral contraceptives on carbohydrate and lipid metabolism in women with recent gestational diabetes: results of a controlled, randomized, prospective study. *Am J Obstet Gynecol* 1990;**163**:1822–7.

31 Skouby SO, Kuhl C, Molsted-Pedersen L, Petersen K, Christensen MS. Triphasic oral contraception: metabolic effects in normal women and those with previous gestational diabetes. *Am J Obstet Gynecol* 1985;**153**:495–500.

32 ACOG Committee Opinion No. 361: Breastfeeding: maternal and infant aspects. *Obstet Gynecol* 2007;**109**: 479–80.

33 Truitt ST, Fraser AB, Grimes DA, Gallo MF, Schulz KF. Combined hormonal versus nonhormonal versus progestin-only contraception in lactation. *Cochrane Database Syst Rev* 2003, Issue 2:CD003988.

34 Smallwood GH, Meador ML, Lenihan JP, Shangold GA, Fisher AC, Creasy GW. Efficacy and safety of a transdermal contraceptive system. *Obstet Gynecol* 2001;**98**:799–805.

35 van den Heuvel MW, van Bragt AJ, Alnabawy AK, Kaptein MC. Comparison of ethinylestradiol pharmacokinetics in three hormonal contraceptive formulations: the vaginal ring, the transdermal patch and an oral contraceptive. *Contraception* 2005;**72**:168–74.

36 Radberg T, Gustafson A, Skryten A, Karlsson K. Oral contraception in diabetic women. A cross-over study on serum and high density lipoprotein (HDL) lipids and diabetes control during progestogen and combined estrogen/progestogen contraception. *Horm Metab Res* 1982;**14**:61–5.

37 Pelkman CL, Chow M, Heinbach RA, Rolls BJ. Short-term effects of a progestational contraceptive drug on food intake, resting energy expenditure, and body weight in young women. *Am J Clin Nutr* 2001;**73**:19–26.

38 Espey E, Steinhart J, Ogburn T, Qualls C. Depo-Provera associated with weight gain in Navajo women. *Contraception* 2000;**62**:55–8.

39 Mangan SA, Larsen PG, Hudson S. Overweight teens at increased risk for weight gain while using depot medroxyprogesterone acetate. *J Pediatr Adolesc Gynecol* 2002;**15**:79–82.

40 Xiang AH, Kawakubo M, Kjos SL, Buchanan TA. Long-acting injectable progestin contraception and risk of type 2 diabetes in Latino women with prior gestational diabetes mellitus. *Diabetes Care* 2006;**29**:613–7.

41 Xiang AH KM, Buchanan TA, Kjos SL. A longitudinal study of lipids and blood pressure in relation to methods of contraception in Latino women with prior gestational diabetes mellitus. *Diabetes Care* 2007;**30**:1952–8.

42 Stage E, Norgard H, Damm P, Mathiesen E. Long-term breast-feeding in women with type 1 diabetes. *Diabetes Care* 2006;**29**:771–4.

43 Cheng L, Gulmezoglu AM, Piaggio G, Ezcurra E, Van Look PF. Interventions for emergency contraception. *Cochrane Database Syst Rev* 2008, Issue 2:CD001324.

44 RHEDI. *Quick Start Algorithm*. New York: The Center for Reproductive Health Education in Family Medicine at Montefiore Medical Center, 2008.

45 Trussell J, Ellertson C, Stewart F, Raymond EG, Shochet T. The role of emergency contraception. *Am J Obstet Gynecol* 2004;**190** (Suppl 4):S30–8.

24 Long-term implications for the mother with hyperglycemia in pregnancy

Jorge H. Mestman

Departments of Medicine and Obstetrics and Gynecology, Keck School of Medicine, University of Southern California, Los Angeles, CA, USA

PRACTICE POINTS

- Gestational diabetes mellitus (GDM) may be the first manifestation of subsequent Type 2 diabetes; the cumulative incidence of diabetes ranges from 2.6% to 70%, increasing steeply within the first 5 years after delivery.
- Epidemiologic comparisons are confounded by different oral glucose loads, differing durations of follow-up and, in the US, the use of different diagnostic criteria during and following pregnancy.
- Women with GDM should undergo repeat glucose testing postpartum and receive appropriate counseling on their risk of future diabetes and of the need for lifestyle changes and weight management. At the time of the diagnosis of Type 2 diabetes, a significant number of patients have already developed micro- and macro-vascular complications; therefore, close follow-up after the diagnosis of GDM is of utmost importance in order to prevent complications.
- Clinicians and other healthcare providers have a great opportunity to improve the lives of women with history of GDM and their families by applying recent knowledge regarding the early detection, prevention, and management of hyperglycemia and other cardiovascular risk factors.

CASE HISTORY

A 39-year-old woman presented to her physician with a 6-month history of polyuria, nocturia, 5 lb (2.3 kg) weight loss and vaginal itch. She was overweight at 168 lb (76 kg) for her height of 5 feet 4 inches (163 cm) (body mass index [BMI] 29) and smoked 10 cigarettes per day. Blood pressure was 138/88 mmHg. A random blood glucose was raised at 14.4 mmol/L (260 mg/dL) with a repeat fasting glucose of 10 mmol/L (180 mg/dL) the following day, confirming the diagnosis of diabetes. A spot early

morning urine test for microalbumin was negative. Fasting lipids showed a total cholesterol of 5.7 mmol/L (220 mg/dL), triglycerides 3.3 mmol/L (294 mg/dL), low-density lipoprotein (LDL) cholesterol 2.9 mmo/L (111 mg/dL), and high-density lipoprotein (HDL) cholesterol 0.9 mmo/L (36 mg/dL). Ophthalmologic evaluation revealed early signs of non-proliferative diabetic retinopathy in the left eye.

She had four previous children. Her last pregnancy, 8 years prior to the current pregnancy, had been complicated by GDM, diagnosed on screening at 28 weeks, for which she was treated with diet initially and subsequently insulin from 34 weeks of gestation. Her weight gain during that pregnancy was 45 lbs (20.4 kg). She delivered a 4400-g healthy infant by cesarean section at 38 weeks of gestation. Her insulin was discontinued at delivery. Six weeks postpartum, she was informed that her fasting plasma glucose was normal and she was advised to have the test repeated in 1 year. She breastfed for 4 months and managed to loose 30 lb (13.6 kg) in the first 6 months postpartum through lifestyle changes. At her request a tubal ligation was performed 9 months after delivery. Contrary to advice she was subsequently lost to review until she represented with classical hyperglycemic symptoms.

Once the diagnosis of diabetes mellitus was confirmed, she expressed concern about her 21-year-old daughter who was diagnosed with GDM at week 28 of her first and only pregnancy. She asked if her daughter was also at risk of developing overt diabetes in the future, and if so, were there any possibilities for prevention?

- Why was the patient asked to return one year after delivery, in spite of a normal 6 weeks postpartum?
- What would you advise the patient's daughter following the birth of her own child in order to prevent the development of diabetes mellitus 2?

A Practical Manual of Diabetes in Pregnancy, 1st Edition.
Edited by David R. McCance, Michael Maresh and David A. Sacks.
© 2010 Blackwell Publishing

BACKGROUND

It was recognized more than 100 years ago that hyperglycemia in pregnant women may disappear after delivery but return years later.[1] In the late 1940s and early 1950s, several retrospective studies demonstrated a high perinatal morbidity and mortality in infants of mothers who developed diabetes years later. These findings stimulated the investigation of carbohydrate metabolism in pregnancy with the use of oral and intravenous glucose tolerance tests, in order to detect hyperglycemia with the aim of improving maternal/fetal outcome.

The development of hyperglycemia years after the diagnosis of what is known today as GDM was first recognized by Duncan in 1892.[2] He made three remarkable statements in the conclusion of his pioneer article on "Diabetes and pregnancy":

- Diabetes may come on during pregnancy
- Diabetes may occur only during pregnancy and be absent at other times
- Diabetes may cease with the termination of pregnancy, recurring some time after delivery.

In the decades between 1930 and 1950, it was shown that at the diagnosis of diabetes mellitus, women frequently gave an obstetric history of macrosomic infants, unexplained intrauterine deaths, and neonatal morbidity and mortality.[3–5] A perinatal death rate of 15.4% was reported in the 5 years preceding the diagnosis of diabetes compared with a perinatal mortality rate of 6% in women delivering 5–12 years before the diagnosis of diabetes.[4]

The first study of the use of an oral glucose tolerance test (OGTT) in pregnancy was by Wilkerson and Remein in Boston.[6] The aim of the study was "to evaluate the effect of insulin treatment on the outcome of pregnancy in women with abnormal carbohydrate tolerance to determine if such treatment would:

- Result in a lower rate of fetal wastage and other complications of pregnancy
- Delay the onset of diabetes in pregnant women in the prediabetic stage
- Decrease the chance of diabetes occurring in the live births".

O'Sullivan and Mahan,[7] using the same material collected by Wilkerson and Remein, established the criteria for the diagnosis of GDM, based not on perinatal outcome, but on the cumulative incidence of future diabetes in women with GDM; they reported an incidence of 67% of diabetes at 5½ years following delivery. In 1960 Jackson[8] from South Africa suggested that a "temporary"

diabetic state or significant impairment of glucose tolerance during pregnancy indicated a state of potentially permanent diabetes in the mother.

Since this first observation of overt diabetes developing years after the diagnosis of GDM, several clinical studies have confirmed these findings. Mestman et al[9] followed 360 mostly Latina GDM women for up to 5 years after delivery. Of 51 women with an elevated fasting blood glucose of greater than 5.5 mmol/L (100 mg/dL) during pregnancy, only four reverted to a normal OGTT 6 weeks postpartum. Of 181 women with an abnormal OGTT but normal fasting blood glucose in pregnancy, 23 (12.7%) developed overt diabetes (fasting blood glucose >5.6 mmol/L [100 mg/dL]) and 59 (32.6%) of them developed impaired glucose tolerance (IGT). Other investigators confirmed the above findings.[10–12]

Based on these findings, the routine use of an OGTT 4–8 weeks postpartum was recommended. Currently, those women with positive tests are referred to healthcare professionals for long-term follow-up, including diabetes education, lifestyle modification, screening, and management of cardiovascular risk factors in order to prevent or delay the deterioration of carbohydrate intolerance and reduce the risk of future cardiovascular disease. This approach is supported by a number of studies in the last two decades which have shown the effectiveness of aggressive lifestyle modification, physical activity, and pharmacologic therapies in the prevention of Type 2 diabetes. It is the responsibility of healthcare professionals caring for women with GDM to encourage them to have an OGTT in the first few weeks after delivery and to make provision for their proper education and long-term care.

RISK FACTORS FOR THE DEVELOPMENT OF TYPE 2 DIABETES IN WOMEN WITH GESTATIONAL DIABETES MELLITUS

Kim et al[13] presented a systematic review of 28 articles published between 1965 and 2001 on GDM and risk of future Type 2 diabetes. All women were examined 6 weeks to 28 years postpartum, and the cumulative incidence of diabetes ranged from 2.6% to 70%. The authors made several interesting observations.

- Once diagnosed with GDM, women from mixed or non-white cohorts seemed to progress to Type 2 diabetes at similar rates.
- The progression to Type 2 diabetes increased steeply within the first 5 years after delivery and then appeared to plateau.

- Women of white ethnicity converted at a similar rate to the other ethnic groups, but it was difficult to assess this because of the relatively few studies in this population.
- Elevated pregnancy fasting glucose before 24–26 weeks of gestation predicted Type 2 diabetes, except when more specific measures of pancreatic beta cell function were concomitantly examined, such as insulin secretion.
- Other risk factors had inconsistent or little predictive value after adjustment for other variables, such as BMI, maternal age, previous history of GDM, family history of diabetes, and parity. In many studies reviewed by the authors, some of the above risk factors were associated in univariate analyses, but not in multivariate analysis.

Kjos et al[14] studied 671 Latino women with GDM, all of whom had a normal OGTT 4–16 weeks postpartum. The subjects underwent at least one OGTT within the following 7.5 years. Life table analysis revealed a 47% cumulative incidence rate of Type 2 diabetes 5 years after delivery. They identified four variables as independent predictors for the development of Type 2 diabetes:

- Glucose area under the postpartum OGTT (4–16 weeks) curve (933 ± 189 mmol/L/min)
- Gestational age at the time of the diagnosis of GDM (28.1 ± 0.3 weeks)
- Glucose area under the pregnancy OGTT (1744 ± 277 mmol/L/min)
- Highest fasting serum glucose concentration (6.2 ± 1.5 mmol/L) (111.7 ± 27.0 mg/dl) during pregnancy.

The area under the postpartum OGTT, however, provided the best discrimination between high-risk and low-risk individuals.

Peters et al[15] in a group of Latino women with GDM reported that an additional pregnancy increased the risk of developing Type 2 diabetes (RR 3.34, 95% Cl 1.80–13.8) as well as weight gain within 7.5 years after delivery (RR 1.95, 95% Cl 1.63–2.33).

Not only are women with GDM at higher risk of developing overt diabetes but those with a slight elevation in blood glucose during a screening oral glucose challenge test (OGCT) or a diagnostic OGTT are at similar risks.[16–18] In a retrospective study[17] women with an abnormal OGCT and one abnormal glucose value during the OGTT were followed for a median period of 8.8 years. Type 2 diabetes was ascertained by ICD-9 codes or pharmacy or laboratory data. The higher the elevation in glucose values during pregnancy, the greater the risk for subsequent development of Type 2 diabetes. The above find-

Table 24.1 Predictors of gestational diabetes mellitus (GDM) and Type 2 diabetes.

GDM	Type 2 diabetes
Obesity	Obesity
Family history of Type 2 diabetes	Family history of Type 2 diabetes
Waist-to-hip ratio	Waist-to-hip ratio
Previous history of GDM	Previous history of GDM
Ethnic background	Ethnic background
Hypertension	Hypertension
Previous history of macrosomia	Dyslipidemia
Advanced maternal age	Low birthweight
Cigarette smoking	Physical inactivity
	Polycystic ovarian syndrome
	Cigarette smoking

ings are supported by studies showing a decrease in beta cell function in women with one abnormal value in the OGTT compared to women with a *negative* OGTT.[18] Furthermore, it was reported that isolated hyperglycemia at 1 hour during an OGTT is associated with postpartum hyperglycemia, insulin resistance, and beta cell dysfunction.[19]

As shown in Table 24.1 risk factors for developing GDM are very similar to those for Type 2 diabetes.

LONG-TERM CARDIOVASCULAR COMPLICATIONS IN WOMEN WITH GESTATIONAL DIABETES MELLITUS

Women with diabetes mellitus are at increased risk of developing cardiovascular disease with a mortality higher than in men.[20] A possible explanation for this observation is that women are less likely to receive the same aggressive treatment for lipids, hypertension, and hemoglobin A1c (HbA1c) than men.[21,22] In one of the earliest studies,[23] 89 women with GDM were interviewed 12–18 years after their pregnancies; 58 (65.2%) of them had developed overt diabetes. The incidence of hypertension was 44.8% in the GDM group *versus* 12.9% in the control group. Five women had had a stroke, four a myocardial infarction, and two were on chronic dialysis. In a preliminary analysis of the Boston Gestational Diabetes Study, O'Sullivan[24] showed that during 26 years of follow-up, postpartum rates of mortality, hypertension, and dyslipidemia were significantly higher in the GDM group compared with controls. He also reported more electrocardiogram (ECG) abnormalities in the GDM women with three- to five-fold more cases of myocardial infarction and angina.

Carr et al[25] studied 994 parous women with Type 2 diabetes, who had a first-degree relative with Type 2 diabetes, 29.9 years after the index pregnancy (range 1.2–74.0). Three hundred and thirty-two women (33.4%) gave a history of GDM, and 662 (67.6%) had no history of GDM. BMI, race, and ethnicity were similar between the two groups with each composed of about one-third Caucasians, African Americans, and Latinas. The mean age at the time of the study was 52.4 years in women without a previous history of GDM and 48.6 years in those with a history of GDM (p < 0.001). Women with previous GDM were more likely to have developed Type 2 diabetes, to have been diagnosed with the metabolic syndrome, and to have suffered a cardiovascular disease (CVD) event compared with women without prior GDM.

Shah et al[26] identified 8191 women diagnosed with GDM in Ontario, Canada between 1994 and 1997, and 81 262 women who had a live birth without GDM, with a median follow-up of 11.5 years. Diabetes, mostly Type 2, developed during follow-up in 27% of the women with GDM and 3.2% of the women without GDM. The authors concluded that women with GDM had a substantially increased risk for CVD events (HR 1.71; 95% CI 1.08–2.69) in later life compared with women without GDM. Much of this increased risk was attributable to the subsequent development of Type 2 diabetes.

RELATIONSHIP BETWEEN GESTATIONAL DIABETES MELLITUS AND METABOLIC SYNDROME

The similarities in risk factors for the development of GDM and Type 2 diabetes have been recognized for the last three decades (Table 24.1). In addition to insulin resistance, compensatory hyperinsulinemia and beta cell dysfunction, abnormalities in lipid metabolism, hypertension, and obesity are present in both clinical entities. It has been suggested that both conditions are the same disorder.[27,28] Women with a history of previous GDM, studied at the time of normal glucose tolerance, present the hallmarks of insulin resistance and hyperinsulinemia.[29]

The metabolic syndrome or insulin resistance syndrome is a predictor for development of cardiovascular complications,[30] with a prevalence of 20–40% in an American adult population.[31] The diagnostic criteria suggested by the National Cholesterol Education Program (NCEP) expert panel[32] require the presence of three of

five of the following for diagnosis: (1) blood pressure 130/85 mmHg or greater; (2) HDL cholesterol less than 1.03 mmol/L (40 mg/dL) in men and 1.29 mmol/L (50 mg/dL) in women; (3) serum triglycerides greater than 1.69 mmol/L (150 mg/dL); (4) abdominal obesity defined as a waist circumference greater than 40 inches (100 cm) in men and 36 inches (92 cm) in women; and (5) a fasting *serum* glucose of greater than 5.5 mmol/L (100 mg/dL). Hyperinsulinemia is a constant feature. Other manifestations of the metabolic syndrome are:

- Hyperuricemia and gout
- Acanthosis nigricans
- Sleep apnea
- Polycystic ovary syndrome
- Fatty liver disease with steatosis, fibrosis, and cirrhosis.

The International Diabetes Federation (IDF) proposed in 2004[33] the following criteria:

- Increased waist circumference
- Serum triglycerides greater than 1.7 mmol/L (150 mg/dL) or treatment for elevated triglycerides
- HDL cholesterol less than 1.03 mmol/L (40 mg/dL) in men and less than 1.29 mmol/L (50 mg/dL) in women, or treatment for low HDL cholesterol
- Systolic blood pressure greater than 130 mmHg, diastolic blood pressure greater than 85 mmHg, or treatment for hypertension
- Fasting plasma glucose greater than 5.5 mmol/L (100 mg/dL), or previously diagnosed Type 2 diabetes.

In a study in the US, the IDF criteria categorized 15–20% more adults with the metabolic syndrome than the NCEP criteria.[34]

Type 2 diabetes develops in subjects with defects in insulin secretion in the presence of insulin resistance. Women with a history of GDM have been studied at different times following the index pregnancy to determine insulin action and insulin resistance in the presence of a normal glucose tolerance test.[29,35] In spite of having a normal glucose tolerance, these women were found to have defects in both insulin secretion and insulin action.

Kjos et al[36] studied lipid metabolism in a group of Latina women with GDM followed for 36 months. At 6–12 weeks postpartum, serum triglycerides were higher and HDL cholesterol lower in those women who later developed diabetes mellitus as compared with women who did not develop diabetes. This is consistent with findings in prediabetic patients.[37]

Birthweight is inversely related to subsequent risk for Type 2 diabetes, insulin resistance, and other features of the metabolic syndrome.[38] Both low birthweight (<2500 g) and high birthweight (>4500 g) are associated with the future development of GDM and Type 2 diabetes (the latter phenomenon is most likely explained by the presence of obesity and hyperglycemia during pregnancy).[39]

Clark *et al*[40] hypothesized that GDM could manifest many of the characteristics of the metabolic syndrome. They compared the metabolic profile in 179 women (91 African American, 81 Caucasian, and seven of other ethnic groups), 52 of whom had a history of GDM while 127 did not, as determined by a normal 1-hour glucose screen. Women with GDM had a higher prepregnancy BMI, c-peptide, insulin levels fasting and at 2 hours postprandially, and fasting free fatty acid, and a lower HDL cholesterol during pregnancy (16–33 weeks). The authors suggested that GDM might be viewed as a component of the metabolic syndrome. It also provides an excellent model for study and prevention of Type 2 diabetes in a relatively young age group.

Launeberg *et al*[41] studied a population of women, mean age 43 years, with prior diet-treated GDM, 75% of whom were of Danish origin, with the aim of estimating the prevalence of the metabolic syndrome 9.8 years (range 6.4–17.2 years) after the index pregnancy; the control group comprised 1000 women (95% Danish). The main outcome measures were BMI, glucose tolerance, blood pressure, lipids, and insulin resistance, measured by fasting insulin levels. The prevalence of the metabolic syndrome was 40% in women with prior GDM, three times higher than in the control group.

The above studies strongly support the hypothesis that GDM has many features in common with the metabolic syndrome. These observations have very important implications not only for the detection of patients at risk at a young age, but also as they offer the potential to prevent diabetes in the offspring of women with GDM. As stated by Norbert Freinkel[42] in the opening address of the First International workshop on GDM, "… with GDM women, we may be able to unmask a population at greater risk for permanent diabetes than under nongravid conditions and use it to evaluate the efficacy of preventive measures".

PREVENTION OF TYPE 2 DIABETES

Since it is known that most women with a history of GDM are at higher risk for the development of Type 2 diabetes, simple and practical measures in early detection of prediabetes and prevention of Type 2 diabetes should have a major impact on decreasing cardiovascular morbidity and mortality. One of the barriers is the lack of

perception and understanding after delivery on the part of the women (and perhaps also that of the healthcare providers) of the seriousness and consequences of diabetes mellitus. Among a selected group of 217 mostly white, affluent, and well-educated women with a previous history of GDM, 7% believed that they had almost no chance of developing diabetes, 35% a slight chance, 41% a moderate chance, and 16% a high chance; only 31% reported engaging in lifestyle modification.[43] Therefore, patient education in lifestyle modification and encouragement to return for glucose testing at regular intervals are important tools for the healthcare professional in the subsequent follow-up of women with GDM.

Physical inactivity and obesity are well-known risk factors for the development of Type 2 diabetes. It was postulated that lifestyle modification, including weight loss, decreasing the total amount of ingested calories, increasing the amount of fiber in the diet, and increasing daily physical activity could delay or prevent the development of Type 2 diabetes in those subjects at higher risk.[44,45] In the study by Helmrich *et al*[45] among a group of women, the incidence of Type 2 diabetes was reduced by a third through vigorous exercise independent of a family history of diabetes.

In the Diabetes Prevention Program,[46] 3234 subjects of both genders aged over 25 years with a BMI of 24 or higher and a fasting serum glucose concentration of 5.3–6.9 mmol/L (95–125 mg/dL]) or a 2-hour value of 7.8–11.0 mmol/L (140–199 mg/dL) after a 75-g glucose load were eligible for the study. The subjects were assigned to four different groups:
- Intensive lifestyle changes under strict supervision with the aim of reducing weight by 7% with diet and 150 minutes of weekly exercise
- Metformin 850 mg twice a day, combined with a meal plan and physical activity advice
- Troglitazone (but this arm was discontinued due to drug toxicity)
- A control group.

The incidence of diabetes was reduced by 58% with lifestyle intervention and by 31% with metformin compared with placebo. The average follow-up of the study was 2.8 years. In the intensive lifestyle group, 50% of the participants had achieved the goal of weight loss of at least 7% or more at the end of 24 weeks; 74% of the participants met the goal of at least 150 minutes of weekly exercise by 24 weeks. The adherence to metformin was 72%. The average weight loss was 0.1, 2.1, and 5.6 kg in the placebo, metformin, and lifestyle intervention groups, respectively (p < 0.001). These effects were similar in men and women and in all racial and ethnic groups. Metformin was more effective in younger individuals.

In Finland,[47] 552 middle-age overweight subjects with impaired glucose tolerance were randomly assigned to either an intervention or a control group. In the former, individual counseling aimed at reducing weight by decreasing intake of dietary fat, increasing intake of dietary fiber, and increasing physical activity was given. The cumulative incidence of diabetes after 4 years was 11 % (95% CI 6–15%) in the intervention group and 23% (95% CI 17–29%) in the control group. During the trial, the risk of diabetes was reduced by 58% in the intervention group and was directly associated with changes in lifestyle.

Drug therapy is also an important tool in preventing or delaying the onset of Type 2 diabetes. The TRIPOD study[48] involved Latino women with previous GDM and no diabetes at entry. They were followed for 30 months and compared with a placebo group matched for age, BMI, and parity. The treated group of 133 women received troglitazone 400 mg a day. However, the study was terminated after 30 months because of withdrawal of the drug from the market due to hepatotoxicity. The incidence of diabetes was 12.1% in the control group and 5.4% in the treated group (p < 0.01). The protection from diabetes persisted for 8 months after the drug was stopped and it was associated with preservation of pancreatic beta cell function assessed by an intravenous glucose tolerance test. This beneficial effect appeared to be mediated by a reduction in the secretory demands placed on the beta cell by chronic insulin resistance. Other studies, summarized by Gerstein,[49] showed the beneficial effect of other drugs in reducing the incidence of Type 2 diabetes in persons with prediabetes (Fig. 24.1).

The natural history of Type 2 diabetes is shown in Fig. 24.2. Individuals with insulin resistance maintain normal glycemia because they produce more insulin. Even with normal glucose levels, a significant proportion of them suffer from asymptomatic hypertension, dyslipidemia, and central obesity. If insulin resistance is not corrected, the pancreas is unable to maintain normoglycemia and postprandial hyperglycemia develops (the prediabetic state). Many of these women will develop GDM while

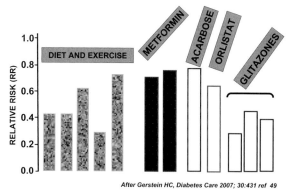

After Gerstein HC, Diabetes Care 2007; 30:431 ref 49

Fig. 24.1 Pharmacologic and non-pharmacologic measures to delay or prevent the onset of Type 2 diabetes. (After Gerstein[49].)

Fig. 24.2 Natural history of Type 2 diabetes. (A) Hyperinsulinemia with normal glycemia (insulin resistance). Hypertension, dyslipidemia, and central obesity are present in a significant number of individuals. (B) Decrease in the production of insulin with gradual increase in glycemia, both fasting and postprandial (prediabetes). (C) Further decrease in insulin secretion, diabetes diagnosed; macro- and micro-vascular complications present in 10–30% of patients. Onset of hyperglycemia occurs between 5 and 10 years before the diagnosis of diabetes. ECG, electrocardiogram; ED, erectile dysfunction.

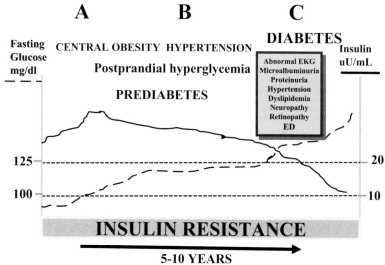

others are alternatively diagnosed on admission to hospital after significant stress, such as a myocardial infarct or stroke. With time, the production of insulin further decreases and fasting hyperglycemia develops. At the time of diagnosis of Type 2 diabetes macro- and microvascular complications are present in 10–30% of individuals.[50,51]

CONCLUSIONS

The case history demonstrates the natural history of GDM, the silent but serious consequences of the undiagnosed prediabetic state, and the potential opportunity for prevention of diabetes and its cardiovascular complications. The patient developed GDM necessitating treatment with insulin during pregnancy, a risk factor in itself for recurrent GDM (estimated to range from 30% to 84%)[52] and for the future development of Type 2 diabetes. Her fasting serum glucose was normal when repeated in the postpartum period. A 2–hour, 75-g glucose load is a better test for diagnosing prediabetes than the fasting serum glucose, because it detects a higher number of prediabetic patients. She was asked to return for a glucose test, but defaulted from review. It is possible that the importance of close follow-up was not emphasized to her or the consequences of developing diabetes mellitus were not discussed.[43] At diagnosis of diabetes, she was noted to have background retinopathy, borderline raised blood pressure and dyslipidemia (low HDL cholesterol and high triglycerides levels).

Both micro- and macro-vascular complications are present in a significant number of persons at the time of the diagnosis of Type 2 diabetes.[51,52] It takes an average of 4–10 years from the onset of hyperglycemia to the diagnosis of Type 2 diabetes. This window of time offers a unique opportunity for the healthcare professional to offer education regarding lifestyle modification and for close follow-up and prevention of both future diabetes and cardiovascular disease (Table 24.2).[53]

Table 24.2 Management of prediabetes.

- Weight loss of about 5–10% of the baseline weight
- At least 30 minutes/day of moderate intense physical activity
- Dietary therapy:
  - Low intake of saturated fats, *trans* fats, cholesterol, and simple sugars
  - Increase intake of fruits, vegetables, and whole grains
- Drugs: metformin?

REFERENCES

1 Mestman JH. Historical notes on diabetes and pregnancy. *Endocrinologist* 2002;**12**:224–42.
2 Duncan JM. On puerperal diabetes. *Trans Obstet Soc Lond* 1882;**24**:256.
3 Miller HC. The effect the prediabetic state on the survival of the fetus and the birth weight of the newborn infant. *N Engl J Med* 1945;**233**:376–8.
4 Herstein J, Dolger H. The fetal mortality in women during the prediabetic period. *Am J Obstet Gynecol* 1946;**51**:420–2.
5 Moss JM, Mulholland HB. Diabetes and pregnancy with special reference of the prediabetic state. *Ann Intern Med* 1951;**34**:678–91.
6 Wilkerson HLC, Remein QR. Studies of abnormal carbohydrate metabolism in pregnancy. *Diabetes* 1957;**6**:324–9.
7 O'Sullivan JB, Mahan CM. Criteria for the oral glucose tolerance test in pregnancy. *Diabetes* 1964;**13**:278.
8 Jackson WPU. Diabetes, pre-diabetes, mothers and babies. *South Afr Med J* 1953;**27**:795–7.
9 Mestman JH, Anderson GV, Guadalupe V. Follow up study of 360 subjects with abnormal carbohydrate metabolism during pregnancy. *Obstet Gynecol* 1972;**39**:421.
10 Metzger BE, Bybee DE, Freinkel N, *et al.* Gestational diabetes mellitus: Correlation between the phenotype and genotype characteristics of the mother and abnormal glucose tolerance during the first year postpartum. *Diabetes* 1985;**2**:111.
11 Stowers JM, Sutherland HW, Kerridge DF. Long range implications for the mother. *Diabetes* 1985;**34**:106–10.
12 Oats JN, Beischer NA, Grant PT. The emergence of diabetes and impaired glucose tolerance in women who had gestational diabetes. In: Weiss PAM, Coustan DR (eds). *Gestational Diabetes.* New York: Springer-Verlag, 1988:199–207.
13 Kim C, Newton KM, Knopp RH. Gestational diabetes and the incidence of type 2 diabetes. *Diabetes Care* 2002;**25**:1862–8.
14 Kjos SL, Peters RK, Xiang AH, Henry OA, Montoro M, Buchanan TA. Predicting future diabetes in Latino women with gestational diabetes. *Diabetes* 1995;**44**:586–91.
15 Peters RK, Kjos SL, Xiang AH, Buchanan TA. Long term diabetogenic effect of single pregnancy in women with previous gestational diabetes mellitus. *Lancet* 1996;**34**:227–30.
16 Corrado F, D'Anna R, Cannata ML, *et al.* Positive association between a single abnormal glucose tolerance test value in pregnancy and subsequent abnormal glucose tolerance. *Am J Obstet Gynecol* 2007;**186**:339.
17 Carr DB, Newton KM, Utzscneider KA, *et al.* Modestly elevated glucose levels during pregnancy are associated with a higher risk of future diabetes among women without gestational diabetes mellitus, *Diabetes Care* 2008; **31**:1037.
18 Ergin T, Lembet A, Duran H, *et al.* Does insulin secretion in patients with one abnormal glucose tolerance test value mimic gestational diabetes mellitus? *Am J Obstet Gynecol* 2002;**186**:204–9.

19 Retnakaran R, Qi Y, Sermer M, *et al.* Isolated hyperglycemia at 1 hour on oral glucose tolerance test in pregnancy resembles gestational diabetes mellitus in predicting postpartum metabolic dysfunction. *Diabetes Care* 2008;**31**:1275–81.

20 Gregg EW, Gu Q, Cheng YJ, *et al.* Mortality trends in men and women with diabetes, 1971 to 2000. *Ann Int Med* 2007;**147**:149–155.

21 Ferrara A, Mangione CM, Kim C, *et al.* Sex disparities in control and treatment of modifiable cardiovascular disease risk factors among patients with diabetes. *Diabetes Care* 2008;**31**:69–74.

22 Gouni-Brthold I, Berthold HK, Mantzoroas CS, *et al.* Sex disparities in the treatment and control of cardiovascular risk factors in type 2 diabetes. *Diabetes Care* 2008;**31**:1389.

23 Mestman JH. Follow up studies in women with gestational diabetes mellitus. The experience at Los Angeles County/University of Southern California Medical Center. In: Weiss PAM, Coustan DR (eds). *Gestational Diabetes.* New York: Springer-Verlag, 1985:191–8.

24 O'Sullivan JB. Subsequent morbidity among gestational diabetic women. In: HW Sutherland, JM Stowers (eds). *Carbohydrate Metabolism in Pregnancy and Newborn.* Edinburgh: Churchill Livingstone, 1984:174–80.

25 Carr DB, Utzscneider KA, Hull RL, *et al.* Gestational diabetes mellitus increases the risk of cardiovascular disease in women with a family history of type 2 diabetes. *Diabetes Care* 2006;**29**:2078–83.

26 Shah BR, Retnakaran R, Booth GL. Increased risk of cardiovascular disease in young women following gestational diabetes. *Diabetes Care* 2008;**31**:1668–9.

27 Pendergrass M, Fazioni E, DeFronzo R. NIDDM and GDM: same disease, another name? *Diabetes Rev* 1995;**3**:566–83.

28 Csorba TR, Edwards AL. The genetics and pathophysiology of type II and gestational diabetes. *Crit Rev Clin Lab Sci* 1995;**32**:509–50.

29 Ward KW, Johnson CLW, Beard JC, *et al.* Insulin resistance and impaired insulin secretion in subjects with histories of gestational diabetes mellitus. *Diabetes* 1985;**34**:861–9.

30 Lakka HM, Laaksonen DE, Lakka TA, *et al.* The metabolic syndrome and total and cardiovascular disease mortality in middle-aged men. *JAMA* 2002;**288**:2709–16.

31 Ford ES, Giles WH, Dietz WH. Prevalence of the metabolic syndrome among US adults: Findings from the Third National Health and Nutrition Examination Survey. *JAMA* 2002;**287**:356–9.

32 National Institutes of Health: Executive summary of the third report of the national cholesterol education program (NCEP) expert panel on detection, evaluation and treatment of high blood cholesterol in adults (Adult treatment panel III). *JAMA* 2001;**285**:2486–97.

33 Alberti KG, Zimmet P, Shaw J. The metabolic syndrome – a new worldwide definition. *Lancet* 2005;**366**:1059.

34 Adams RJ, Appleton S, Wilson DH, *et al.* Population comparison of two clinical approaches to the metabolic syndrome: Implications of the new International Diabetes Federation consensus definition. *Diabetes Care* 2005;**28**: 2777.

35 Ryan EA, Imes S, Liu D., McManus R, Finegood DT, Polonsky KS, Sturis J. Defects in insulin secretion and action in women with a history of gestational diabetes. *Diabetes* 1995;**44**:506–12.

36 Kjos SL, Buchanan TA, Montoro M, Coulson A, Mestman JH. Serum lipids within 36 months of delivery in women with recent gestational diabetes. *Diabetes* 1991;**40**:142–6.

37 Haffner SM, Stern MP, Hazuda HP, Mitchell BD, Patterson JK. Cardiovascular risk factors in confirmed prediabetic individuals. Does the cloak for coronary heart disease state ticking before the onset of clinical diabetes? *JAMA* 1990;**263**:2893–8.

38 Phillips D. Birth weight and the future development of diabetes: A review of the evidence. *Diabetes Care* 1998;**21**:B150–B155.

39 McCance DR, Pettitt DJ, Hanson RL, Jacobsson LTH, Knowler WC, Bennett PH. Birth weight and non-insulin-dependent diabetes. "Thrifty genotype", "thrifty phenotype", or "surviving small baby genotype"? *Br Med J* 1994;**308**:942–5.

40 Clark CM, Qui C, Amerman B, *et al.* Gestational diabetes: Should it be added to the syndrome of insulin resistance? *Diabetes Care* 1997;**20**:867–71.

41 Lauenorg J, Mathiesen E, Hansen T, *et al.* The prevalence of the metabolic syndrome in a Danish population of women with previous gestational diabetes mellitus is three-fold higher than in the general population. *J Clin Endocrinol Metab* 2005;**90**:4004–10.

42 Freinkel N. Gestational diabetes 1979: Philosophical and practical aspects of a major public health problem. *Diabetes Care* 1980;**3**:399–401.

43 Kim C, McEwen LN, Piete JD, *et al.* Risk perception for diabetes among women with histories of gestational diabetes mellitus. *Diabetes Care* 2007;**30**:2286.

44 Eriksson KF, Lindgarde F. Prevention of type 2 (non-insulin dependent) diabetes mellitus by diet and physical; exercise: the 6 year Malmo feasibility study. *Diabetologia* 1991;**34**:891–8.

45 Helmrich SP, Ragland DR, Leung RW, *et al.* Physical activity and reduced occurrence of non-insulin dependent diabetes mellitus. *N Engl J Med* 1991;**325**:147.

46 Diabetes Prevention Program Research Group: Reduction in the incidence of Type 2 diabetes mellitus with lifestyle intervention or metformin. *N Engl J Med* 2002;**346**: 393–403.

47 Tuomilehto J, Lindstrom J, Eriksson JG, *et al.* Prevention of type 2 diabetes mellitus by changes in lifestyle among subjects with impaired glucose tolerance. *N Engl J Med* 2001;**344**:1343–50.

48 Buchanan TA, Xiang AH, Peters RK, *et al.* Preservation of pancreatic [beta]-cell function and prevention of type 2 diabetes by pharmacological treatment of insulin resistance in high risk Hispanic women. *Diabetes* 2002;**51**:2796–803.

49 Gerstein HC. Point: If it is important to prevent type 2 diabetes, it is important to consider all proven therapies within a comprehensive approach. *Diabetes Care* 2007;**30**: 432–4.

50 Harris MI, Klein R, Welborn TA, Knuiman MW. Onset of NIDDM occurs at least 4–7 years before clinical diagnosis. *Diabetes Care* 1992;**15**:815–19.

51 UK Prospective Diabetes Group : UK Prospective diabetes Study (UKPDS). VIII. Study design, progress and performance. *Diabetologia* 1991;**34**:877–90.

52 Kim C, Berger DK, Chamany S. Recurrence of gestational diabetes mellitus. A systematic review. *Diabetes Care* 2007;**30**:1314–19.

53 England LJ, Dietz PM, Njoroge T, *et al.* Preventing type 2 diabetes: public health implications for women with a history of gestational diabetes mellitus. *Am J Obstet Gynecol* 2009;200:**365**:e1–8.

25 Long-term implications for the baby of the hyperglycemic mother

David J. Pettitt

Sansum Diabetes Research Institute, Santa Barbara, CA, USA

PRACTICE POINTS

- Rates of diabetes in pregnancy are increasing in all populations.
- The diabetic intrauterine environment affects the offspring of women with all types of diabetes mellitus.
- Offspring of women with diabetes during pregnancy are at higher risk of developing obesity and Type 2 diabetes at young ages.
- Offspring of women with diabetes during pregnancy are at higher risk of developing hypertension and other cardiovascular disease.
- The diabetic intrauterine environment represents a vicious cycle with the offspring being at risk of developing gestational diabetes or diabetes at a young age.

CASE HISTORY

Maria is a 34-year-old Hispanic woman who is pregnant for the fourth time. She has two living children. Her first pregnancy was uneventful but her second pregnancy ended in miscarriage and her third baby, who weighed over 5 kg, was delivered by cesarean section. During the latter pregnancy she had sought medical care late in the third trimester and was diagnosed with gestational diabetes that was treated with insulin. That child, who is now 2½ years old, has done well, but has remained above the 97th centile for weight. Following the third pregnancy Maria was tested for diabetes at her 6-week check-up and was found to have normal glucose tolerance. During the present pregnancy she first saw her physician late in the first trimester and was again diagnosed with gestational diabetes that responded to diet and exercise until early in the third trimester at which time insulin was added. Maria's general health has been good but she

had excessive weight gain during each pregnancy, which she never lost. She currently has a body mass index (BMI) of 39 kg/m^2.

Family history is remarkable in that she has two sisters with diagnosed diabetes and her mother, who is no longer living, is thought to have had diabetes but only while pregnant. Maria's aunt also has diabetes. Maria describes everyone in her family as "heavy".

Maria has recently heard that her diabetes may not be good for her unborn child and has many questions for her doctor:

- Doctor, will my baby be born with diabetes?
- Will my baby be affected by my diabetes?
- Is there anything I can do to assure her health?
- Can I keep her from experiencing the same problems I've had?

BACKGROUND

Once the care of the newborn is over and the ostensibly "healthy" baby of a mother with hyperglycemia during pregnancy is discharged to his/her devoted family, the long wait begins. It is now 25 years since it was clearly established that children of diabetic Pima Indian women who had diabetes during pregnancy were themselves more likely to become obese[1] and to develop diabetes.[2] This phenomenon had been established previously in animal models[3] and was soon observed in children of women with either Type 1 diabetes or gestational diabetes.[4,5]

OBESITY

Among the Pima Indians of Arizona, a population with high rates of Type 2 diabetes, the weight centiles and the rates of obesity were significantly higher among offspring

A Practical Manual of Diabetes in Pregnancy, 1st Edition.
Edited by David R. McCance, Michael Maresh and David A. Sacks.
© 2010 Blackwell Publishing

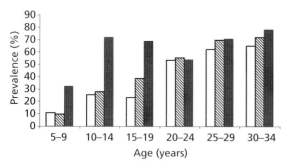

Fig. 25.1 Prevalence of severe obesity (weight ≥140% of age–sex–height-specific standard) by mother's diabetes during and following pregnancy in 5–34-year-old Pima Indians. Open bars, offspring of non-diabetic women; hatched bars, offspring of women who were normal during pregnancy and later developed diabetes; solid bars, offspring of women with diabetes during pregnancy. (Reproduced with permission from Dabelea et al[7].)

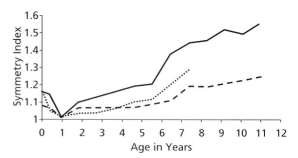

Fig. 25.2 Symmetry index (age–sex-specific weight centile divided by age–sex-specific height centile) in offspring of diabetic women from the Diabetes in Pregnancy Center in Chicago (dotted line) and the Pima Indian study (solid line). Also shown is the symmetry index offspring of non-diabetic Pima women (dashed line). (Reproduced with permission from Pettitt[10].)

whose mothers had had diabetes during pregnancy than among offspring whose mothers either had not developed diabetes or developed it after the pregnancy (Fig. 25.1).[1,6,7] Although offspring of diabetic women were, on average, larger for gestational age at birth than were offspring of women without diabetes or of women who developed diabetes later in life, large birthweight was not a prerequisite for the development of obesity by 5–9 years of age. Even normal birthweight offspring of diabetic women were likely to be obese throughout childhood.[8] This is in contrast to a study in predominantly Caucasian children from Rhode Island who were aged 4–7 years.[9] Normal birthweight offspring of women with gestational diabetes were, if anything, less likely to be overweight than controls, while large for gestational age offspring were more obese by age 4 years and became increasingly obese by age 7 years. Data from Chicago demonstrated that offspring of women with Type 1 or gestational diabetes had a faster than expected growth during the first 7 years of life.[4] A direct comparison of data from the Pima and Chicago studies showed that, after the age of 2 years, even though the Pima children were heavier for their height, the two populations of children exposed in utero to maternal diabetes grew at similar rates (Fig. 25.2).[10] After the age of about 5 years, the offspring of diabetic women in the Chicago study were heavier for height than the Pima children who had not been exposed in utero.

Among the Pima Indians, a fairly linear relationship between maternal glucose in the mother during pregnancy, even when in the normal range, and infant birth-

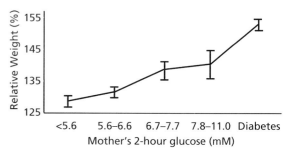

Fig. 25.3 Relative weight for height in 10–14-year-old offspring of Pima Indian women according to maternal glucose 2 hours after a 75-g glucose load during pregnancy. (Adapted from data included in Pettitt et al[13].)

weight was seen.[11] This finding was confirmed recently in a sample of 25 000 women followed in the Hyperglycemia and Adverse Pregnancy Outcome Study (HAPO).[12] On follow-up of Pima children, a relationship between maternal glucose and both childhood obesity (Fig. 25.3) and childhood glucose tolerance (Fig. 25.4) was found across the full spectrum of glucose,[13] and follow-up of children whose mothers were enrolled in the HAPO study should determine if a similar relationship emerges in other populations.[14] Evidence suggesting that this may occur comes from the Early Bird Study.[15] In that study, insulin resistance measured in the mothers 5 years following pregnancy, a value likely to be highly correlated with insulin resistance and fasting glucose during pregnancy, was directly related to the child's weight.[15]

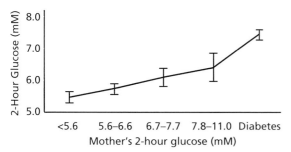

Fig. 25.4 Glucose concentration 2 hours after a 75-g glucose load in 10–14-year-old offspring of Pima Indian women according to maternal glucose 2 hours after a 75-g glucose load during pregnancy. (Adapted from data included in Pettitt et al[13].)

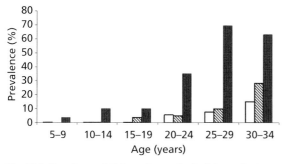

Fig. 25.5 Prevalence of diabetes by mother's diabetes during and following pregnancy in 5–34-year-old Pima Indians. Open bars, offspring of non-diabetic women; hatched bars, offspring of women who were normal during pregnancy and later developed diabetes; solid bars, offspring of women with diabetes during pregnancy. (Reproduced with permission from Dabelea et al[7].)

ABNORMAL GLUCOSE TOLERANCE

Compared with infants of non-diabetic Pima women, infants of Pima women who had Type 2 diabetes during pregnancy themselves developed Type 2 diabetes at younger ages, resulting in higher rates of diabetes throughout childhood.[2] This finding was subsequently extended to age 34 years (Fig. 25.5) and remained significant.[6,7] In an attempt to control more completely for shared environment and genetics, sibling pairs who were discordant both for Type 2 diabetes and for their exposure *in utero* to a diabetic pregnancy were analyzed. In three-quarters of cases, the sibling who was born later, and who was therefore exposed to diabetes *in utero*, was the sibling with diabetes.[16] A similar analysis of sibling

pairs, whose father had diabetes that developed after the first sibling but before the second sibling was born, showed no tendency for the second sibling to be affected more often than the first sibling.[16]

Maturity-onset diabetes of the young (MODY) is the phenotypic manifestation of a monogenic autosomal dominant mutation. Physiologically it is characterized by a defect in insulin secretion accompanied by normal insulin resistance. There are six known monogenic subtypes of MODY, of which that resulting from a mutation of the *HNF-1α* gene is one of the most common. Those born after their mother's MODY was diagnosed manifested their glucose intolerance at a significantly younger age than those who were born before their mother's disease developed (15.5 ± 5.4 *vs* 27.5 ± 13.1 years, respectively; $p < 0.0001$).[17] A younger paternal age of onset of MODY was not associated with a younger age of onset in subjects who inherited MODY from their fathers. This again provides evidence that the diabetic intrauterine environment is associated with a younger age of onset of diabetes over and above genetic and other environmental factors.

By age 16 years, few of the children from the Chicago study, whose mothers had had either Type 1 or gestational diabetes during pregnancy, had themselves developed diabetes. However, almost 20% had impaired glucose tolerance.[5] This was about 10-fold the rate of impaired glucose tolerance found in a control sample of children from the same population whose mothers had been normal during pregnancy.

More recently, examination of a cohort of young adults from Denmark confirmed the findings of the Chicago study in that offspring of women with Type 1 diabetes had rates of Type 2 diabetes and prediabetes (impaired glucose tolerance or impaired fasting glucose) about three-fold that in the background population (11% *vs* 4%, respectively) and equal to rates among offspring of women with identifiable risk factors for gestational diabetes.[18] Unlike the Chicago study, however, the Danish study found even higher rates of abnormal glucose tolerance among offspring of women with diagnosed gestational diabetes (21%) than among offspring of women with Type 1 diabetes.

The phenomenon of diabetes in pregnancy resulting in more diabetes, or an earlier age of diabetes onset, in the offspring, represents a vicious cycle (Fig. 25.6).[6,19] Many young women who were exposed to diabetes *in utero* have become obese and have developed diabetes by the time they enter their child-bearing years, thus perpetuating the cycle. The vicious cycle is also enhanced by

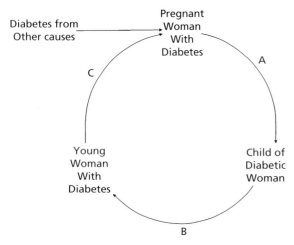

Fig. 25.6 Vicious cycle of diabetes in pregnancy. Potential points of intervention are: A – to reduce the effect of the diabetic pregnancy on the offspring; B – to reduce the incidence of obesity and diabetes in the offspring of the diabetic woman; C – to control the diabetes prior to and during pregnancy to lessen the impact of the diabetes throughout gestation.

new cases of diabetes in pregnant women because of other risk factors for gestational or pregestational diabetes. This can be seen most clearly in Type 2 diabetes among populations such as the Pima Indians. However, in MODY diabetes due to an *HNF-1α* gene mutation,[17] a younger age of onset of diabetes means the young women will be more likely to have developed their disease by the time they have children, thus exposing the next generation to the diabetic intrauterine environment. Those offspring who have also inherited the *HNF-1α* mutation will then be at risk of an earlier age of onset of MODY diabetes. In the Chicago study,[5] if further follow-up had been possible, it is likely that children with impaired glucose tolerance whose mothers had Type 1 or gestational diabetes would have developed diabetes or gestational diabetes by their early 20s, and thus exposed their offspring to diabetes *in utero*. In the Danish study, although not limited to pregnant offspring, the young adults were all of child-bearing age,[18] so those with abnormal glucose tolerance or Type 2 diabetes constitute the next generation of young affected mothers.

DIABETES TYPES

As seen from the above, the effect of the diabetic intrauterine environment appears to occur in all types of dia-

betes. The Pima Indians have typical Type 2 diabetes, and are anti-insulin antibody, anti-islet cell antibody, and GAD-65 antibody negative. They rarely develop ketoacidosis and usually do not require insulin initially for the control of diabetes symptoms.[6,20] The women in the Chicago study had a mix of either gestational or pregestational diabetes, the latter being primarily Type 1. Although the data were not presented in these two groups separately, the authors state that the offspring of women with Type 1 diabetes developed impaired glucose tolerance at the same rate as the offspring of women with gestational diabetes.[5] In the Danish study, diabetes types were reported separately and, although gestational diabetes placed the offspring at a higher risk for developing abnormal glucose tolerance, rates in the offspring of women with Type 1 diabetes were clearly elevated.[18] Thus, three of the major classifications of diabetes, Type 1, Type 2, and gestational, have been shown to increase the risk for obesity and abnormal glucose tolerance in the offspring. While offspring of women with MODY diabetes who inherited the *HNF-1α* mutation are all likely to develop MODY diabetes at some point, those who were born after their mothers developed symptoms and were therefore exposed *in utero*, developed MODY at a younger age than those who were born before their mothers developed symptoms.[17] The end result will be a longer duration of diabetes and a consequent potential increase in complications. This implies that these offspring carrying the *HNF-1α* mutation will expose their children to diabetes *in utero* who, in turn, will also be at risk of an earlier development of MODY. Findings from studies in animal models that lack any known genetic predisposition to diabetes have been similar to those in humans.[3] Such data strongly support the belief that diabetes and/or obesity in offspring may be a universal consequence of diabetes during pregnancy whether or not a genetic predisposition to diabetes or obesity is present.

DIFFICULTIES WITH COMPARATIVE DATA

When two groups or subgroups with different characteristics are compared, there is always the concern of a Type 1 error resulting in an erroneous inference. A better control for other diabetes risk factors can be achieved by the use of family data, such as sib-pair analyses, and analyses of populations with restricted genetic distributions, such as subjects with MODY or the Pima Indians. However, one of the most convincing arguments for the role of the intrauterine environment is the consistency of the finding across populations and diabetes types,[1,2,4,5,17,18] as well as the excellent supportive animal data.[3,21] The overwhelming magnitude of this finding also strongly implicates the diabetes in pregnancy.

CARDIOVASCULAR DISEASE RISK

Cardiovascular disease is one of the major complications of diabetes and is a significant cause of mortality among persons with diabetes. To date, human studies have been too short to allow a continuous follow-up of the offspring of a pregnancy complicated by diabetes from birth through cardiovascular events in the offspring. However, the problems that are recognized to occur (obesity, insulin resistance, glucose intolerance) are well established risk factors for cardiovascular disease. Since these risk factors develop early in life, they place the offspring of women with diabetes at risk throughout adulthood. A recent review of this subject summarizes the increased rates of the metabolic syndrome among offspring of women with gestational diabetes.[22] Examination of children between ages 5 and 11 years who had normal fasting glucose and insulin revealed that those of women with Type 1 diabetes had more dyslipidemia and high serum markers for vascular disease.[23,24] Thus, in addition to treating more obesity, diabetes, and gestational diabetes in the future, medical personnel may need to be prepared for a resurgence of cardiovascular events as the population ages.

IMPLICATIONS FOR MANAGEMENT AND PREVENTION

The implications for prevention and treatment are far reaching and involve addressing the problem from several sides. If diabetes or impaired glucose tolerance in women can be prevented from developing until after child-bearing age, this will then reduce the problem for their offspring. Alternatively, if a way can be found to control diabetes sufficiently during pregnancy, the developing offspring should be presented with a normal intrauterine environment and be less likely to suffer the adverse effects. Good diabetes control can reduce the rates of macrosomia,[25,26] but whether this degree of control is enough to prevent the long-term complications is an unanswered question. Finally, treatment of the child and young woman at high risk for obesity and diabetes at young ages should prevent the consequences for the child and for subsequent generations. Success at any or several of these points may break the vicious cycle. Several

promising regimes have been proposed[27,28] and shown to be effective in high-risk groups. At present, however, none of these has been approved for use in pregnancy, although studies are currently underway,[29] and so far metformin appears to be safe for the developing fetus.[30] However, there are no results from studies of the long-term effect of metformin on the offspring. Other studies to prevent diabetes before pregnancy have used drugs that have either been removed from the market[31] or are contraindicated in pregnancy.[32]

SUMMARY OF RISKS TO THE OFFSPRING

In answer to the mother's questions, we can be reassuring that neonatal diabetes is extremely uncommon and not associated with maternal diabetes during pregnancy. However, the woman's hyperglycemia is likely to have an effect on her child, placing him/her at high risk of developing obesity, abnormal glucose tolerance, and cardiovascular disease at a young age. While we cannot assure the woman that these problems are preventable, we do know that good diabetes control during pregnancy will lessen the chances of her child being born large for gestational age, suffering from birth trauma, and of having hypoglycemia in the newborn period. Observational studies have demonstrated that lower glucose concentrations during pregnancy are associated with a lower risk for the offspring of becoming obese or developing diabetes later in life. We can and should council the mother to help her child avoid gaining excess weight and to seek early diagnosis if she suspects diabetes.

FUTURE GENERATIONS AND AREAS FOR FUTURE RESEARCH

The world is faced with an alarming increase in childhood obesity and Type 2 diabetes and this trend shows no sign of abating.[33,34] Now, for the first time in over 200 years, the life-expectancy of American children is less than that of their parents.[35] If the data from the Pima Indians can be generalized to other populations, and so far this appears to be the case, then diabetic pregnancy is potentially a major factor responsible for the high rates and marked increase in childhood Type 2 diabetes. Thus, solving this problem needs to be made an international priority or the outlook for the next generation looks bleak.

Limiting the increase in obesity and diabetes are two of the major challenges of the 21st century. The task of clinicians and researchers will be to identify an effective means of breaking the vicious cycle of maternal diabetes leading to diabetes in the offspring. In populations such as the Pima Indians, where maternal diabetes during pregnancy accounts for up to one-third of all diabetes in the population,[36] solving this single problem would have a major impact on reducing the overall burden of diabetes. However, this will not be an easy task. Technology needs to be developed that will absolutely normalize glucose metabolism during pregnancy. Only then will the fetus have the chance to develop normal regulatory mechanisms. At present, however, there is no agreement on what level of glucose intolerance in the mother should be considered abnormal[37–39] and there are very few data on the long-term effects of minor elevations of maternal glucose on the offspring.[13] Future research should establish the universality of the effect of the diabetes in pregnancy on the offspring and determine what level of metabolic control is needed to decrease the prevalence of obesity and diabetes in the offspring to acceptable levels. Data from the HAPO study[12] confirmed findings in the Pima Indians[11] and suggest that the linear relationship between maternal glucose concentration and perinatal complications, without any evidence of a cut-off point, may be universal. Children whose mothers were enrolled in the HAPO study are currently being followed.[14] Studying children at younger ages than are usually considered appropriate for even moderately invasive research may be necessary. For gestational diabetes as well as pregestational diabetes, closed loop glucose regulatory systems[40–42] may be needed to normalize glucose metabolism optimally and these should be evaluated during pregnancy in a wide variety of settings. Finally, very long-term prevention trials will be required to assess the effectiveness of the intervention strategies.

REFERENCES

1 Pettitt DJ, Baird HR, Aleck KA, Bennett PH, Knowler WC. Excessive obesity in offspring of Pima Indian women with diabetes during pregnancy. *N Engl J Med* 1983;**308**:242–5.
2 Pettitt DJ, Aleck KA, Baird HR, Carraher MJ, Bennett PH, Knowler WC. Congenital susceptibility to NIDDM: Role of intrauterine environment. *Diabetes* 1988;**37**:622–8.
3 Aerts L, Van Assche FA. Animal evidence for the transgenerational development of diabetes mellitus. *Int J Biochem Cell Biol* 2006;**38**:894–903.
4 Silverman BL, Landsberg L, Metzger BE. Fetal hyperinsulinism in offspring of diabetic mothers. Association with the subsequent development of childhood obesity. *Ann N Y Acad Sci* 1993;**699**:36–45.
5 Silverman BL, Metzger BE, Cho NH, Loeb CA. Impaired glucose tolerance in adolescent offspring of diabetic mothers. Relationship to fetal hyperinsulinism. *Diabetes Care* 1995;**18**:611–7.
6 Knowler WC, Pettitt DJ, Saad MF, Bennett PH. Diabetes mellitus in the Pima Indians: incidence, risk factors and pathogenesis. *Diabetes Metab Rev* 1990;**6**:1–27.
7 Dabelea, D, Knowler WC, Pettitt DJ. Effect of diabetes in pregnancy on offspring: follow-up research in the Pima Indians. *J Matern Fetal Med* 2000;**9**:83–8.
8 Pettitt DJ, Knowler WC, Bennett PH, Aleck KA, Baird HR. Obesity in offspring of diabetic Pima Indian women despite normal birthweight. *Diabetes Care* 1987;**10**:76–80.
9 Vohr BR, McGarvey ST, Tucker R. Effects of maternal gestational diabetes on offspring adiposity at 4–7 years of age. *Diabetes Care* 1999;**22**:1284–91.
10 Pettitt DJ. Summary and comment of: Silverman BL, Rizzo T, Green OC, *et al.* Long-term prospective evaluation of offspring of diabetic mothers (*Diabetes* 1991;**40** (Suppl 2):121–25). *Diabetes Spectrum* 1992;**5**:39–40.
11 Pettitt DJ, Knowler WC, Baird HR, Bennett PH. Gestational diabetes: Infant and maternal complications of pregnancy in relation to third-trimester glucose tolerance in the Pima Indians. *Diabetes Care* 1980;**3**:458–64.
12 The HAPO Study Cooperative Research Group. Hyperglycemia and adverse pregnancy outcomes. *N Engl J Med* 2008;**358**:1191–2002.
13 Pettitt DJ, Bennett PH, Saad MF, Charles MA, Nelson RG, Knowler WC. Abnormal glucose tolerance during pregnancy in Pima Indian women: long-term effects on the offspring. *Diabetes* 1991;**40** (Suppl. 2):126–30.
14 Pettitt DJ, McKenna S, McLaughlin C, Patterson C, Hadden DR, McCance DR. Glucose tolerance test results during pregnancy and skin fold thickness in offspring at age 2 years: a HAPO ancillary study at the Belfast center. *Diabetes* 2008;**57** (Suppl. 1):A509.
15 Jeffery AN, Voss LD, Metcalf BS, Wilkin TJ. The impact of pregnancy weight and glucose on the metabolic health of mother and child in the south west of the UK. *Midwifery* 2004;**20**:281–9.
16 Dabelea D, Hanson RL, Lindsay RS, *et al.* Intrauterine exposure to diabetes conveys risks for type 2 diabetes and obesity: a study of discordant sibships. *Diabetes* 2000;**49**:2208–11.
17 Stride A, Shepherd M, Frayling TM, Bulman MP, Ellard S, Hattersley AT. Intrauterine hyperglycemia is associated with an earlier diagnosis of diabetes in HNF-1 alpha gene mutation carriers. *Diabetes Care* 2002;**25**:2287–91.
18 Clausen TD, Mathiesen ER, Hansen T, *et al.* High prevalence of type 2 diabetes and pre-diabetes in adult offspring of women with gestational diabetes mellitus or type 1 diabetes. *Diabetes Care* 2008;**31**:340–6.
19 Pettitt DJ, Knowler WC. Diabetes and obesity in the Pima Indians: a cross-generational vicious cycle. *J Obesity Weight Regulation* 1988;**7**:61–75.

20 Dabelea D, Palmer JP, Bennett PH, Pettitt DJ, Knowler WC. Absence of glutamic acid decarboxylase antibodies in Pima Indian children with diabetes mellitus. *Diabetologia* 1999;**42**:1265–6 (letter).

21 Gauguier D, Nelson I, Bernard C, *et al.* Higher maternal than paternal inheritance of diabetes in GK rats. *Diabetes* 1994;**43**:220–4.

22 Vohr BR, Boney CM. Gestational diabetes: the forerunner for the development of maternal and childhood obesity and metabolic syndrome. *J Matern Fetal Neonatal Med* 2008;**21**:149–57.

23 Manderson JG, Mullan B, Patterson CC, Hadden DR, Traub AI, McCance DR. Cardiovascular and metabolic abnormalities in the offspring of diabetic pregnancy. *Diabetologia* 2002;**45**:991–6.

24 McAllister AS, Atkinson AB, Johnston GD, McCance DR. Endothelial function in offspring of type 1 diabetic patients with and without diabetic nephropathy. *Diabet Med* 1999;**16**:296–303.

25 Jovanovic L, Bevier W, Peterson CM. The Santa Barbara County Health Care Services Program: birth weight change concomitant with screening for and treatment of glucose-intolerance of pregnancy: a potential cost-effective intervention. *Am J Perinatol* 1997;**14**:221–8.

26 Bevier WC, Fischer R, Jovanovic L. Treatment of women with an abnormal glucose challenge test (but a normal oral glucose tolerance test) decreases the prevalence of macrosomia. *Am J Perinatol* 1999;**16**:269–75.

27 Diabetes Prevention Program Research Group. Reduction in the incidence of type 2 diabetes with lifestyle intervention or metformin. *N Engl J Med* 2002;**346**:393–403.

28 Xiang AH, Peters RK, Kjos SL, *et al.* Pharmacological treatment of insulin resistance at two different stages in the evolution of type 2 diabetes: impact on glucose tolerance and beta-cell function. *J Clin Endocrinol Metab* 2004;**89**: 2846–51.

29 Simmons D, Walters BNJ, Rowan JA, McIntyre HD. Metformin therapy and diabetes in pregnancy. *Med J Aust* 2004;**180**:462–4.

30 Rowan RA, Hague WM, Gao W, Battin MR, Moore MP, for the MiG Trial Investigators. Metformin versus insulin for the treatment of gestational diabetes. *N Engl J Med* 2008;**358**:2003–15.

31 Buchanan TA, Xiang AH, Peters RK, *et al.* Preservation of pancreatic beta-cell function and prevention of type 2 diabetes by pharmacological treatment of insulin resistance in high-risk hispanic women. *Diabetes* 2000;**51**: 2796–803.

32 Xiang AH, Peters RK, Kjos SL, *et al.* Effect of pioglitazone on pancreatic beta-cell function and diabetes risk in Hispanic women with prior gestational diabetes. *Diabetes* 2006;**55**:517–22.

33 Koplan JP, Liverman CT, Kraak VI (eds). *Preventing Childhood Obesity: Health in the Balance.* Institute of Medicine of the National Academies. Washington, DC: The National Academies Press, 2005.

34 UK Houses of Parliament. *Childhood Obesity.* The Parliamentary Office of Science and Technology, 2003:No. 205:1–4.

35 Olshansky SJ, Passaro DJ, Hershow RC, *et al.* A potential decline in life expectancy in the United States in the 21st century. *N Engl J Med* 2005;**352**:1138–45.

36 Dabelea D, Hanson RL, Bennett PH, Roumain J, Knowler WC, Pettitt DJ. Increasing prevalence of type 2 diabetes in American Indian children. *Diabetologia* 1998;**41**:904–10.

37 National Diabetes Data Group. Classification and diagnosis of diabetes mellitus and other categories of glucose intolerance. *Diabetes* 1979;**28**:1039–57.

38 WHO Study Group. Diabetes mellitus. *WHO Tech Rep Ser* 1985;**727**:1–113.

39 Metzger BE, Coustan DR. Summary and recommendations of the Fourth International Workshop – conference on gestational diabetes mellitus. The Organizing Committee. *Diabetes Care* 1998;**21** (Suppl 2):B161–B167.

40 Matsuo Y, Shimoda S, Sakakida M, *et al.* Strict glycemic control in diabetic dogs with closed-loop intraperitoneal insulin infusion algorithm designed for an artificial endocrine pancreas. *J Artif Organs* 2003;**6**:55–63.

41 El-Khatib FH, Jiang J, Damiano ER. Adaptive closed-loop control provides blood-glucose regulation using dual subcutaneous insulin and glucagon infusion in diabetic swine. *J Diabet Sci Technol* 2007;**2**:181–92.

42 Palerm CC, Zisser HZ, Bevier WC, Jovanovic L, Doyle FJ III. Prandial insulin dosing using run-to-run control. *Diabetes Care* 2007;**30**:1131–6.

Index

A

abruptio placentae   148, 157, 161

acarbose   109, **110**, 111, 113, *247*

accelerated fetal growth   117, 118, 119, 120, 121, 124, 125

"accelerated starvation" in pregnancy   19, 186

ACE (angiotensin-converting enzyme) inhibitors   77, 81, **82**, 86, 142, 143, 146, 149, 153, 155, 158, 159, 162, 208

aceto-acetic acid in urine   38

ACHOIS   *see* Australian Carbohydrate Intolerance in Pregnancy Study (ACHOIS)

acidemia   *see* fetal acidemia

acidosis   119, 185, 186, 188, 189, **190**, **191**, 193, 194

ADA *see* American Diabetes Association (ADA)

adipocyte dysfunction   21

adipokines   21

adiponectin   21

adipose tissue   20

albuminuria   149, **149**, 154, 155, **155**, 235

alpha-feto-protein (AFP)   143

alpha-glucosidase inhibitors   113

American College of Obstetricians and Gynecologists (ACOG)
  combined oral contraceptive (COC) preparations and   236
  folic acid supplement recommendations   97
  screening and diagnosis of gestational diabetes   5

American Diabetes Association (ADA)   5, 57, 58, 59, 60, 61, **101**, 148, 189, 191

amniocentesis   73, 120, 122–124, 204

amniotic fluid
  erythropoietin in   124, **125**
  insulin in   72–73, *73*, 124, **125**

amniotic fluid volume   121–122

analgesia, in labor   205

angiotensin receptor blockers (ARBs)   81, **82**, 86, 143, 146, 150, 151, 153, 159, 160, 162
  nephropathy and   154, 155
  teratogenicity and fetotoxicity   142, 149

anion gap metabolic acidosis   184, 188, 189

antenatal cardiotocography (CTG)   120, **125**, 205, *207*

antenatal care, aims of multidisciplinary   89–90

antenatal fetal surveillance   202

antenatal hypoxia–ischemia   223

antenatal steroids   212–213

antiangiogenic factors, alterations in fetal levels in pregnancy with GDM and T1DM   **28**

antibiotics, ketoacidosis and   193

antihypertensive drugs   142–143, 162
  during breastfeeding   151
  for use before and during pregnancy   149–150

antioxidants   151

Appropriate Blood Pressure Control in Diabetes Trial (ABCD)   169

ARBs   *see* angiotensin receptor blockers (ARBs)

aspart   *see* insulin aspart

aspiration pneumonia   187

aspirin   143, 151

atenolol   **159**
  breastfeeding and   151

Australian Carbohydrate Intolerance in Pregnancy Study (ACHOIS)   13, 66–67, 202

Australian Diabetes in Pregnancy Society (ADIPS), screening and diagnosis of gestational diabetes   **6, 46, 47**

autonomic dysfunction   176, 178, **181**, 182

autonomic nervous system (ANS)   177

autonomic neuropathy in diabetes in pregnancy *see* diabetic autonomic neuropathy (DAN)

B

baby, long-term implications for the baby of the hyperglycemic mother   251–257

bedside biochemical measures   188

Bennewitz, Heinrich   37

beta-agonists, combined use with glucocorticoids   187

beta-blockers   150, 162

beta-sympathomimetics   204, 212

bicarbonate   193

biguanides   **110**, 142

biophysical profile (BPP)   122, **125**

birth injury   220, **221**, 224

birthweight   **244**, 245–246
  odds ratio for birthweight of ≥4.5 kg   **4**

bladder dysfunction   178, **179**

blood glucose monitoring, in neonates   225–226

blood pressure   146, **149**, 162
  management in diabetic nephropathy in pregnancy   159
  normal levels in diabetes in pregnancy   **148**, 148
  retinopathy and   171

blood urea nitrogen (BUN) values   162

brachial plexus injury   203

brain injury   224

bread, low glycemic   **133**

breakfast tolerance tests   61